OCD

2nd Edition

by Laura L. Smith, PhD

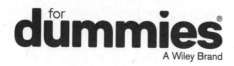

OCD For Dummies®, 2nd Edition

Published by: **John Wiley & Sons, Inc.**, 111 River Street, Hoboken, NJ 07030-5774, www.wiley.com

Copyright © 2023 by John Wiley & Sons, Inc., Hoboken, New Jersey

Published simultaneously in Canada

For general information on our other products and services, please contact our Customer Care Department within the U.S. at 877-762-2974, outside the U.S. at 317-572-3993, or fax 317-572-4002. For technical support, please visit https://hub.wiley.com/community/support/dummies.

Wiley publishes in a variety of print and electronic formats and by print-on-demand. Some material included with standard print versions of this book may not be included in e-books or in print-on-demand. If this book refers to media such as a CD or DVD that is not included in the version you purchased, you may download this material at http://booksupport.wiley.com. For more information about Wiley products, visit www.wiley.com.

Library of Congress Control Number: 2022943430

ISBN 978-1-119-90314-7 (pbk); ISBN 978-1-119-90315-4 (ebk); ISBN 978-1-119-90316-1 (ebk)

SKY10036033_091322

Contents at a Glance

Table of Contents

Introduction

Obsessive compulsive disorder affects about 2 to 3 million American adults. Since the first edition of this book, new research-backed strategies have been introduced for treating OCD. However, the most well-researched standard treatment, exposure and response prevention, has remained essentially the same with only a few minor changes. This book updates the standard treatment and explains some of the newer, emerging strategies.

The introduction to the first edition of this book described the experience of being delayed on a flight. After finishing a movie or a novel, people tended to mindlessly look at the inflight magazines and catalogues. Many of those catalogues were filled with gadgets. Some of those gadgets were for sanitizing devices. Handheld wands were offered for sale that disinfected areas in the plane that others may have touched.

After reading about bacteria, germs, and microbes in the catalogues, the text described the feeling of discomfort one might have on an airplane. That would be especially true when other passengers were sneezing and coughing and the person next to you had bad breath. That experience was somewhat like what people with OCD feel all of the time.

Well, since then, those magazines are no longer in the pockets of the seat in front of you because they could be contaminated. And I wouldn't dismiss someone who was concerned about germs on airplanes. The world changed over the course of a few months in the spring of 2020.

Many people experienced the fear of contamination during those first few months of the worldwide pandemic. And those with OCD tended to suffer the most. In spite of the challenges posed by pandemics, people with OCD can expect to improve with appropriate treatment.

About This Book

This book is about OCD. My goal is to help you understand OCD as well as give you strategies for getting help and getting better. I also tell you what you can do to help a child or someone you care about who has OCD. In addition, I describe the symptoms of other conditions, such as anxiety or depression, that can occur at the same time as OCD. Finally, I explain the differences and similarities of disorders that can be considered related to OCD.

This book covers the primary strategies used to treat OCD, including cognitive behavioral therapy (CBT), metacognitive therapy (MCT), mindfulness, exposure and response prevention (ERP), and medication. The information is based on the latest scientific research.

Throughout the book you'll receive tips on when to consider getting more help from a mental-health professional. I provide sources and ways for you to choose the right person to assist your recovery.

Case examples are used throughout this book to illustrate points. These stories are based on symptoms, thoughts, and feelings from real people with OCD. However, the individual illustrations are composites of people rather than recognizable examples. The case examples leave out or change many details so that privacy and confidentiality are protected. Any resemblance to any person, whether alive or deceased, is entirely coincidental.

This book is full of information, and every word is well worth reading (and recommending to your family and friends). But you really don't have to read every single word, sentence, or chapter to benefit. You can use the table of contents or index to look up what you want to know. There is no predetermined order to the chapters; you can read them in any order you choose. Sometimes, I suggest going back or checking out certain chapters or sections for more information, but that's up to you.

Foolish Assumptions

If you're reading this paragraph, I suspect that you may be holding this book (or device) in your hands (now that was a brilliant deduction). Maybe you're interested in OCD because you think you have some symptoms. Or maybe you worry that someone you care about has OCD. Perhaps you're simply intrigued by this very interesting disorder (possibly having seen it portrayed in movies or on television).

You may be a mental-health professional who wants to find out more about specific treatment options for OCD or look at books that may be helpful to your clients. Or you may be a student of psychology, counseling, social work, or psychiatry hoping to get a clearer picture of this complex problem, without getting bogged down in the weeds of technicalities.

Whatever reason you have for picking up this book, I promise a comprehensive depiction of everything you need to know about OCD.

Icons Used in This Book

TIP

This icon highlights a specific strategy or tool for beating OCD, or an idea that can save you time and effort.

WARNING

Watch out for this icon. It alerts you to information you need to know in order to avoid trouble.

REMEMBER

This icon gives you information that you want to take from the discussion and file away in your brain, even if you remember nothing else. It's also used to remind you of important information that appears elsewhere in the book.

TECHNICAL STUFF

This icon lays out material that I think is rather interesting or cool, but not needed for understanding the essentials.

Beyond the Book

For some quick tips about obsessive compulsive disorder, go to www.dummies.com and type "OCD For Dummies Cheat Sheet" in the search box. There you can access quick information about what is OCD, living with OCD, and the types of OCD.

Where to Go from Here

I expect that reading this book will thoroughly inform you about OCD and related disorders. The book spells out the major treatment strategies for OCD. I hope you find the text interesting and, at times, entertaining.

If you are reading this book to help you overcome OCD, I encourage you to get a notebook or keep a file, write out the exercises, take notes, and reflect upon your efforts.

Unless you're reading this book for your own interest or education (and not because you have OCD), you're likely to want to consult a professional as well. I anticipate that most trained mental-health professionals will welcome the opportunity to work with you on the strategies outlined in this book.

1

The Ins and Outs of OCD

Chapter **1**

Facing Obsessive-Compulsive Disorder (OCD)

Depending on how you define the terms, almost everyone has a few obsessive or compulsive tendencies. *Obsessive* is a word often used to describe someone's intense interest in something. For example, a person could be obsessed with making money, putting money ahead of all other goals in life. Someone could have an intense interest in collecting coins or stamps, spending hours looking through catalogues, dreaming of the next rare find. Some people are obsessed with sports teams, never missing a game. Obsessions are common in everyday life and are not necessarily reflective of a mental health problem.

Compulsive refers to rigid patterns of behavior. For example, someone could be compulsive about always cleaning the house on Saturday — never on Monday, only on Saturday. Another person could compulsively walk the dog on the same route every day. Yet another compulsion could involve never stepping on cracks in the sidewalk. Compulsive behaviors are not deemed abnormal when they don't cause harm or distress.

Thus, some people with ordinary obsessions or compulsions manage quite well. For example, many major-league sports figures have elaborate good-luck rituals that look pretty strange. Some feel compelled to listen to the same song prior to the game; others eat exactly the same food. You've probably watched pitchers straighten their hats, smooth out the dirt on the mound, and spit in the sand before each pitch. Many baseball hitters have elaborate rituals they carry out with their bats. Other athletes have strange beliefs, good-luck charms, or compulsive acts that they must perform, allegedly to help their performance. If you are a major-league sports player making zillions of dollars to play a game, you can indulge in a few weird behaviors. No one will question you.

But mental-health professionals define these terms quite differently. In the mental-health field, obsessions are considered to be *unwanted* thoughts, images, or impulses that occur frequently and are quite upsetting to the person who has them. Compulsions are various actions or rituals that a person performs in order to reduce the feelings of distress caused by obsessions. These obsessions and compulsions consume hours of the day and interfere with essential tasks of life.

REMEMBER

Anyone can have a few obsessions or compulsions, and, in fact, most people do. But it isn't obsessive-compulsive disorder (OCD) unless the obsessions and compulsions consume considerable amounts of time and interfere *significantly* with the quality of your life.

This chapter introduces you to OCD. The disorder debilitates individuals who have it and costs society plenty. The chapter also provides an overview of the major treatment options. With guidance and assistance, much can be done to help those with OCD. Finally, because OCD treatment can be enhanced by the help of friends and family, this chapter offers tips on what you can do to help someone you care about who has OCD.

What Is OCD?

OCD has many faces. Millions of people are held prisoner by the strange thoughts and feelings caused by this disorder. Between 1 and 2 percent of the worldwide population has OCD. Most people with OCD are bright and intelligent. But doubt, uneasiness, and fear hijack their normally good, logical minds.

Whether or not you have OCD, you can probably recall a time when you felt great dread. Imagine standing at the edge of an airplane about to take your first parachute jump. The wind is blowing; your stomach is churning; you're breathing hard. Suddenly the pilot screams, "Stop! Don't jump! The chute is not attached!"

You waver at the edge, terrified, and fall back into the plane, shaking. That's how many people with OCD feel every day. OCD makes their brains believe that something horrible is about to happen. Some people fear that they left an appliance on and the house will burn down. Others are terrified that they may get infected with some unknown germ. OCD causes good, kind people to believe that they might do something horrible to a child, knock over an elderly person, or run over someone with their car.

Those with OCD almost always struggle with one or more of the following concerns: shame; the intense desire to avoid all risks; and constant, nagging doubt. The next three sections describe these issues.

Suffering shame

Because the thoughts and behaviors of those with OCD are so unusual or socially unacceptable, people with OCD often feel deeply embarrassed and ashamed. Imagine having the thought that you might be sexually attracted to a statue of a saint in your church. The thought bursts into your mind as you walk by the statue. Or consider how you would feel if you stood at a crosswalk and had an image come into your mind of pushing someone into oncoming traffic.

However, the frightening, disturbing thoughts of OCD are not based on reality. People with OCD have these thoughts because their OCD minds produce them, not because they are evil or malicious. It is extremely rare for someone with OCD to actually carry out a shameful act.

REMEMBER

Throughout this book you'll see references to the "OCD mind" rather than you or someone you care about with OCD. The purpose of doing that is to emphasize that *you are not your OCD*. You have these thoughts, urges, impulses, and rituals because of a problem with the way your brain works. OCD is not your fault, and it doesn't make you a bad person.

Wrestling with risk

The OCD mind attempts to avoid risks of all kinds almost all the time. That's why those with contamination OCD spend many hours every single day cleaning, scrubbing, and sanitizing everything around them. People with superstitious OCD perform rituals to keep them safe over and over again. Interestingly, most OCD sufferers focus on reducing risks around specific themes such as contamination, household safety, the safety of loved ones, or offending God. But those with contamination fears don't necessarily worry about damnation. And those who worry about turning the stove off usually don't obsess about germs.

Risks of all kinds abound in life. And no one can ever know when something horrible might happen. All people eventually suffer from a variety of risky situations and outcomes such as illness, accidents, tragedy, war, grief, and ultimately death. But the OCD mind tries to create the illusion that almost all risks can be anticipated and avoided.

In truth, OCD doesn't provide significant protection in spite of extraordinary efforts to reduce risks. In chapters to come I give you many ideas about how to accept a certain amount of risk in order to live a full life, no matter how long or short that life is.

Dealing with doubt

Doubt permeates the OCD mind. It's difficult to be 100 percent certain of almost any situation in life. The OCD brain takes advantage of that fact and goes to town. Someone with OCD often has worries such as:

>> Am I sure I locked the door?

>> Is it possible that I might lose control and shout obscenities?

>> Could I actually be sexually attracted to animals?

>> Might this be dirty and make me sick?

>> If I don't count by 3s, will bad luck follow me?

>> If I don't alphabetize my cans, will I be able to function?

>> Am I sure I won't harm my children?

>> Am I positive I won't get sick if I touch that dish?

With thoughts like that, who wouldn't be worried all of the time?

Counting the Costs of OCD

People with OCD suffer. They are more likely than others to have other emotional disorders such as depression or anxiety. Due to embarrassment, they often keep their symptoms secret for years, which prevents them from seeking treatment. Worldwide, it is estimated that almost 60 percent of people with OCD *never* get help.

The pain of OCD is accompanied by loneliness. OCD disrupts relationships. People with OCD are less likely to marry, and, if they do, they are more likely to divorce than others. Those who do hang on to their families often have more conflict.

OCD also costs money. These costs include money spent on treatment, lost productivity on the job, and lost days at work. Costs of treatment are often high in part because many with OCD don't get effective treatment for years. They may enter treatment and be too ashamed to tell the therapist their symptoms. Or well-meaning therapists may not be trained to provide effective OCD treatment.

Someone with fears of contamination may be late for work because they can't get out of the shower quickly enough because of excessive washing. A person who believes that they may have possibly hit someone with their car may circle around multiple times to check, resulting in once again being late for work. Someone else may have to recheck that the door is locked multiple times. A person who has a need for perfection may not be able to turn in completed work in a timely manner because of repeatedly checking for mistakes. And someone else with a need for symmetry may spend endless hours arranging their desk.

OCD and the Media

Media, especially social media, depends on sensationalism to gain viewers. News is mostly negative and dramatic. Human beings are prewired to pay attention to potential threats. And the media takes advantage of that tendency. No wonder people with OCD tend to get worse when the news constantly spews out possible catastrophes.

Pandemic panic

The outbreak of COVID exposed everyone around the world to potential infection, illness, and possible death. The public was advised to wash, sanitize, avoid people, and wear masks. Shaking hands or hugging others became taboo. Touching a doorknob or elevator button were thought to be risky. Even if you didn't have OCD, those early months of the pandemic led most people to feel the fear of contamination.

Imagine the terror caused by COVID to those who already suffered from the type of OCD that fears contamination. OCD tends to get worse when people are stressed. Researchers and clinicians who worked with patients suffering from OCD reported a substantial worsening of symptoms. (See Chapter 13 for specific recommendations about dealing with OCD during a pandemic.)

Disgusting filth

OCD is not a new disorder. However, you can't help but think that the appetite for sensation in the media accelerates OCD concerns. Recently, a television special featured people buying used mattresses. Reporters used special lights and took cultures to find all sorts of horrible matter (bed bugs, fecal matter, and body fluids) still clinging to supposedly refurbished bedding. In another show, zealous reporters burst into hotel rooms armed with petri dishes and black lights to help them find filth and grime on the glasses left in the room, as well as on the carpet and bedding

Furthermore, the sales of cleaning products, sanitizers, personal hygiene products, and mouthwash have soared. You can find antibacterial ingredients in products designed to clean your refrigerator, mop your floors, scrub your body, and disinfect your toilets. Antiviral ingredients fly off the shelves, especially during a pandemic.

Yet, try and find solid evidence about deaths from refurbished mattresses, less-than-pristine hotel rooms, and homes not cleaned with every antibacterial and antiviral ingredient known to humans, and you'll come up wanting. In fact, a clever study conducted by researchers at Columbia University in Manhattan provided households with free cleaning supplies, laundry detergent, and hand-washing products. All the brand names were removed. Half of the households were given products with antibacterial properties, and the other half was provided supplies without antibacterial properties. The researchers carefully tracked the incidence of infectious diseases (runny noses, colds, boils, coughs, fever, sore throats, vomiting, diarrhea, and conjunctivitis) for almost a year. They found no differences between those who used antibacterial cleaning agents and those who did not.

WARNING

If you spend loads of time cleaning and using antibacterial disinfectants, you may be doing yourself more harm than good! Scientists now believe that excessively clean environments may actually be causing an increase in allergies and asthma. Furthermore, excessive use of antibiotics appears to run some risk of encouraging the development of new, resistant bacteria.

No, people should not stop washing their hands, especially in hospitals! And plenty of evidence supports the long-term dangers posed by prolonged exposure to air pollution, insecticides, and toxic chemicals. Furthermore, a dirty hotel room or a well-used mattress seems pretty disgusting. At the same time, the media and advertisers have shown a disturbing obsession with issues involving excessive cleanliness and minimal exposure to low-level risks.

GERMS: RESISTANCE IS FUTILE

Some people with OCD spend hours vacuuming in hopes of defeating dust and dirt in their homes. Household vacuum cleaners not only may spread germs throughout the house, but also may be a safe haven for accumulating bacteria. Vacuum brushes apparently harbor fecal material, mold, and even E. coli. What to do about this situation? One recommendation has been to spray antibacterial disinfectant on your vacuum brushes after every use. Another solution is to buy a new breed of vacuum that purportedly kills bacteria and germs through the use of an ultraviolet, germicidal light.

Other researchers have found bacteria and fecal matter in ice machines at restaurants and on restaurant menus. Therefore, some suggest not using ice machines, not allowing a menu to touch your plate, and washing your hands after selecting your food from the infected menu.

The problem with these studies and recommendations is that no one has proven that any of these sources cause significant amounts of illness or disease. Though reasonable precautions are always a good idea, you can easily start down the disinfectant road and never return. Bacteria and germs exist everywhere. You cannot eliminate all of them, and you can spend huge amounts of time and money trying.

Exploring Treatment Options for OCD

If you had OCD during the Middle Ages, you very well may have been referred to a priest for an exorcism. The strange, violent, sexual, or blasphemous thoughts and behaviors characteristic of OCD were thought to derive from the devil. If you had OCD during the dawn of the 20th century, you may have been sent for treatment based on Freudian psychoanalysis, which purportedly resolved unconscious conflicts from early development. For example, if your OCD involved sexual obsessions or compulsions, you were assumed to have unconscious sexual desires for your mother or father. In fact, the common use of the word "anal" to describe people who are overly rigid, controlled, and uptight came from the Freudian idea that strict, early toilet training caused children to grow up with excessive concerns about neatness and rules.

However, neither exorcism nor psychoanalysis ultimately proved to have much impact on OCD. Only in the last half century or so have effective treatments evolved for OCD. And some of these treatments have only become widely available quite recently.

The next few sections provide an overview of the major treatment options for OCD that have shown significant promise based on scientific studies. For clarity, sections are divided into the categories of cognitive behavioral therapy (CBT), metacognitive therapy (MCT), mindfulness, exposure and response prevention (ERP), medications, and deep brain stimulation. In reality, rarely are any of these therapies used as a single, exclusive treatment for OCD. For example, a patient may start out taking medications while getting cognitive behavioral therapy; another could receive exposure and response training as well as training in mindfulness.

Changing the way you think with CBT

Cognitive therapy was developed by Dr. Aaron Beck in the early 1960s and is a major component of the broader category, cognitive behavioral therapy (CBT).

Originally, this approach was used to treat depression. Cognitive therapy is based on the idea that the way you feel is largely determined by the way you think or the way you interpret events. Therefore, treatment involves learning to identify times when your thoughts contain distortions or errors that contribute to your misery. After you've identified those distortions, you can learn to think in more adaptive ways. Soon after it was adopted for treating depression, cognitive therapy was applied quite successfully to anxiety disorders and, ultimately, to a dizzying array of emotional problems, including eating disorders, oppositional defiant disorder, and even schizophrenia.

In the early years, cognitive therapy was not applied to OCD, perhaps because of the success of exposure and response prevention (ERP) (described in the section "Modifying behavior through ERP"). However, in recent years, the cognitive therapy component of CBT has been found to be quite effective in treating OCD. Usually, CBT includes at least some elements of ERP. Some practitioners believe that applying cognitive strategies first may make the application of ERP somewhat more comfortable and acceptable to the person contemplating that approach. See Chapters 8, 9, and 10 for more information about the various subtypes of CBT.

Thinking about thinking: Metacognitive therapy

Metacognitive therapy takes a step back from cognitive therapy. Instead of going after specific thought distortions, metacognitive therapy involves finding a new way to look at thinking in general. It teaches that thoughts are simply thoughts. When people engage in patterns of anxious brooding, anxiety and obsessive thinking increases. Those with OCD tend to fixate on their brooding. Metacognitive therapy helps people develop new ways of controlling attention and relating to thoughts. See Chapter 9 for more about metacognitive therapy.

Approaching OCD mindfully

The OCD mind focuses on possible future calamities. The predictions almost never come true. Yet, the obsessive thoughts keep coming and demanding attention.

>> I worry about shouting obscenities, so maybe someday I'll lose control and do it in church.

>> Maybe my thoughts of death will cause harm to someone I love.

>> Perhaps touching that doorknob will make me sick.

When it isn't thinking about the future, the OCD mind dwells on possibilities from the past. The mind fills with thoughts about what might have occurred.

>> Maybe I left the stove on.

>> Maybe I ran that person over with my car.

>> Perhaps I was poisoned by that tuna fish sandwich.

Furthermore, the OCD mind judges people, the world, and even OCD itself harshly.

>> A bad thought is just the same as doing something bad.

>> Having OCD thoughts means that I'm crazy.

>> I am a weak person for having these thoughts.

Mindfulness is the practice of existing in the present moment without judgment or harsh evaluations. Thus, as you acquire a mindful approach to OCD, you understand that thoughts are truly just that — thoughts. Thoughts do not make someone good or bad. See Chapter 9 for more information about how to apply mindfulness to your life and your OCD. As you do, you will become more self-accepting and better able to quiet your OCD mind.

Modifying behavior through ERP

A true breakthrough in the treatment of OCD occurred in the mid-1960s when Victor Meyer tested a treatment called exposure and response prevention (ERP) with two patients suffering from severe cases of OCD. These patients had not improved with shock therapy, supportive therapy, or medication. The drastic measure of brain surgery was even being considered. One of the patients was obsessed with cleaning. Dr. Meyer and a nurse exposed this patient to dirt and did not allow her to clean (ergo, the term "exposure and response prevention"). This radical treatment was the first to help decrease the patient's symptoms. The other patient was obsessed with blasphemous thoughts. She was told to purposefully rehearse those thoughts without doing the rituals that she had used to decrease her obsessions. Like the first patient, this woman was helped by ERP after years of other unsuccessful therapies.

ERP resulted in a substantial reduction in both patients' OCD. The mental-health profession took notice because OCD treatments previously had shown little ability to help those with this disorder. Suddenly, the prognosis for OCD turned from utterly grim to quite hopeful.

However, ERP requires patients (and sometimes therapists) to get down-and-dirty — literally. Thus, patients may be asked to

» Not check the door locks

» Refrain from cleaning up

» Repeat blasphemous thoughts over and over

» Say the number "13" over and over again

» Shake hands

» Stop arranging their closets in certain ways

» Touch grimy surfaces

You may wonder whether carrying out ERP causes some distress. Indeed, it does. Perhaps that's why the strategy took quite a while to be embraced by large numbers of mental-health professionals. However, the discomfort is worth it because ERP is very effective. You can read all about this strategy in Chapter 10.

Controlling OCD with medications

Medications given for OCD had shown almost no effectiveness until Anafranil (Clomipramine) was found to work in 1966, a date roughly corresponding to when ERP was first tested. Thus, prior to 1966, about the only known strategy for treating OCD was psychosurgery, a rather radical approach involving the cutting of certain connections in the brain. Such surgery sometimes left the patient with devastating side effects, such as an inability to function normally. Obviously, psychosurgery was reserved for the most severe cases. Others were left to fend for themselves.

Today, some of the same medications used for depression (specifically, selective serotonin reuptake inhibitors or SSRIs) frequently work for OCD. However, they are thought to work in a different manner for OCD than they do for depression. The good news is that if medication is going to work, it will work fairly quickly for OCD.

The bad news is that a substantial number of people do not seem to benefit from medications for their OCD. And those who do benefit find that they relapse quickly if they discontinue the medication. Furthermore, side effects can be significant. For more information about the pros and cons of taking medication for OCD, see Chapter 11.

Sending signals deep into the brain

Prior to the discovery of effective treatments of OCD, severe cases were some-times referred for brain surgery to get relief. Severe OCD can be excruciatingly painful, so there were some takers. Although there were success stories, other patients were left with little improvement and permanent brain damage. Not a good option unless as a last resort.

However, in 2018, the United States Food and Drug Administration approved deep transcranial magnetic stimulation (dTMS) as an effective treatment for OCD. Unlike brain surgery, dTMS is non-invasive; in other words, no scalpels are involved. (See Chapter 11 for more information on dTMS.)

Helping People with OCD

If you're reading this book because your child, a family member, or a close friend has OCD, there is much you can do to help. Here are a few points to keep in mind if you want to do more good than harm:

>> **Don't try to be a therapist.** Generally speaking, those with OCD should consult a mental-health professional. Those with a very mild case may want to try some of the techniques described in this book on their own. However, treatment plans should either be designed by a professional and/or the person with OCD. At the most, you can make a few suggestions. Even if you are a professional therapist, you don't want to take on that role for a friend or family member.

>> **Understand OCD.** Even if you're not taking on the role of a therapist, knowing a lot about this disorder helps a great deal. Understanding OCD can help you

feel compassion and acceptance for the one you care about. You will also know that your family member, child, or friend didn't ask for OCD. No one wants to have this problem.

>> **Encourage; don't reassure.** You want to encourage the one you care about to participate in treatment. At the same time, you don't want to do what seems natural — reassure the person that everything will be okay. Please read Chapter 22 to find out how to devise alternatives to giving reassurance.

>> **Don't get sucked into rituals and compulsions.** Those with OCD often try to elicit help with their rituals and compulsions. For example, they may ask someone to recheck that the doors are locked or that the oven is turned off. Though complying with the request may seem caring, doing so only makes matters worse.

Chapter **2**

Understanding What OCD Is All About

Although it goes by a single name, obsessive-compulsive disorder (OCD) is actually a diverse disorder with multiple presentations. OCD can manifest itself as quirky behavior, exaggerated fears, or seriously disturbed thinking. Thus, in one instance, the diagnosis of OCD may be assigned to someone with the odd habit of hanging clothes exactly 1.2 inches apart in the closet, whereas in someone else, OCD may show up as excessive worries about germs and constant hand-washing. Alternatively, OCD could cause someone to check and recheck to see whether the windows and doors are locked, not once or twice but dozens and dozens of times.

You may be surprised to know that *everyone* occasionally has a few signs of OCD. And some symptoms of OCD are perfectly normal. For example, you may worry about whether you turned off the coffeepot, remembered to pack all the right clothes, brought along your passport, or left a light on as you rush off to the airport for an important business trip. Your mind tells you to stop your car and turn around to check. But, usually, you don't because you realize that the odds are pretty much in your favor that your worries are exaggerated.

Occasionally feeling compelled to count steps, knock on wood, or arrange items on your nightstand in a particular pattern is also normal. These actions, although possibly unwanted or a little strange, are common. Just because you have one or more symptoms of OCD doesn't mean that you have the disorder.

This chapter explains OCD in plain words and provides clear examples of its symptoms, and then it sorts out what's normal and what's OCD. OCD has two components — *obsessions* and *compulsions*. First, obsessions and compulsions are detailed and differentiated. The next section discusses how people with OCD cycle through obsessions, worry, and compulsions. Then, the wildly divergent mutations of OCD are introduced.

WARNING

OCD can steal the minds and dismantle the lives of those affected. Therefore, this book takes a serious and respectful approach to reviewing the diagnosis and treatment of OCD. At the same time, let's face it, the OCD brain can come up with some wild thoughts and strange actions. These thoughts and behaviors may look downright bizarre, and occasionally funny, but they are real, often exquisitely painful, and serious. Although nothing is funny about having OCD, taking a lighthearted approach to the disorder can help at times. A bit of humor can reduce the stigma, decrease the anxiety, and help those with OCD face the hard work of getting better.

Seeing the Two Sides of OCD

Technically, OCD involves either obsessions or compulsions, or a combination of both. In reality, almost everyone with OCD has both obsessions and compulsions. Distinguishing between obsessions and compulsions can seem a little tricky, but here goes.

The difference between an obsession and a compulsion is that obsessions are *intrusive mental events* that make a person feel upset. Compulsions, on the other hand, are behaviors or actions someone engages in either mentally (like counting or repeating words) or physically (like washing hands) *in order to feel better*. In other words, obsessions start in the mind and then create a negative emotional response, while compulsions are actions (either mental or physical) targeted to soothe negative emotions.

The next two sections examine the nature of obsessions and compulsions in more detail.

Obsessing about obsessions

Obsessions are like uninvited houseguests who refuse to leave. They barge into your mind like mental terrorists. Obsessions make you feel uncomfortable, uneasy, angry, and sometimes frightened. Obsessions come in three forms:

>> **Thoughts:** Thoughts are the words that clang around in your head. For example, if you touch something dirty, you may have the thought "I'm sure to get sick if I don't do something immediately." Other obsessional thoughts come in the form of doubting whether you've locked the doors or concerns about things not being arranged correctly.

>> **Urges:** These are feelings, impulses, or worries that you're going to do something inappropriate or undesirable. For example, you may have an urge to harm someone you care about or a need to have everything in a very specific, "just so" order. Other examples of obsessive urges include worries that you may shout out obscenities during a religious ceremony or that you may turn your car into oncoming traffic.

>> **Images:** These are uninvited pictures that form in your mind, often depicting violent, horrifying, morally reprehensible, weird, and unwanted scenes. Disturbing images may include scenes involving inappropriate sexual activities, child abuse, or gruesome murder.

Obsessive thoughts, urges, or images seem to pop into the mind without warning. When they do appear, they cause a lot of distress if you have OCD. Lonnie's story illustrates how an obsession is experienced by someone who suffers from OCD.

Lonnie forces themself to attend their niece's wedding. Lonnie's not particularly close to family and finds themself seated at a table with seven elderly aunts. The reception has barely started, and they're already anxious to get home.

The best man toasts the bride and groom, and Lonnie's mind wanders. Suddenly, Lonnie looks around at their tablemates, and a picture of what they would look like naked pops into their mind. Lonnie's mind envisions seven women, over 75, with sagging breasts, wrinkled faces, and much worse. Horrified, Lonnie gulps the sweetly spiced punch in front of them. "My God," they think, "Why do I have thoughts like these all the time? I must be a sick pervert!"

Just as suddenly, Lonnie's mind suggests a slow, sensual dance with an 85-year-old aunt seated next to them. Then, a second later, comes an image of a steamy hotel room scene with the elderly aunt. I won't give you the details of the rest of Lonnie's imagery. Lonnie has a sudden urge to shout out, "Baby, you are so hot!"

"Ick, what's wrong with me? Am I losing my mind?" Lonnie blushes with embarrassment and almost jumps out of their skin when an aunt touches their arm and asks kindly, "Lonnie, are you okay? You look flushed; is there anything I can do for you?"

Lonnie experienced intrusive, unwanted thoughts, impulses, and images. These are obsessions. Lonnie's rather strange incident is not an uncommon example of an obsession. Lonnie's thoughts represent the *essential characteristics* of obsessions (as opposed to normal, mildly worrisome thoughts and doubts). The thoughts Lonnie associates with their obsession are

>> **Disconnected:** The obsessive thoughts, urges, or images jump into conscious awareness. They seem disconnected to what the person had been doing or thinking. These are not pleasant daydreams; people don't willfully ask for obsessions.

>> **Unacceptable:** The thoughts are unwanted and unacceptable to the person who has them. Obsessions involve actions or thoughts that are totally uncharacteristic, morally upsetting, violent, or uncomfortable.

>> **Uncontrollable:** The thoughts capture attention. Wow, do they! When an obsession comes along, it's difficult to think about anything else. Thus, they interfere with whatever a person was trying to think about or get done. Obsessions overpower the mind and feel uncontrollable.

>> **Highly upsetting:** Feelings after the obsessive thoughts, images, or urges are highly upsetting. Worry, guilt, fear, anger, disgust, or sadness often follow obsessions.

>> **Frequently reoccurring:** An obsession tends to reoccur often. People who have obsessions work hard to suppress them. They may avoid situations that they associate with their thoughts or perform rituals to keep their thoughts at bay. Untreated, obsessional thoughts spread like unchecked weeds, choking out healthy, adaptive thinking and increasing the distress of their victims.

This final characteristic, "frequently," truly separates the "obsessions" (that is, mild worries) almost everyone occasionally has from obsessions experienced by people with OCD. For those who suffer from OCD, the frequency of the obsession is what makes life miserable.

TECHNICAL STUFF

The informal use of the word "obsession" often conveys a positive, enthusiastic focus on something pleasant or desirable such as a passion for fishing, coin collecting, a new relationship, or art. The word "obsession" as used in OCD has nothing to do with such positive interests.

Considering compulsions

Compulsions are actions people feel driven to complete in order to deal with obsessions. These actions take the form of behaviors, such as handwashing or repeatedly checking locks, or rituals, such as lining up everything in a cupboard in an unusually precise manner. Unlike obsessions that merely heighten anxiety and distress, compulsions are intended to neutralize obsessions or reduce distress. Compulsions can also come in the form of mental acts (such as counting or repeating phrases).

Compulsions are attempts to

>> **Reduce anxiety:** For example, after suffering from an obsessional worry that the doors are unlocked (thus inviting unwanted intruders) a person may feel compelled to return and recheck their door locks. Once they've done so, they feel briefly relieved. But then they leave the house again, and the obsession returns, thus compelling them to go back to check. This cycle may continue numerous times before they're able to let go and continue with their day.

>> **Respond to an urge:** After using the public restroom a person may obsess about possible germs, contamination, and sickness. They may feel an irresistible urge to scrub their hands. They carry a powerful disinfectant and spend 30 minutes washing their hands, even though they're red, raw, and oozing from all the washing they do.

>> **Decrease discomfort:** Some compulsions appear out of a need to feel more comfortable or "just so." For example, a person may have a ritual they feel compelled to perform in order to go to bed. They arrange items on their nightstand over and over until they feel "just right." In addition, they touch their shoulders five times each and repeat these touches until they feel comfortable. Only then can they allow themself to go to bed.

>> **Seek certainty:** A person may have an obsession that they might run someone over in their car. Almost every time the car goes over a bump in the road they start to worry. They often feel compelled to turn the car around to check. Even then, sometimes they drive off and feel they must return to check again to be absolutely certain they did not injure someone. This compulsion consumes hours of their time each day.

>> **Obtain reassurance:** A 10-year-old may worry obsessively that their parents might not still love them. So, every night, after they've been put to bed, they get up and go to their parents' bedroom and asks if they still love them. They feel compelled to repeat this ritual many times seeking this reassurance. Before they stop, the parents become upset and irritated. But they always give them the reassurance they ask for.

>> **Increase a sense of safety or well-being:** Someone may have frequent obsessional worries that their thoughts might cause harm to their family. So, if they have the slightest negative image or thought about anyone in their family, they feel compelled to repeat the words "Hail Mary; I love my family so much," 50 times in their mind. Sometimes they lose count and have to start over.

Coming to Terms with OCD

People with OCD have obsessions and/or compulsions. Well, duh! How's that for stating the obvious? These obsessions and compulsions can vary in both intensity and content over time. Thus, someone may have a terrible problem with compulsive handwashing for two hours every day. After a year or so passes, the handwashing may fall off, but compulsive rituals involving excessive cleaning of the house and arranging the furniture precisely emerge in its place.

TECHNICAL STUFF

For decades, OCD used to be considered as one of the anxiety disorders (which include generalized anxiety disorder, phobias, and panic disorder, among others). That's because people with OCD usually complain of *feeling* anxious, uneasy, or distressed. This feeling is often brought on by obsessive fears, thoughts, or images. See the latest edition the book *Anxiety For Dummies* (Wiley) for more information about anxiety disorders. However, OCD involves more than anxiety. It also includes distorted thinking, as well as repetitious urges and impulses. Therefore, more recent diagnostic categories list OCD and related disorders separately from anxiety disorders.

The OCD worry cycle

In OCD, an obsessive thought, urge, or image occurs, sometimes out of the blue and other times triggered by an event. For example, consider a person who has extreme obsessions about the possibility of hitting someone with their car. While driving, they perceive a slight bump in the road. An image of a lifeless body suddenly flashes in their head. They feel a strong urge to turn the car around and check for a body. Their logical mind is overwhelmed with uneasiness. They give in to the impulse and turn the car around and return to the area they just passed. Seeing no body, they are temporarily relieved and return to driving. But just as they start to move forward, their OCD mind produces another scenario. The image of a body on the side of the road creeps into their mind. When they checked the first time, they did not look along the edges. They cannot tolerate not being sure, so once again they circle back. This time they get out of their car to look on both sides of the road. Again, they have a brief sense of relief. Unfortunately, completing the compulsion results in only a short period of relief, which, in turn, actually increases the likelihood that the compulsion will be turned to again. To illustrate this OCD worry cycle, consider the following example of Cyan.

> **Cyan** is a bookkeeper who worries excessively about getting AIDS from touching anything that other people may have touched. Thus, they avoid touching doorknobs, shaking hands, and using public restrooms. They work at home to avoid unnecessary contact with germs. They carry hand sanitizer and disinfectant in their bag. Even at home they disinfect countertops and telephones dozens of times each day. They worry that germs float in the air and invade their home.

Whenever an obsessional worry about contamination pops into their mind, Cyan believes that they are at high risk for acquiring AIDS or some other serious illness. Their overestimation of risk leads Cyan to feel intense anxiety and overwhelming dread. That distress causes Cyan to immediately wash their hands with sanitizer and disinfect their computer keyboard, kitchen countertops, and phones. After they have done "enough" cleaning, they feel greatly relieved, but only for a short while. The power of that relief keeps the cycle going. Their obsessive thoughts soon return.

Cyan's cycle is common in OCD and is depicted in Figure 2-1.

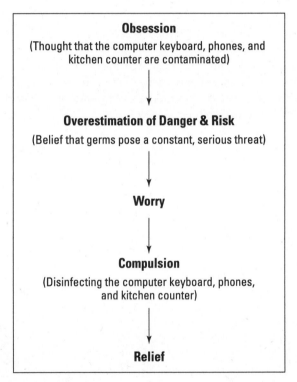

FIGURE 2-1: Cyan's OCD worry cycle.

Cyan's obsession about getting contaminated leads to anxiety. Their cleaning rituals reduce anxiety. However, thoughts about germs keep coming back.

This worry cycle is a continuous loop. Obsessions are interpreted as serious dangers, which lead to anxiety and a compulsion to do something to reduce the risk in order to alleviate the anxiety. But OCD is actually more complicated, and the symptoms often appear to involve more than feelings of anxiety. A couple other culprits need to be considered in the quest to understand OCD. People with OCD have problems with the way they think and with their ability to control urges and impulses.

Thinking and believing

OCD is really a disorder of belief or thinking. People with OCD lack complete insight into the truth of their obsessions or compulsions. They may be able to admit that their obsessions or compulsions are unreasonable. But they don't fully believe the obsessions or compulsions are completely irrational because their minds are full of doubt.

For example, a person with OCD may believe that putting soup cans in a certain order on their shelves protects their children from getting sick. That is not an especially logical thought. If you ask that person what evidence they have that their ritual protects their children, they don't have much to tell you. But they have enough doubts that they feel compelled to continue with their compulsive ritual. After all, they want to keep their kids safe.

Or someone with OCD may worry about the possibility of leaving the stove on. They may admit in a calm discussion that their beliefs are not completely consistent with reality. They've never actually left the stove on, even though they've checked hundreds of times. But they continue to act as if their beliefs about needing to check are true. They have just enough doubt to continue checking again and again.

Delusional thinking

OCD thinking sometimes goes to such extremes that it appears delusional or completely out of touch with reality. For example, some cases of OCD involve worries like becoming contaminated and infected by molecules emanating from things made out of stainless steel. Other sufferers may feel compelled to perform an elaborate ritual involving counting and precisely arranging items — firmly believing that if the ritual is not performed correctly, a loved one will die. When OCD thinking becomes this distorted, treatment and diagnosis becomes more complex.

WARNING

Because the OCD mind can come up with some pretty weird thoughts, some people who have OCD are misdiagnosed as psychotic. That leads to inappropriate treatment and poor outcomes. If you or a loved one has bizarre thoughts that seem out of touch with reality, be sure to get a diagnosis from a mental health professional with experience in diagnosing and treating both psychosis and OCD.

Extreme doubting

People without OCD also experience doubt. They demand certainty in what is almost always an uncertain world. For example, how certain can you be that the sun will come up tomorrow? Almost 100 percent certain, but there is an extremely remote possibility that the sun will implode. For people with OCD, that doubt may keep them up at night. Thus, the remote chance that a door is unlocked, even though a person recalls locking it, would nag at a person with OCD and literally cause a desperate need to recheck repeatedly.

Uncertainty simply can't be completely eliminated. Consider the common superstition that knocking on wood after stating something positive will ward off bad things happening in the future. Is it really true that knocking on wood keeps someone safe? Where is the evidence? Have there been studies about not knocking on wood? Most people would agree that the superstition is sort of silly. Yet, many people continue to knock on wood. Why not, just in case, right?

Those who continue to engage in wood knocking technically have a disorder of thinking and believing, but it's hardly a serious one. At least I hope it isn't serious, because many perfectly sane people are wood knockers on occasion.

REMEMBER

What makes wood knocking okay and *not* a compulsion are two characteristics that make OCD a disorder:

» The first characteristic of OCD is that when a compulsion is blocked, there is a great deal of distress. However, "wood knockers" don't usually get too upset when they can't find wood to knock on (besides, a head, plastic, or wood laminates will do in a pinch!).

» The second aspect of OCD that makes it different from wood knocking is that it interferes with life and takes huge amounts of time. Most people don't spend hours each day knocking on wood.

Inspecting impulses

Some people have described their OCD like a "brain itch" or a "brain hiccup." In other words, OCD can feel impossible to suppress. An obsessive thought intrudes into the mind like a bolt of lightning. A compulsive action, such as arranging food alphabetically in the refrigerator, can feel as necessary as breathing. The impulse often involves an intense feeling or need for things to be just right.

WHEN YOUR EAR HAS WORMS: READ THIS SIDEBAR AT YOUR OWN RISK!

If you have attended a wedding in the last few decades, you can probably conjure up the melody to "Y.M.C.A." or, worse, "Macarena." Can you recall the jingle that starts with "I love my baby back, baby back . . ." or how about the song on the ride at Disneyland with the lyrics, "It's a small world. . . ." Have I ruined your day?

Scientists study and label everything. So, they've come up with a term for getting a song stuck in your mind. That term is "earworm." Now, think about an earworm, a slimy parasite, digging into your brain. What does it look like? Imagine one crawling through your ear. Yuck!

When you consider these musical annoyances, the earworm has many of the same characteristics of an obsession. Segments of songs, like obsessional images and thoughts, flood your mind over and over and feel both unwanted and obnoxious. The more you try to get rid of the melody, the more entrenched it becomes. Like obsessions, earworms occur more often in people who worry a lot.

So, how do you get rid of the nuisance? That's the bad news. To date, no sure and successful earworm exterminators have been found. Some people try to substitute one song for another. Others get unstuck by passing the worm onto someone else. Here I go, I'll try passing this one along that's been bugging me since I started writing this sidebar . . . Y.M.C.A. . . .

For some people, this driven impulsivity seems to underlie their OCD more than anxiety or worry. That's why some experts suggest that problems such as trichotillomania (uncontrollable hair-pulling) and tics (uncontrollable jerking, body movements, or sounds) are related to OCD. See Chapter 3 for more information about OCD's relatives.

Categorizing the Types of OCD

Unlike depression and some other disorders, OCD is variegated. People who suffer from depression look a lot alike. Although their symptoms differ somewhat, most depressed folks feel sad and gloomy, have low energy, and lack enthusiasm. By contrast, OCD looks more like breeds of dogs that differ in appearance the way that Dachshunds, Great Danes, Cocker Spaniels, Goldendoodles, and Yorkshire Terriers do. In other words, OCD shows up in very different forms from person to person.

Experts have struggled to come to an agreement on the various breeds of OCD and have so far failed to reach a consensus. Thus, a certain amount of uncertainty remains about how to categorize OCD. Unfortunately, people with OCD typically crave certainty.

Therefore, the following sections reveal a reasonably comprehensive list of OCD subtypes. Although not every expert would fully agree that this list is definitive, you're likely to find the most common types of OCD listed and even a few that are rather rare:

>> Checking and doubting

>> Contamination

>> Inappropriate, disturbing, or shameful thoughts

>> Superstitions

>> Symmetry or perfection

>> Parenting OCD

>> Obsessive feelings and sensations

TECHNICAL STUFF

Each subtype of OCD can occur by itself or in concert with other categories of obsessions and compulsions. It is not unusual to have a mix of symptoms or for OCD to morph and change over time. Having a mix of symptoms can make treatment a little more challenging, but certainly not impossible.

Doubts, fears, and uncertainties

Doubt and uncertainty plague the minds of those with the "checking" form of OCD. Some experts even call OCD a "disease of doubt." When doubts show up, the person goes back to check over and over again. A slight amount of uncertainty always remains even after checking, so the person does it yet again. Sometimes it takes an awful lot of rechecking before the person is able to stop. Doubts involve the following types of concerns:

>> **Forgetting to do important tasks like**

- Closing doors, windows, and blinds correctly

- Turning appliances off

- Locking doors

- Saving documents

- Turning the water off

>> **Fear of making mistakes, such as**

- Forgetting appointments

- Turning in imperfect school or work assignments

- Being late

- Balancing your checkbook incorrectly

>> **Needing reassurance that**

- Loved ones are safe

- You haven't offended anyone

- Loved ones still care

- Your appearance is okay

- Your home is safe

Each time people with this problem check on a concern, they feel momentary relief. That relief is short-lived as uncertainty begins to creep in again. Some people with obsessions and compulsions regarding checking spend hours each day worrying and futilely checking and rechecking. See Chapter 14 for more information about this form of OCD and its treatment.

Contamination, germs, and dirt

Obsessions about contamination, germs, and dirt plague more sufferers with OCD than any other issue. Some worry about getting ill from dirt or germs; others believe they may become contaminated and sickened by garbage, other people, chemicals, radiation, asbestos, insects, sticky substances, animals, bodily waste or secretions, or pesticides.

The OCD mind greatly exaggerates real risks. Although dirt is well, dirty, it is not dangerous unless you eat large quantities, or it's actually contaminated with toxins. Getting sick from the vast majority of dirty areas is unlikely. People with fears about becoming contaminated by dirt will repeatedly clean and sanitize to reduce risk. Cleaning rituals sometimes consume much of the day. The exaggerated fears about germs and contamination often lead to one or more of the following:

>> Avoiding items that have touched other items imagined to be contaminated

>> Avoiding people or places thought to be contaminated

>> Avoiding public restrooms

- Hours of daily cleaning with harsh disinfectants and chemicals
- Hours of handwashing every day causing raw, bleeding skin
- An inability to eat outside of the home
- Throwing away clothes or other items imagined to be contaminated
- Washing dishes in a particular order and manner — a ritual that must be repeated if not done "properly"
- Creating clean and dirty areas in the home

Fear of contamination is the most common type of OCD. Some contamination fears are pretty wild. The OCD mind develops strange fears such as being contaminated by the following:

- Any random word
- Sap from a tree
- Bad thoughts from other people
- Sticky, messy food like avocados or oranges

TIP

The COVID pandemic made contamination fears soar. And it became more complicated to treat those with contamination OCD. See Chapter 13 for more information.

Shame, embarrassment, and inappropriate thoughts and behaviors

This type of OCD involves a host of concerns about the possibility of doing something humiliating or grossly inappropriate. As with most categories of OCD, the specifics of these concerns can vary greatly from one person to the next. Following, you find a multitude of flavors.

Religious obsessions and compulsions (scrupulosity)

Scrupulosity describes someone's excessive concern with sin and morality as well as fears about offending God. The word scrupulosity comes from the Latin word "scrupulus" and means sharp stone, suggesting the feeling of stabbing pain that results from acts against the conscience. People with this type of OCD have extreme concerns about not pleasing God or dread that they will be dammed and rejected. They often spend hours praying or performing complicated rituals.

Religious obsessions can come in the form of blasphemous thoughts. Some people with OCD worry that they might shout out swear words during a religious ceremony. Others have repeated sexual images of contemporary spiritual leaders or even historical religious figures. Some have repeated phrases, such as "god damn," popping into their thoughts throughout the day. These obsessions are accompanied by feelings of profound dread and shame. The person tries to neutralize or undo the feelings of intense guilt by resorting to compulsive prayers or rituals.

The compulsions that follow religious obsessions typically don't make logical sense. The following example of Cade illustrates how illogical these compulsive rituals can be.

> **Cade** is obsessing about displeasing God. Cade constantly worries when profane words come into their mind because they believe that having such thoughts greatly offends God. In order to deal with distress, they have developed a compulsion designed to undo the obsession.
>
> Cade's compulsion involves walking a few blocks to their church, day or night. Then Cade climbs the stairs and stands by the door. They count to 45, and then say 45 prayers. If they are interrupted or distracted, they must start the routine over until it feels just right. Cade's compulsion may seem strange and silly to others, but Cade believes that they must do this in order to show God that they are worthy. When finished, Cade feels better for a while, but the obsessions and compulsions always return.
>
> As you can see, Cade's counting and praying compulsions don't make a great deal of sense. Nonetheless, they believe that the compulsions somehow rectify their standing with God.

Sexual and aggressive obsessions and compulsions

People with this type of OCD dwell on the possibility, no matter how slight, that they might harm others or engage in sexual acts that they feel would be abhorrent and repugnant. See Chapter 15 for more information about sexual and aggressive forms of OCD, as well as treatment strategies for dealing with them. There, you also see that those with this type of OCD *almost never* do the things they gravely fear they'll do.

A fairly common variant of sexual obsessions has to do with intrusive thoughts that one's sexual orientation is incorrect. For example, someone who identifies as being gay may have intrusive thoughts that they should be transgender; another person who identifies as heterosexual obsesses about being gay. These people may spend hours worrying and have compulsive rituals to check on the validity of their beliefs and obsessions. This particular form of OCD is extremely difficult to diagnosis because many people without OCD wonder about their own sexuality. That's perfectly normal, especially during adolescence.

WARNING

OCD about sexual orientation is associated with high rates of suicidal thoughts. Therefore, obsessions and compulsions about confused sexuality should be taken seriously. Again, it is imperative to have knowledgeable, experienced, professional help.

Another sexual obsession concerns worry that one might be a pedophiliac (someone who sexually abuses children). These obsessions are abhorrent to those who have them and are highly distressing. Those with this fear may compulsively avoid any contact with children. Unfortunately, parents can have these obsessions with their own children. The shame of such repugnant thoughts can lead to major disruptions in parenting. See the later section "Parenting OCD."

Other people with OCD become concerned that they will harm or hurt someone. Here are a couple of common obsessions and compulsions with this theme:

>> While walking on a busy sidewalk, a person worries that they may push someone next to them into oncoming traffic. They are abhorred by this image and try to block it by repeating "God, save me," 17 times to themselves.

>> A teacher has sudden images of throwing their desk at students. They feel horribly guilty for having that thought and begin doubting that they belong in the classroom. They try to keep the image out of their mind but can't.

TECHNICAL STUFF

Sometimes OCD in one category can easily overlap with OCD themes from another category. Thus, those with sexual and aggressive OCD obsessions and compulsions commonly have concerns about the religiously inappropriate nature of their thoughts.

Other disturbing obsessions and compulsions

The OCD mind can create an infinite variety of obsessions and corresponding compulsions. For example, a few people have endless loops of wondering about what their purpose in life is. This is not just a typical adolescent existential crisis, but a continuous stream of unanswerable anxiety producing questions that lead to compulsive quests for reassurance. Others may have obsessive thoughts and fears that what they are experiencing is not reality, that there is somehow another world that exists. They, too, may constantly and compulsively search and ask for reassurance from others.

TECHNICAL STUFF

Although theoretical physicists and theologians ponder similar issues, they are curious and undisturbed by their queries and speculations. Thus, they don't suffer from OCD.

Superstitions and rituals

Superstitions involve beliefs that various events, circumstances, and happenings have extraordinary significance with ominous implications. The ultimate concern of most superstitions involves fear of death. Thus, one with superstitious OCD may attach great meaning to the power of

>> **Numbers:** Those with superstitious OCD may feel they must do everything in sets of five or some other special number, or something horrific will occur. Hotels typically skip the 13th floor because so many people believe it's unlucky. However, folks with that concern only have superstitious OCD if they spend lots of time worrying excessively about certain numbers.

>> **Anything related to death:** Here, special significance is attached to having passed a hearse, cemetery, or funeral home. Sometimes these obsessions and compulsions have only a superficial, subtle connection to death. For example, a person with this type of OCD may avoid sitting in a chair previously owned by a now-dead person.

>> **Words:** Sometimes the superstitions concern the special power and meaning of specific words. For example, a person with this type of OCD may feel compelled to say "Bingo!" whenever they end a sentence because they fear that someone will die if they don't.

Again, these categories of OCD are somewhat arbitrary. Superstitions permeate many of the earlier categories of OCD.

Symmetry and perfectionism

A driven need for symmetry, slowness, and precision are common themes in an OCD category sometimes called the "just so" or the "just right" type of OCD. As with most OCD categories, "just so" OCD frequently accompanies other types of OCD. Some examples include:

>> Feeling compelled to order books alphabetically by the second word in the title and align them exactly one-half inch from the bookshelf's edge

>> Spending hours each day making sure the fringe on floor rugs is lined up perfectly

>> Rewriting class notes in perfect calligraphy each day

Joey is a 10-year-old child who worries about their parents' safety. Joey's story illustrates OCD with a checking component along with a need for rituals to be "just so."

> Joey gets up several times each night to check on their parents. Joey also believes that they must follow a special bedtime routine involving reading a special story, putting pajamas on in a certain way, smoothing out the bed perfectly, placing the pillow diagonally from the left bedpost, and demanding that both parents say "I love you" three times. Otherwise, Joey believes that their parents will die during the night. Joey spends hours on these routines until they get a feeling that they've done everything "just right."

Joey's story demonstrates how "just so" OCD has no real logic to it. People with this form of OCD believe that the feeling of "just so" has some kind of special importance and significance. See Chapter 16 for more information, illustrations, and treatment strategies for this type of OCD.

Parenting OCD

When parents first take on the responsibilities of parenthood, they usually experience mixed feelings. Hopefully and generally, new parents feel great joy and love. But parents are also likely to feel a significant amount of fear. Most new parents report having strange, unwanted thoughts such as the following:

>> What if I drop my baby?

>> What if I lose my temper and yell at the baby?

>> Is it safe to give my baby a bath; what if I slip and the baby drowns?

>> What if I grab a knife and stab my baby?

>> What if the baby stops breathing?

>> Am I sexually attracted to my baby?

>> What if I hurt my baby?

Parents are horrified by these thoughts. But the thoughts are perfectly normal and common among new parents. They are not obsessions at all if the new parent simply dismisses the thought as weird and carries on with life.

However, for a few new parents, the random thoughts take on great importance. These parents try to block the thoughts or begin new behaviors to protect the baby from harm. A small percentage of new parents form pathological obsessions and compulsions, almost always about the fear of harming their newborn.

Usually referred to as perinatal OCD, this disorder is found in both moms and dads. If left untreated, it can interfere with bonding and care of the infant. A mom might avoid giving the infant a bath out of fear of drowning them. A dad may start checking the locks on doors and windows repetitively to keep intruders from harming the baby. Dad may spend so much time checking that they miss the baby's bedtime routine. The bad news is that parents usually suffer in silence because they feel intense shame about their unacceptable thoughts. The good news is that once identified, perinatal OCD responds well to treatment.

REMEMBER

Everyone has weird, nasty thoughts from time to time, especially sleep-deprived new parents. It doesn't necessarily mean that you have OCD. These unwanted thoughts of harming your baby do not mean that you are at greater risk of hurting your baby. However, if the thoughts occur frequently, don't feel ashamed, but certainly check it out with your health care provider.

Obsessive feelings and sensations

Imagine if you paid close attention to every time you blink. Each time you blink brings your awareness to the feeling in your eyes. Start counting your blinks. Most people blink about one thousand times an hour. Now that you're paying attention to blinking, how long can you keep that up? How would you feel if hours a day you were hyperaware of your blinking?

People with upsetting preoccupations with normal body processes or physical states suffer from sensorimotor obsessions. People with this type of disorder become overly focused on a specific aspect of functioning and believe that they are unable to change their focus. The following are some of the more common obsessions and what is obsessed about:

>> **Breathing:** how deep, shallow, rapid, slow, or how the breath feels going in and out

>> **Swallowing:** how many times, how much saliva is in the mouth, the feeling of swallowing in the mouth and throat

>> **Blinking:** frequency of blinking, the feeling of the eyes when the blink occurs, and the visual changes a blink can make

>> **Background noise:** the hum of a heater, air conditioner, refrigerator, traffic noise

>> **Specific noises:** the sound of a song, throat clearing, sniffing, a particular voice

>> **Physical urges:** feelings of hunger, urges to urinate or defecate, yawns

>> **Pulse or heartbeat:** listening to the sound, often occurs when attempting to fall asleep

>> **Position in space:** where one puts hands when sitting or standing, the feeling of sitting on a specific surface, standing posture

The obsession is being overly focused. The discomfort can be severe. People feel out of control. So, what are the compulsions that follow? Those with sensorimotor obsessions try desperately to distract themselves from focusing on their sensations. Their compulsions include the following:

>> Mental checking to see whether they are still aware

>> Chanting or praying

>> Asking others for reassurance they are normal

>> Seeking medical help

>> Avoiding certain areas that are associated with the sensation

>> Using substances to numb the feelings

>> Repeating or counting the bothersome sensation

HEARING TOO MUCH: MISOPHONIA

Some people are extremely sensitive to certain sounds. When triggered, this sensitivity to sound can result in anger outbursts, irritability, fear, arousal, subjective pain, and/or anxiety. Misophonia can occur in children or adults. Sounds like swallowing, throat clearing, chewing, and sniffing are relatively common culprits. Sometimes disturbing sounds like a certain person's voice, background noise, paper rustling, barking dogs, birds singing, and so on can cause symptoms.

Misophonia can result in significant impairment. Children and adolescents may have tantrums or angry outbursts when confronted with the sound that upsets them. Many people avoid places or situations in which they might encounter the particular sound that upsets them.

(continued)

(continued)

Although this disorder has not yet been classified as an official diagnosis, many clinicians have seen those who suffer misophonia in their offices. Friends, colleagues, and family members are often dismissive of misophonia. They often tell those with the disorder to just get over it. Unfortunately, that attitude makes about as much sense as telling someone with a broken leg to just get over it.

Like other rare disorders, misophonia lacks research to determine the best treatment strategies. However, treatment such as exposure and response prevention, psychoeducation, and distress tolerance training have been used successfully in individual cases.

Separating OCD from Normal Worries

Are you obsessively wondering whether you have OCD? Table 2-1 is a simple little quiz that can help you gain some insight on the matter. Check the appropriate "Yes" or "No" box next to each question. (Each question is representative of a symptom of OCD.)

Did you check "yes" to two or more items in Table 2-1? You did? Good! That means you answered honestly. But no matter how many items you checked yes or no, this quiz doesn't say much at all about whether you suffer from OCD.

Studies tell us that almost everyone has *occasional* unwanted thoughts (obsessions) or engages in a *few* actions designed to reduce tension or distress (compulsions) just like the ones in Table 2-1. Yet the "symptoms" in Table 2-1 look pretty much like the obsessions and compulsions that make up OCD. The operative words are *occasional* and *few*.

More than 90 percent of people report occasionally experiencing some of the *exact same kinds* of obsessive thoughts, urges, and images that someone with OCD may have (and you've got to wonder if the other 10 percent are telling the truth!). For example, most people have occasionally imagined physically hurting someone in a terrible way. Maybe you've walked by the knife holder and had a brief disturbing image of pulling one out and stabbing your child. You are not alone! Occasional imaginings like this are neither rare, nor an indication you have OCD.

REMEMBER

Someone with OCD, on the other hand, *frequently* experiences unsettling images, truly worries about acting out those images, and feels *enormously upset* by them.

TABLE 2-1   ## Could You Have OCD?

Yes	No	Have you . . .
		Counted the stairs as you walk up them?
		Carried a lucky charm?
		Knocked on wood?
		Had a horrible image of hurting someone you care about?
		Felt a need to clean your house more than usual?
		Gone back to recheck the locks in your house?
		Had a bad feeling you may have left the coffeepot on?
		Wondered whether you might be gay?
		Avoided stepping on cracks?
		Worried that your house might burn down?
		Struggled to throw out things you don't need?
		Had an inappropriate, unwanted sexual image in your mind?
		Worried that you may have committed a sin?
		Worried that you may have offended someone?
		Had a minor physical symptom that your mind blew up into a serious illness?
		Felt dirty for no good reason and had a strong urge to wash your hands?

OCD and Diversity

OCD occurs around the world. Similar themes occur across cultures. People all over the world tend to get OCD at about the same rate (1 to 2 percent). The themes of OCD regarding fear of contamination, need for symmetry and order, worries about having inappropriate thoughts, and fear of harming oneself or others are consistent globally.

However, specific differences can be observed, depending on cultural experiences. For example, some cultures have more prevalence of scrupulosity (fears regarding sin and morally inappropriate thoughts); other countries have more people with OCD obsessions regarding violent actions; and still others have a higher prevalence of contamination OCD.

The United States is a diverse nation. Diversity includes not only racial, cultural, and ethnic difference, but religious diversity, gender diversity, economic diversity, and ability/disability diversity. Although research suggests that different groups in the United States tend to have different presentations of OCD, the rates across groups are similar. However, there is not equal access to treatment. Some barriers to treatment add a burden to many diverse people seeking help such as:

>> **Cost:** A significant number of Americans are uninsured or underinsured. Mental health treatment can be out of reach for many in diverse communities.

>> **Stigma:** Unfortunately, there continues to be a great deal of stigma related to admitting to having a mental health problem. In some cultures, mental health problems may seem like a sign of moral weakness.

>> **Lack of access:** Poor or inadequate transportation and lack of available professionals make finding appropriate help difficult. These challenges are more prevalent for people with limited resources.

>> **Language and ability differences:** It may be difficult to find trained professionals who speak the language of those seeking services. For example, people who are deaf or hard of hearing may require a professional competent in American Sign Language. Uncertainty of immigration status may also be a barrier to seeking help.

>> **Lack of confidence in treatment:** Some groups have been denied or given inadequate or inappropriate treatment in the past. They may believe that offered treatment will not work.

Getting to a Diagnosis of OCD

To be officially diagnosed as having OCD, three factors must be present:

>> The person must frequently experience either obsessions, compulsions, or both.

>> Except for children, at one time or another, the person must at least *partially* recognize that the symptoms are illogical or unreasonable.

>> Dealing with the symptoms must take up lots of time and interfere with life in a significant way.

Insight or awareness of the "unreasonable" nature of OCD varies widely from person to person. If you talk with most adults who suffer from OCD, usually they know at some level that their obsessions and compulsions don't make a whole lot of sense. For example, people who fear becoming contaminated by touching doorknobs probably know that their fear is overblown. But ask a man with this fear to touch a doorknob, and you'll encounter surprising resistance and emotional upset at the very thought.

Children sometimes have almost no insight or awareness that their OCD is irrational. They sometimes think that their rituals or obsessive thoughts are quite plausible and necessary. For example, a child may truly believe that they must repeat "Thank you, God, for my family" 20 times in order to keep everyone safe — and if they don't say it just right, they must keep repeating the phrase, or someone in their family will die.

Sometimes people with OCD even worry that they're losing their minds. OCD takes over so much of their lives that they feel totally helpless and incapacitated. At its worst, OCD can take many hours of a person's time every single day. OCD interferes with jobs, relationships, school, achievements, and ordinary household chores.

TIP

Although OCD can be quite serious, the problem is definitely treatable. If you or someone you care about has OCD-like symptoms, seek help. See Chapter 7 for more on finding appropriate treatment for OCD.

REMEMBER

OCD takes away joy, productivity, time, and relationships while giving back worry, doubt, uncertainty, and misery. If you spend an hour or so each day worrying about and trying to solve your financial problems while teetering on the edge of bankruptcy, that's not OCD. That's realistic concern. But if you're sitting on a six-million-dollar stash of cash fretting for hours each day whether you'll have enough to retire, you just may be showing signs of OCD.

Avoiding self-diagnosis

WARNING

Please do not attempt to diagnose OCD in yourself or others. This book gives you general guidelines so that you can know enough to get any such concerns checked out by a professional. OCD is complex and should be evaluated by a professional who is experienced with this disorder. See Chapter 7 for information on finding qualified professionals who can diagnose and help you.

Avoiding misdiagnosis

OCD often is missed or misdiagnosed by doctors and counselors. Quite a few people go from professional to professional before receiving a correct evaluation. According to the International Obsessive Compulsive Foundation, people with

OCD take up to 9 years to obtain an accurate diagnosis and an average of 17 years to receive appropriate treatment. One of the reasons it takes so long is that many of those with OCD keep their symptoms secret, especially the more bizarre symptoms. So be open with your mental-health professional and be sure you go to someone well-qualified in diagnosing OCD.

Chapter **3**

Meeting the Associates and Relatives of OCD

O bsessive-compulsive disorder (OCD) has many associates and relatives. Associates of OCD are disorders or emotional problems that often accompany OCD but are not thought to be directly related to the disorder. They don't always occur, but OCD sufferers are at greater risk of succumbing to them.

Relatives of OCD are disorders that look somewhat like OCD but are not necessarily OCD. These related disorders all involve difficult-to-repress, repetitive urges, thoughts, images, impulses, and/or behaviors. These impulses are often difficult to control, even though people find them quite disturbing and disruptive to their lives.

This chapter first describes the co-occurring mental health conditions that increase the suffering of those with OCD. Next, closely related disorders are discussed. Finally, more distantly related disorders are introduced.

REMEMBER

Mental health professionals diagnose their patients with various disorders. It is important to do that in order to communicate with other providers regarding care, to keep records of improvement, to bill insurance, and to conduct research. However, when you are suffering, it doesn't matter as much whether your particular diagnosis is OCD or something similar. You want to feel better. A good mental health provider will treat your symptoms and not be overly worried about nailing down your specific diagnosis.

Recognizing the Guests or Associates of OCD

People with OCD often have emotional problems such as anxiety or depression that occur along with OCD but are not considered part of the OCD spectrum. Thus, they do not involve the same repetitive, irresistible obsessions and compulsions found in OCD. Those with OCD are at higher risk of having these emotional disturbances than those without OCD. In fact, OCD commonly is accompanied by one or more of these or other emotional disorders.

When anxiety and OCD hang out together

Those with OCD are at higher risk than other people for having anxiety disorders. Common anxiety disorders include generalized anxiety disorder, panic disorder, specific phobia, social anxiety disorder, agoraphobia, and anxiety disorders related to medication or medical conditions. Symptoms of anxiety disorders include the following:

>> Avoidance of people and places

>> Excessive worry

>> Fears of losing control

>> Feeling spacey

>> Feelings of impending doom

>> Restless agitation

>> Frequent feeling of being on edge

>> Hyper alertness

>> Intense fears

>> Problems sleeping

>> Irritability

>> Panic attacks

>> Tension

WARNING

If you experience symptoms of an anxiety disorder, you should get them checked out. Left untreated, anxiety disorders can lead to problems with health, relationships, and work. For a more thorough review of anxiety disorders, see the latest edition of *Anxiety For Dummies* (Wiley).

Moods and OCD

Studies suggest that at least a quarter of people diagnosed with OCD also have a disturbance of mood. Mood disorders come in two major types: depression and mania.

>> **Depression:** Depression involves intense, prolonged feelings of sadness and low mood. Symptoms can include a lack of interest or pleasure in things, insomnia, hypersomnia (sleeping too much), poor or excessive appetite, feelings of worthlessness, problems concentrating, feelings of hopelessness, and fatigue.

>> **Mania:** Mania involves inflated self-esteem, decreased need for sleep, distractibility, racing thoughts, rapid speech, increased energy, excessive indulgences in high-risk behaviors (such as foolish business endeavors, sexual acting out, gambling, illegal drug use), and lack of judgment. Although some with mania report extremely high moods, most people with mania do things that are not in their best interests. And they usually crash at some point. Bipolar disorder involves alternations between manic and depressive states.

WARNING

If you experience symptoms of a mood disorder, you should get them checked out by a mental health professional. Left untreated, mood disorders can lead to serious problems. For a more thorough review of mood disorders, see *Depression For Dummies* and *Bipolar Disorder For Dummies* (both published by Wiley).

Meeting the Close Relatives of OCD

A rainbow contains a spectrum of colors. Although each color is distinct, the colors are all formed by reflected sunlight within the same rainbow. Scientists continue to engage in robust arguments about whether or not OCD and its related disorders can be thought of as a spectrum of closely related disorders sharing certain common features as opposed to a single distinct disorder. In fact, recent studies on the neurobiology of OCD–related disorders suggest that they have some common genetic and biological roots.

What OCD and its related disorders all have in common is an inner need, impulse, or urge to do something to meet a perceived craving. These needs are dealt with compulsively. People with compulsive disorders feel compelled to do something. Compulsions in OCD are repetitive behaviors designed to bring relief by decreasing distress. By contrast, some of the related disorders involve repetitive urges driven by a need to maximize stimulation or pleasure. These compulsions are stimulating and done with little thought about safety or risk, as opposed to relieving discomfort.

Body dysmorphic disorder (BDD): A seriously distorted self-image

Probably everyone has at least one or more minor things they don't like about their appearance or body, but it's ultimately no big deal. On the other hand, people with body dysmorphic disorder (BDD) believe something is horribly wrong with their appearance or bodies. They obsess about minor flaws in their appearance and engage in compulsive actions to reduce the discomfort they feel. BDD often occurs in people with a diagnosis of OCD and shares many of the same features. Common obsessive thoughts associated with BDD include worries about having

>> A complexion with mild discoloration

>> A crooked nose

>> A head that's too big or too small for the body

>> A small facial scar

>> A thin mouth

>> A weak jaw

>> Bumps on the face

>> Eyes that are too small

>> Hair that's too curly or too thin, or too much hair

>> Mild acne

>> Protruding ears

>> Wrinkles

Other concerns involve the size of one's sex organs or other body parts. The list is endless. The defects that concern people with BDD are greatly exaggerated and rarely (if ever) noticed by others.

The concerns of those with BDD may change from one aspect of the sufferer's appearance to another. Symptoms may ease up for a while and then get worse.

BDD involves much more than normal preoccupation about one's looks. People with BDD feel that they are deformed, ugly, and defective. In order to feel better, BDD sufferers engage in compulsive behaviors, such as the following:

>> Asking for frequent reassurance from others

>> Becoming housebound because of embarrassment

- » Checking themselves constantly in the mirror

- » Digging or picking at imagined deformities (causing infections, skin irritations, and scars)

- » Washing or shaving excessively

- » Visiting dermatologists frequently

- » Having extensive cosmetic surgery

- » Keeping the head down or combing hair across the face

- » Wearing excessive make-up to hide the perceived flaw

- » Wearing hats or clothes to camouflage the imagined defects

One could make the argument that BDD is actually a specific type of OCD, one that has an exclusive focus on the issue of appearance. On the other hand, BDD is a little different from the usual OCD in that behaviors like getting plastic surgery or wearing a wig don't occur repeatedly throughout each day like compulsions associated with most OCD (see Chapter 2 for more information about OCD and compulsions).

WARNING

BDD can result in severely disabling depression, isolation, and even suicide. If you or someone you know has symptoms of BDD, have an evaluation by a professional experienced with this disorder and get help.

Hoarding disorder

Children begin "hoarding" hobbies at young ages. Kids like to collect coins, bottle caps, and pinecones. Collections are a normal developmental process unless the collecting goes awry and spirals out of control. Hoarding usually starts in adolescence with a normal amount of stuff, but evolves into perpetual, driven squirrels. They find themselves collecting a wider and wider variety of things. Eventually, some hoarders discover that they can't throw out much of anything.

Characteristics of a hoarding disorder include the following:

- » People accumulate huge quantities of possessions that have trivial value. At the same time, they may mix items into their piles of junk that do have value — jewelry, legal papers, and so forth. But it is the piles of items without real value that define this characteristic.

- » Homes become so cluttered that the living areas can no longer be used for their original purposes (such as dining, watching television, bathing, or cooking).

>> Those who acquire these possessions either feel distressed by the effects of their hoarding, or they show signs of impaired ability to work or carry out their lives in a normal manner.

Note that the third characteristic involves either distress or impairment — thus, one can have a hoarding disorder without actually feeling distressed about it. And not feeling concerned about the problem is quite common. The lack of distress is surprising, though, because hoarding causes substantial disability.

The consequences of having hoarding OCD can be quite harsh and severe; some hoarders are found dead or injured as a result of malnutrition or poor home safety conditions. The clutter and resulting unsanitary conditions can result in high risk for

>> Chronic breathing problems

>> Fire

>> Gas or water leaks

>> Insect and rodent infestations

>> Tripping and falling

Hoarders eventually stop inviting people to their homes. The stove may stop working, but they fear calling an appliance repairman because someone entering their house might alert health or welfare officials. Even a pizza delivery could result in a report to the police.

Sometimes homes suffer structural damage because of leaky water faucets, insects or rodents feed on rotting food, or feces and urine, which often accumulate from rodents, large numbers of animals, or the unusual act of hoarding one's own excrement. If someone turns a hoarder in, officials may hospitalize or evict them. Cleanup when hoarders are discovered can be extremely costly — and is usually covered by tax dollars.

Perhaps not surprisingly, hoarders tend to be single. They develop an attachment to "stuff" rather than people. Those who do marry have a high divorce rate.

Those afflicted with hoarding often show profound signs of various other disabilities. They have an increased occurrence of depression, anxiety, and most other emotional problems. They miss more work than most people, and they often have many other health problems.

THE TRAGIC HOARDING OF THE COLLYER BROTHERS

One of the strangest and saddest stories of hoarding involves the reclusive brothers Langley and Homer Collyer. Their story was covered by newspapers throughout the world. Sons of a doctor and an opera singer, the Collyer brothers inherited a 12-room townhouse in New York City. They had both graduated from Columbia University. Homer worked for a time as a lawyer, and Langley became increasingly reclusive. At some point, Homer became blind, apparently from various health issues. He was unable to work and was totally dependent on Langley for his care. They filled their home with newspapers, magazines, broken furniture, thousands of books, 14 pianos, and junk. They kept their doors locked. Eventually utilities were turned off because of unpaid bills.

The brothers became increasingly paranoid and set booby traps so that anyone breaking in would be crushed by the rubble. Someone called the police in 1947 because of a horrible smell. A single officer was unable to get in — he faced a solid wall of broken furniture and newspapers. It took a squad of seven men to finally get through; they discovered Homer dead from cardiac arrest, likely caused by malnutrition and dehydration. It took several weeks to find Langley. Police speculated that he'd been attempting to deliver food and water to his invalid brother when he was crushed by one of his own booby traps. More than 100 tons of hoarded stuff were cleared from the four-story building, which had to be demolished.

Trichotillomania: Pulling your hair out

Trichotillomania involves repetitively pulling hair out of one's body and sometimes eating the hair. The hair can be pulled from anywhere on the body — the scalp, the eyebrows, other parts of the face, the underarms, the stomach, or even the pubic area. Hair-pulling can occur sporadically and briefly throughout the day, or it can go on for hours. In order to have this diagnosis, a person must exhibit noticeable hair loss.

Besides hair loss, other effects of trichotillomania can include skin infections, social isolation, tendonitis, muscle strains (from repetitive movements of the wrist, head, or neck), and even gastrointestinal problems from ingesting hair. Some hair-pullers stroke pulled hairs, inspect them, or slide them between their teeth (causing wear of tooth enamel). People who have this disorder often go to great lengths to disguise their problem by combing over, using cosmetics, wearing wigs, or pulling hair from areas usually covered by clothing.

OBSESSIVE-COMPULSIVE DOGS

Studies suggest that OCD may exist in the animal kingdom as well as in humans. Acral canine lick is a skin disorder in dogs that involves repetitive licking, scratching, or grooming. Dogs who are bored, left alone, or suffer from separation anxiety begin excessively licking an area, resulting in irritation and hair loss. This behavior may temporarily reduce tension but usually results in discomfort, infection, and sometimes nerve damage. The similarity to OCD and other impulse control disorders is that the behavior is repetitive, impulsive, and probably originally intended by the dog to decrease anxiety or distress. That's why many veterinarians consider Acral canine lick to be the OCD of dogs. Interestingly, the same class of antidepressant medication that has been found to be helpful in treating OCD and trichotillomania has helped dogs with this disorder. But, please, don't ever give any of your medication to your pets. Take them to the vet to get their own dosage prescribed.

Some people with trichotillomania report feeling pleasure when they pull hair. Others report feeling an overwhelming urge to pull out hair, followed by a reduction of the urge and tension after they have pulled their hair for a while. While anxiety can increase hair-pulling, anxiety seems to play a less important role in trichotillomania than it does in OCD.

Like OCD, impulses or urges are repetitive. Rituals or compulsions can be involved with the hair-pulling. Hairs are sometimes chosen because they feel just right, are a particular color, or are in a certain location. After hairs are pulled, they can be eaten, stored or preserved in ritualistic ways, or brushed against the face. See Chapter 19 for some ideas on reducing symptoms of trichotillomania.

Skin-picking: Excoriation disorder

Almost everyone occasionally picks at the skin on their hands or face to a limited degree at one time or another. This behavior is especially common when a scab forms, a rough patch of skin appears, or some other minor anomaly emerges on the scalp, nails, or skin. However, for some people, nail-biting and skin-picking develop into a serious disorder that causes scarring, bleeding, sores, infections, and considerable tissue destruction.

Skin-picking and nail-biting are surprisingly common. Although precise statistics are not available, some researchers have reported as many as 5 percent of a sample of college students picked at their skin for over an hour per day. Those with this problem report great shame and worry about reactions from other people.

Typically, skin-picking seems to be driven by strong urges and a sense of temporary relief once the act is completed. Anxiety may not play quite as large of a role with skin-picking as it usually does with OCD, but skin-picking shares the repetitive, difficult-to-control aspects of OCD. Furthermore, those who skin-pick have higher than average rates of OCD.

TIP

Skin-picking and nail-biting sometimes occur because a person has body dysmorphic disorder (see the section on BDD earlier in this chapter). Thus, a person with BDD may perceive a slight imperfection on their face and pick at the area in an attempt to remove the imperfection. Unfortunately, the skin-picking associated with BDD usually start with an attempt to improve appearance and end up making things worse — sometimes much worse.

Distant Cousins of OCD

The following disorders share some characteristics of OCD but are not thought to be closely related. However, each share some similarities. Those similarities and differences are discussed in the following sections.

Obsessive-compulsive personality disorder

People with healthy personalities have satisfying relationships and live meaningful lives. They can handle stress effectively and solve most problems of daily living. For the most part, they understand their feelings and those of others. They tend to be resilient and flexible.

On the other hand, people with personality disorders demonstrate a wide variety of longstanding, rigid patterns of behavior and problems relating to others. These patterns interfere with living, relationships, work, and play. These problems are quite wide-ranging, and most people with a personality disorder have only some of them.

Obsessive–compulsive personality disorder (OCPD) is a somewhat common type of personality disorder. You may assume that most of those with OCD would also suffer from OCPD. Although those with OCD do have an elevated risk of OCPD, most people with OCD do not also have OCPD.

People with OCPD tend to

>> Be excessively dedicated to work and productivity

>> Be perfectionists

>> Be preoccupied with control

>> Be self-righteous

>> Demonstrate excessive frugality and fear of spending money

>> Exhibit rigid, rule-bound thinking

>> Have a reduced need for friendships and leisure versus work

>> Have an excessive need for orderliness and rules

>> See recreation as serious work

In other words, OCPD has a plodding, chronic pattern of general rigidity, orderliness, righteousness, and perfectionism. Although this list of OCPD tendencies may seem a little like OCD, OCPD does not include specific obsessions or compulsions. (See Chapter 2 for more information about obsessions and compulsions.) Most importantly, people with OCPD differ from those with OCD in that they are usually perfectly content with their condition.

Smelling bad: Olfactory reference disorder

People with olfactory reference disorder believe that they smell bad. Not only do they believe that they smell bad, but they also believe that those around them notice their putrid smell and are disgusted and offended.

This is not just a temporary feeling that many people experience after sweating in a hot or humid place or after working out. This belief is fixed and pervasive. People with this disorder may engage in compulsive showering, excessive deodorant use, and even surgical intervention to remove sweat glands. Those with this disorder report extreme distress, shame, and even suicidal thoughts related to their problem.

The disorder has not been studied sufficiently to determine whether or not it fits as part of the OCD spectrum. That may be because those with olfactory reference disorder rarely seek mental health treatment.

Tics and Tourette's syndrome: Involuntary sounds and movements

Everyone demonstrates a few behaviors from time to time that look a lot like tics. For example, who hasn't drummed fingers, tapped a pencil, or experienced a sudden body jerk? However, those behaviors don't quite qualify as tics. That's because tic disorder involves movements or sounds that occur against a person's will, suddenly, repeatedly, and irresistibly. Tourette's syndrome includes multiple movements with sounds.

WARNING

If you or someone you care about has signs of tics or Tourette's syndrome, obtaining a complete neurological examination is important. Other types of neurological conditions can mimic tics and/or Tourette's syndrome. Such conditions include Sydenham's chorea, which is related to rheumatic fever; autism, which is a complex developmental disorder; and pediatric autoimmune neuropsychiatric disorders associated with streptococcal infections (also known as PANDAS). These other conditions may require different treatment approaches.

Tic disorders

Simply put, tics are rapid, repetitive movements or vocalizations that a person can only temporarily suppress. Tics usually get worse when someone is under stress and improve when the person is completely absorbed by an activity (such as video games, playing the piano, giving a lecture, or even performing surgery). Tics usually abate during sleep. Common motor tics (involving body movements) include the following:

>> Blinking

>> Facial gestures

>> Facial grimacing

>> Grooming

>> Hand gestures

>> Jumping

>> Shoulder-shrugging

>> Sniffing

>> Stamping

>> Touching something

Common vocal tics (involving noise) include the following:

>> Barking

>> Clicks with the tongue or teeth

>> Grunting

>> Making screeching sounds

>> Repeating words

>> Snorting

>> Throat-clearing

Tics show up in young children as early as the age of two. Often the sounds or gestures can be rather subtle and almost unnoticeable. Other times, they can appear dramatic and disruptive to others. Tic symptoms usually worsen between the ages of nine and fifteen. Over time, symptoms wax, wane, and shift from one type of tic to another.

Tourette's syndrome

The diagnosis of Tourette's syndrome (TS) is given when a person exhibits multiple motor tics along with at least one vocal tic. This distinction between tics and TS seems somewhat arbitrary. For example, someone with many motor tics would not receive the diagnosis of Tourette's syndrome, but someone else with two motor tics and one mild vocal tic would be deemed as suffering from TS.

TIP

Good news. No one knows why for sure, but many people with either tic disorders or TS discover that their symptoms significantly improve over the years. And even if the symptoms don't improve, treatments can help (see Chapter 19 for information about treating tic disorders and TS).

So how are tic disorders and TS like OCD? Tics feel irrepressible and uncontrollable just like compulsions feel for most people with OCD. And after a tic has been carried out, sometimes people report feeling slightly better for a while. Compulsions in OCD have an explicit intent to reduce anxiety or distress. By contrast, no clear goals are associated with tics, and they seem automatic and reflexive.

WHEN TOURETTE'S SYNDROME IS MISUNDERSTOOD

Tourette's syndrome is often confused or miscategorized by the public and media who are familiar with one of Tourette's more noticeable sub-types, coprolalia. Those with the misfortune of having this type of verbal tic find themselves uncontrollably shouting out obscenities. Sometimes teachers, coaches, and friends think that this symptom is under the sufferers' control and incorrectly blame them for their seemingly inappropriate behavior.

Interestingly, some people with OCD greatly fear that they will shout out obscenities in public. However, they almost never actually do what they fear. Those with coprolalia unfortunately do experience uncontrolled shouting and swearing.

Fortunately, most people with Tourette's syndrome do not experience the symptom of coprolalia. Estimates vary, but experts contend that only about 10 to 15 percent of those with Tourette's syndrome have coprolalia. Furthermore, many of those with tic disorder or TS have fairly mild tics that often go undiagnosed for many years. Getting a diagnosis can be useful because then treatment can be sought for the disorder (and tics and TS are treatable). However, some people's symptoms are sufficiently mild and do not greatly interfere with their lives; for them, treatment may seem unnecessary.

Although tics, TS, and OCD appear to be a little different from each other, it is common to suffer from both tics and OCD at the same time. Scientists theorize that tics, TS, and OCD have genetic links.

Somatic symptom disorder: I think I'm really sick

People with somatic symptoms disorder (commonly known as hypochondriasis) have deep fears and are preoccupied with the idea that they suffer from a serious illness. These fears are usually based on misinterpretations of vague bodily sensations, and they persist even after medical evaluations confirm that nothing is wrong. Often those who suffer from this disorder seek multiple medical tests, make frequent trips to the doctor's office, and repeatedly change medical professionals. Somatic symptom disorder significantly interferes with vocational and interpersonal functioning.

WARNING

Vague physical symptoms can be signs of real, treatable illnesses. If you or someone you care about experiences pain or new, undiagnosed symptoms, see your primary care doctor or other medical expert for an evaluation. If you receive a diagnosis of somatic symptom disorder, it will be important for your mental-health provider and your healthcare provider to communicate closely with one another.

What makes somatic symptom disorder similar to OCD? First, the over-concern and attention to physical complaints are uncontrollably obsessional. These worries exist in the mind of the sufferer. People with somatic symptom disorder ask for repeated reassurance from caregivers and family. Second, they engage in repetitive checking for bodily symptoms, like unusual coloration or consistency of their stools and minor aches and pains. Normal results of lab tests are typically doubted, and they ask for tests to be repeated.

TIP

It is, of course, possible that someone exhibiting symptoms of somatic symptom disorder or hypochondriasis suffers from a real, undiagnosed illness and that a doctor will eventually discover the problem. However, people with somatic symptom disorder and OCD of other types function better if they can learn to live with a certain degree of uncertainty.

Eating disorders: Intense fear of fat

Most eating disorders share the issue of obsessive concern with appearance found in those with body dysmorphic disorder (BDD; see earlier section). In addition, research has shown that roughly 20 to 30 percent of those who have eating disorders also have OCD.

ATTENTION DEFICIT DISORDERS (ADD)

The various attention deficit disorders involve problems with attention, impulsivity, and/or hyperactivity. Attentional problems include trouble staying focused, making careless errors, losing everyday items, forgetfulness, and distractibility. Little kids with hyperactivity can't stay in their seats at school; whereas adults with hyperactivity may remain seated but look physically restless and have problems staying with a single activity. People with impulsivity talk before they think, have trouble waiting in line, and often interrupt others.

People diagnosed with OCD frequently receive an additional diagnosis of one of the attention deficit disorders. And, undoubtedly, sometimes this diagnosis is accurate. However, clinically I have seen people whose obsessions and compulsions have interfered with their ability to focus, perform their jobs, or complete assignments. In other words, OCD consumes lots of attentional resources. In some of those folks, treating the OCD is likely to greatly alleviate what appears to be ADD.

Eating disorders occur in various forms but share an obsessional concern about weight. Sufferers intensely fear gaining weight and frequently have a distorted view of their body and shape. People with eating disorders sometimes

>> Exercise to excess in order to lose weight

>> Have highly restricted diets

>> Overuse laxatives as a weight-loss strategy

>> Self-induce vomiting to purge their bodies of calories consumed

>> Use diuretics and enemas to lose weight

WARNING

Eating disorders can result in brain damage, loss of tooth enamel, erosion of the esophagus, malnutrition, abnormal heart rhythms, hormonal imbalances, and even death. If you or someone you care about exhibits any of the symptoms of an eating disorder, please see a specialist in eating disorders to receive an appropriate diagnosis and treatment plan. You may also want to check out *Eating Disorders For Dummies* (Wiley).

Impulse control disorders: unstoppable bad habits

Impulse control disorders share the concept of repetitive urges found in OCD. However, with impulse control disorders, the urges are not as clearly about needing to reduce distress or anxiety. Rather, the impulses seem more related to increasing a sense of pleasure or excitement. Impulse control disorders include

>> **Kleptomania:** Kleptomaniacs can't resist the impulse to steal things that they don't even really need. They feel tense before stealing and experience pleasure and excitement following the act.

>> **Compulsive buying:** Compulsive shoppers have problems similar to kleptomaniacs in the sense that they can't resist things they don't need. But in this case, they at least pay for the items. Their compulsive shopping frequently leads to serious financial problems.

>> **Gambling:** Those with this problem often get themselves into serious trouble with finances, relationships, and even illegal behavior. They have recurrent, obsessive thoughts about gambling. Logically, they have some insight into the futility of their pursuits, but they cannot stop themselves from going after the next big win.

» **Paraphilias:** People with paraphilias are drawn to sexually arousing fantasies and various sexual activities that are typically considered unacceptable or deviant (see the sidebar "Sexual obsession versus acting out").

» **Pyromania:** People with pyromania are fascinated and obsessed by fires. They feel tension prior to setting fires and excitement following the act. They do not set fires for financial gain or revenge. Nonetheless, their behavior often lands them in jail.

SEXUAL OBSESSION VERSUS ACTING OUT

Paraphilias are quite different from sexual obsessions experienced by some who have OCD (see Chapter 2). Sexual obsessions associated with OCD are deemed to be highly inappropriate by the person who experiences them. Those with OCD sexual obsessions obsess about whether they might have a paraphilia, but they actually do not. Thus, those with OCD sexual obsessions almost never act out their obsessions.

On the other hand, those with paraphilias derive considerable pleasure from their fantasies and often act them out. Just a few paraphiliac fantasies and activities include the following:

- **Exhibitionism:** Exposing one's genitals to strangers
- **Fetishism:** Using various non-living objects, such as underwear or shoes, to stimulate masturbation
- **Frotteurism:** Touching or rubbing against a non-consenting person
- **Pedophilia:** Sexual activity with underage children

Chapter **4**

Blaming the Brain for OCD

Just a few hundred years ago, many people believed that obsessive-compulsive disorder (OCD) symptoms were signs of demonic possession. People prayed over, exorcised, or scorned OCD sufferers. Life for those with OCD improved only slightly when Sigmund Freud came along and blamed OCD on hidden desires or early traumatic experiences. Neither approach was very helpful.

Today, OCD is considered a disorder involving brain function, emotions, and behavior; there may even be a link between OCD and some infections. What all this means is that OCD can appear in well-adjusted, smart, normal people without a history of trauma or deep-seated emotional problems. This chapter describes how the brain plays a critical role in the development of OCD.

Looking at the Brain's Role in OCD

The brain governs perception, thinking, memory, behaviors, and emotions. Thus, the brain plays a major role in all emotional disorders, including OCD. But saying the brain is heavily involved with OCD isn't quite the same as saying that OCD is a brain disease and nothing more. In actuality, you can't really separate the brain, behavior, thoughts, and the environment. All of these contributors interact in intricate ways, and they can't be considered as operating in isolation, independently from one another.

Every single thought that you have is generated by neurons communicating inside some portion of your brain. Medications that change the way the brain functions also change the way people think. Alternatively, therapies designed to change the way people think have been shown to change the way the brain functions as well.

To date, no one can point to specific biological processes that *directly cause* OCD (infections are an exception — see the sidebar "PANDAS: Part of the puzzle," later in this chapter). However, brain circuitry appears to work a little differently in those with OCD versus those who do not have OCD. It's the classic chicken and the egg question. No one knows for sure whether biological processes, learning, genetics, or environmental events contribute the most to that circuitry going awry. Or, for that matter, which comes first.

Connecting genetics with OCD

Biological and genetic factors that impact the brain clearly assume some of the blame for OCD, as these factors significantly increase the risk of developing the disorder. Many studies support a genetic predisposition for OCD, that is, the idea that OCD runs in families. If several members of your family have OCD, you run a risk of developing symptoms. If you have an identical twin with OCD, your risk is even higher. However, the particular way the disorder is inherited is not yet clear.

OCD has many faces, and the face shown by OCD in a parent may differ from that seen in a child. For example, a parent who has the kind of OCD in which they check door locks can give birth to a son who is obsessed about germs and a daughter with no signs of OCD.

OCD seems to be biologically or genetically linked to Tourette's syndrome (tics involving sudden movements such as grimacing, eye-blinking, grunts, or throat-clearing). OCD sufferers are much more likely to develop tics, and people with tics are more likely to develop OCD. This holds true for families as well as individuals. Families in which OCD is prevalent are more likely to also have family members with tic disorder (for more information on tics, see Chapter 3).

Getting inside your head

Knowledge of the brain — its structures, functions, and biochemical processes — has accumulated rapidly since the last century. In part, that's because there are highly sophisticated, safe ways of observing the brain at work. These imaging assessment methods have allowed scientists to increasingly understand the ways in which the OCD brain works both before and after treatment. At this time, OCD is not diagnosed via brain scans, but scans do enable us to see how treatments affect the brain.

Interesting research has looked at what the brain does when someone with OCD is presented with an image that might set off a compulsive reaction. This research suggests that differences exist between how the brain works in people with OCD versus those without the disorder.

TIP

Feel free to skip this material if you're a brain surgeon. (I'm guessing you already know this stuff.) Or you can skip it if you're a regular person who simply doesn't like anatomy and physiology. You can understand OCD pretty well without knowing the intricacies of brain circuitry and chemistry.

Choosing a Path to OCD

Think of the brain as an orchestra with a variety of sections coordinating their parts to produce a pleasant-sounding symphony. If the sections of the orchestra don't communicate well because the conductor isn't doing a good job, the entire performance collapses. However, in the orchestra of OCD, not only is the conductor having problems, but the musicians are also not always following the score. For those with OCD, some of the musicians are daydreaming, others are playing too loud, and some are playing off key. The following material explains the unharmonious result.

Note: This is not an attempt to describe neuroanatomy and neurophysiology in depth. The descriptions of brain functioning will be limited to what you need to know to understand what goes awry in the OCD brain.

You don't need to memorize these terms, but brain structures will be discussed as they relate to OCD. Here are some brief, simple descriptions:

>> **Thalamus:** The relay station of the brain processes information coming from all of the senses and sends it to other structures of the brain.

>> **Amygdala:** Processes emotional information, which just happens to be most of what makes life feel fulfilling and meaningful. The amygdala also sounds an alarm when threatening events occur — even before you consciously know what's going on.

>> **Cortex:** The thinking part of the brain *interprets* information coming from all parts of the brain. The cortex takes in what you sense, see, hear, and feel and makes decisions or evaluations. It also generates thoughts based on memories.

>> **Hippocampus:** The hippocampus is involved in retrieving and storing memories. It also sends information to the amygdala, especially when memories are triggered by similar past events.

The brain is highly complex and adaptable. Many years ago, when I was learning neuropsychology, I recall my mentor telling me that it's not as important to determine exactly where something is happening in the brain as it is to see the effects on individual functioning. Is a brain injury or dysfunction impacting the individual in carrying out responsibilities such as taking care of themselves, having meaningful relationships, driving safely, or achieving vocational goals? In other words, if you have OCD, it may help you understand the various possible pathways in the brain that lead to your problems, but the main concern is how you are coping in everyday life.

Taking information in

The brain is essential for awareness of your surroundings as it orients you to sights, sounds, and sensations. For example, if your ears hear a shout behind you, your brain tells you to turn around and look for the source. If you feel a burning sensation in your foot, your brain directs you to pick up your foot and see what's going on. If your eyes tell you that you're walking on hot coals, you know to jump.

The *thalamus* is the part of the brain that receives, interprets, and integrates information from multiple sites in the brain, including those involved with hearing, seeing, touching, feeling, tasting, and smelling. The thalamus sends this information on to other regions in the brain.

The amygdala and the cortex are two structures in the brain that the thalamus sends information to and are most critical in understanding OCD. The thalamus sends immediate information first to the amygdala and then to the cortex. See Figure 4-1 for how these structures communicate.

The thalamus has been shown to be overly active and even larger in size in some studies of OCD sufferers compared to those without OCD. Other studies have demonstrated that the thalamus appears to normalize after treatment with either medication (see Chapter 11) or therapy (see Chapters 8, 9, and 10).

Selecting the shortcut

The quickest path to responding to potential danger is a direct line from the thalamus to the amygdala. The amygdala processes emotional information. It reacts to threatening events almost instantly. People who suffer damage to the amygdala lose much of the ability to process emotions — good or bad — along with the early warning system.

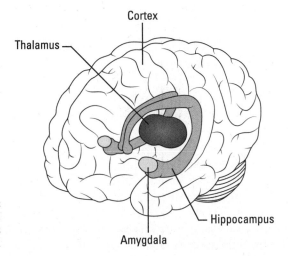

FIGURE 4-1:
Primary Brain
Structures
Involved in OCD.

The amygdala is the first responder to danger. It activates a series of physiological changes in the body that gets you ready to fight for your life, run for your life, or (when overcome with fear) simply freeze. The problem with the amygdala is that it sometimes responds with the fight, flight, or freeze response when there is nothing dangerous going on.

It's the amygdala responding to a sudden loud noise or a shadow that frightens you. This quick processing has advantages. When real danger occurs, your body responds immediately. Your heart pounds, and you begin breathing faster, sending energy to the large muscles. You're ready to jump into action. You scan the environment looking for danger.

Those with OCD have sensitive amygdalas, and they respond with alarm when the threat may not really be threatening. For example, a pillow may be out of order on the couch and someone with OCD immediately feels intense distress. Or a dirty tissue is on the floor, and the brain responds with a flood of fear regarding possible contamination.

Picking the high road

There is another path from the thalamus that takes a few more milliseconds to process than the signal that goes directly to the amygdala. That process goes directly from the thalamus to the cortex. The cortex, the thinking part of the brain, takes that original signal and decides what to do.

This is where the possible danger is analyzed. The cortex decides:

>> Is that shadow an attacking bear or a tree blowing in the wind?

>> Is that a gunshot or a car backfiring?

>> Should I run, duck, cover, or fight?

>> Or would it be better to take a deep breath, realize nothing is wrong, and proceed with my life?

A good working cortex is able to come up with a reasonable plan that fits the threat. It takes that immediate information and chooses an action that responds to potential danger or dismisses it as a false alarm.

However, the cortex can also sound a false alarm. Those with OCD often spend lots of time obsessively thinking of possible dangers without strong signals from the actual world. Instead of relying on information from the thalamus, the OCD cortex conjures up worries about uncertainty, doubt, or risk. Some of these worries are based on memories that are stored in the hippocampus. These fears or worries take a detour back to the amygdala that then begins to pump up the body's response to danger. In fact, research has shown that people with OCD have difficulty recognizing errors in thinking, tend to overreact, and have difficulty stopping their resulting compulsions.

The normal brain puts out a few false alarms too but manages to detect and repress the response to them. An OCD brain has a reduced capacity to inhibit or put brakes on the reaction to false alarms. The following two stories about Ben and Brad illustrate the normal brain's response to false alarms versus the response of the OCD brain.

Ben wakes up at 3 a.m. and thinks, "I think I left the stove on; maybe I need to go check. I'd hate to burn the house down." Ben's cortex sends a mild signal of alarm throughout his brain. However, Ben's amygdala doesn't go into high gear. Various parts of Ben's brain process the information, and Ben concludes, "Well, it's pretty darn unlikely that I left the stove on. I never have before. I'm pretty comfortable right now; it doesn't seem worth getting up. Besides, I have smoke detectors." Ben turns over and goes back to sleep.

Brad wakes up at 3 a.m. and has the same thought as Ben, "Gosh, I think I might have left the stove on; maybe I need to go check. I'd hate to burn the house down." Brad has OCD and Brad's cortex screams a message to Brad's amygdala. Brad's heart races and his entire body fills with dread. Brad jumps out of bed to check the stove. Brad feels relief when he sees that it's turned off. Brad returns to bed. Then Brad thinks, "Maybe I didn't really check the stove carefully enough. Did I check all the burners?" The cycle reactivates and sends Brad scrambling to check the stove again. The entire process is repeated many times before Ben can settle down and go back to sleep.

The contrasting stories of Ben and Brad illustrate how the brain circuitry in people with OCD differs from that of non-sufferers. They both experience a worrisome thought, but Ben's brain responds in a realistic manner, whereas Brad's OCD brain makes him feel that the house is in imminent danger.

Additional evidence supporting the idea that these brain structures and the ways they communicate are involved with OCD can be found in the fact that injury to any of these areas sometimes results in OCD-like symptoms. Even more intriguing is the fact that surgery designed to cut the connections between some of these brain structures appears to improve OCD symptoms. As discussed in Chapter 11, this approach to OCD is reserved for extremely severe cases that have repeatedly failed to respond to numerous other treatments — not something to be tried at home.

Communication within the Brain

The brain is an amazing collection of cells and connections intertwined with a vast network of blood vessels. The average adult brain weighs around three pounds. Within those three pounds are two types of cells: neurons and glia.

>> **Neurons:** The brain has about 100 billion neurons (give or take). Neurons are the cells that communicate with one another. They order muscles to move and generate thoughts. They congregate in groups. Each group communicates within itself as well as with other neuronal groups in the brain.

>> **Glia:** Your brain has about ten times as many glia cells as it does neurons. Glia cells help out by protecting and nourishing the neurons as well as keeping the house clean by removing waste and dead neurons.

Neurons and glia come in many specific forms depending upon the type of work they are called upon to do. They form the basic structures of the brain.

TECHNICAL STUFF

Brain neurons communicate with each other through a sophisticated system that involves both energy and chemistry. Neurons have a cell body and projections that assist in communication. Axons are the projections that transmit information from the cell body toward the next cell. Dendrites are the projections that collect information from other cells. Axons and dendrites transmit their information across something known as a *synaptic cleft*. The cleft is a small space between axons and dendrites.

Electricity and chemicals

Communication among brain neurons starts with an electrical impulse in the cell body that is transmitted down the axon toward another cell. When the impulse arrives at the presynaptic ending (or terminal), substances known as neurotransmitters are released. These neurotransmitters function as chemical messengers between cells.

Neurotransmitters are released from one neuron and travel across the synaptic cleft. There, most are vacuumed up by a receiving neuron at the postsynaptic receptor site. From the postsynaptic receptor site, an electrical impulse travels down the dendrite toward the receiving cell body. Some of the neurotransmitters don't make it to the receiving cell and return to the sending cell. See Figure 4-2 for an illustration of how this process works.

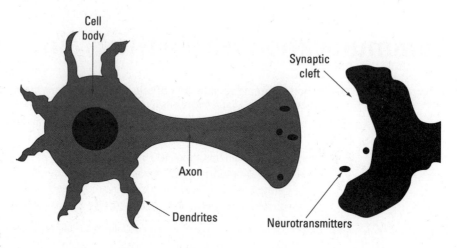

FIGURE 4-2: The cellular method of carrying on a conversation.

PRESYNAPTIC NERVE   POSTSYNAPTIC NERVE

Serotonin, dopamine, and glutamate

Scientists continue to discover new types of neurotransmitters. Currently, three transmitters, serotonin, dopamine, and glutamate seem to be particularly related to the brain functioning of people with OCD. These transmitters follow circuits through different regions of the brain and are thought to be central to mood, energy level, memory, learning, and behavior. Although much remains to be determined about how and why these systems cause problems in the brain, the following has been discovered:

>> **Serotonin:** This neurotransmitter is involved in wakefulness and mood. Disruptions in serotonin are related to OCD, anxiety, depressed moods, eating disorders, tics, aggression, and impulsivity.

Medications that increase the availability of serotonin have been found to help most people with OCD. Some report that they continue to have obsessive thoughts, but are able to cope with their feelings without responding with compulsions. (See Chapter 2 for more about obsessions and compulsions.)

>> **Dopamine:** This transmitter is involved in the reward system of the brain and seems to be related to addictions. Parkinson's disease, a condition in which people experience tremors and muscle rigidity, is associated with decreased availability of dopamine. Schizophrenia, a disorder that involves disorganized thinking, is related to too much dopamine. OCD and Tourette's syndrome (see Chapter 3) also appear to involve disruption in the dopaminergic system.

Drugs that block dopamine have been found to be effective in treating tics as well as repetitive behaviors. Drugs that increase dopamine can induce tics and symptoms of OCD. See Chapter 11 for more information about medication and OCD.

>> **Glutamate:** This chemical messenger is involved in regulating learning and memory. Decreased levels of glutamate are found in people with insomnia, poor concentration, and fatigue. Excess glutamate result in toxicity and neuronal death and has been associated with Alzheimer's disease. There is some evidence that glutamate dysfunction is evident in OCD, however far more research is needed to determine the effects and potential treatments using medication to change concentrations of glutamate in the brains of people with OCD.

TIP

People check the oil level in their cars by using a dipstick to see whether more is needed. No dipstick equivalent exists to check the levels of neurotransmission in the brain. That's why sometimes multiple medications that target these areas need to be tried before the right one is found. (See Chapter 11 for more information about medication.)

PANDAS: PART OF THE PUZZLE

So what do Chinese bears that eat bamboo have to do with OCD? Nothing, really. PANDAS is the abbreviation for Pediatric Autoimmune Neuropsychiatric Disorders Associated with Streptococcal Infection. Whew. No wonder they're called PANDAS.

PANDAS describe children or teens who suddenly develop OCD symptoms or tics (see Chapter 3 for more on tics and Tourette's syndrome) following a strep throat. Other infections, such as a complication of rheumatic fever called *Sydenham's chorea* and some types of encephalitis, also can result in these or similar symptoms. Symptoms develop rapidly, almost overnight. Kids usually have tics, obsessions, compulsions, and lots of irritability. This sudden onset of symptoms generally improves unless another strep throat comes along.

Researchers believe that PANDAS occur when the body produces antibodies to combat the strep infection. These antibodies do a good job of fighting off the infection. However, sometimes, in some kids, the good guys (antibodies) go after the wrong bad guy. In PANDAS, the antibodies attack the basal ganglia in the brain, which in turn leads to OCD and/or tics.

The use of antibiotics for the treatment of PANDAS is currently being investigated and shows some promise. If antibiotics work, they may work quickly or take a longer time than usual; otherwise, treatment of PANDAS is conducted in the same way as for other types of OCD and has about the same effectiveness. Refer to Chapters 20 and 21 for more on OCD and kids.

Chapter **5**

Developing and Living with OCD

How does obsessive-compulsive disorder (OCD) begin, and why does it develop in some people and not others? OCD symptoms often start in childhood and get worse without treatment. But the disorder can also manifest in adults. Chapter 4 discusses the biological basis for OCD. But biology and the brain are not the only culprits in its development. The environment, experiences, and thinking styles are also important in the genesis and maintenance of OCD.

OCD becomes more entrenched through the innocent encouragement or reinforcement of others. It can also worsen because of wrong thinking patterns exhibited by OCD sufferers.

This chapter reveals childhood experiences that may contribute to the development of OCD. It describes how OCD is maintained and reinforced by giving in to its demands. Finally, the chapter runs down the problems worsened by the way the OCD mind thinks.

REMEMBER

An obsession is an intrusive thought, urge, or image. Compulsions are repetitive mental acts or behaviors intended to reduce the distress associated with obsessions. The cycle of obsessions and compulsions cause mental distress because they are unwanted, time-consuming, and feel completely unacceptable to the sufferer.

More often than for other emotional disorders, such as anxiety and depression, the origins of OCD usually can be traced to childhood where both nature and nurture play roles. Parents are usually quite well-intentioned, but sometimes their efforts to protect or teach their kids go too far and provide fertile ground for the development of OCD.

But OCD can also crop up in adulthood for a number of reasons. In most instances, OCD occurs in adults who have shown some predisposition or symptoms of OCD in childhood. However, OCD can also occur in adults who have no such obvious predispositions but who have suffered a serious infection, head injury, trauma, or major life change. This section examines potential roots of OCD in childhood and looks at some of the likely triggers for adult-onset OCD.

Developing OCD Early

Have you ever observed the bedtime routines of typical two-year-old children? Many have elaborate rituals that they insist their parents follow. These patterns of behavior are rigid and serve to ease children into sleep.

Most children have some anxiety over separating from their mothers or fathers at nighttime. Having rituals helps young children make that separation from awake during the day to asleep at night more securely. In the following example, Alaina illustrates a normal, albeit time-consuming, bedtime routine.

> Two-year-old **Alaina's** mom starts the process of getting her ready for bed shortly after dinner. "Time for your bath; let's pick up your toys," she tells her. Alaina insists on lining up all of her stuffed animals and dolls on a bench in her room. She places each one carefully in an order only she understands. If her mom moves one, she gets upset and rearranges them so that they're just right.
>
> Other toys are tossed into a toy chest. Next comes the bath. Again, she has certain toys for the water. She allows her mom to wash her but remains busy in a pattern of play, singing a song, and carefully arranging her water toys in order on the edge of the tub. After the bath and getting into her pajamas, Alaina chooses three books. Her mother must read them in a certain order.
>
> Then to bed. The comforter must be placed with a certain pattern showing. She has a blanket that she holds onto and three stuffed bears that sleep next to her. The closet door must be completely closed and the blinds up one inch so that a

little light from the street shines through. A family picture sits on the nightstand, angled so that Alaina can see it from her bed. Alaina likes to have her mom sit with her for a couple of minutes. Then there's a short prayer, a kiss, and mom says "Good-night, I love you forever."

Does Alaina have OCD? Not likely. Alaina's rituals are cute and perfectly normal for a two or three-year-old child. Rituals and conventions help children feel cozy and secure. However, if these rituals persist well into middle childhood, they can also point to the first signs of impending OCD. The change from normal to OCD is thought to happen due to unknown mixtures of biology and early experiences (nature and nurture).

Childhood experiences can involve well-intentioned but misguided parenting, trauma, stress, or other negative events. They can also involve a child modeling or adopting the behaviors of a parent who suffers from OCD.

REMEMBER

If family members have OCD, the probability of a child having OCD is higher. This increased probability could be a result of children learning OCD behaviors from their parents. But this increased risk could also be due to genetics. See Chapter 4 for more info on genetics and biological causes of OCD. In fact, in one person, OCD may be entirely the result of genetics, in another it may be entirely the result of the environment, and in a third it may be due to a combination of the two. Pinning down the cause of OCD in any individual case is pretty much impossible.

Good intentions; bad results

Early childhood experiences shape personalities and can set the stage for the development of later emotional difficulties, such as OCD. Parents have tremendous influence over their children. They generally mean well and want only what's best for their kids. The concepts they may introduce their children to are intended to have a positive effect. If taken too far, however, these intentions may boomerang and contribute to a child's OCD.

REMEMBER

Misguided or bad parenting is not the primary cause of OCD. OCD is a complicated disorder that involves the brain as well as learning. However, experiences do influence the occurrence of OCD symptoms and how severe OCD becomes. See Chapters 20 and 21 for more information about OCD in children.

Giving too much information

Good parents warn their children about dangers. But sometimes children are exposed to information that they're not ready to handle. For example, three-year-old children should never be left unsupervised. Sternly warning them to stay away from strangers because people they don't know might steal or kidnap them is not really necessary if they are closely watched over by caring adults. A three-year-old who hears this information may develop intense fear of any unknown person. This fear can lead to obsessional thinking about various dangers in the world.

Exposing children to inappropriate media

Kids spend considerable time watching screens. In fact, recent surveys indicate that kids between 8 and 12 average 4 to 6 hours a day, and teenagers are occupied by screens up to 9 hours a day. Understandably, many busy parents have little idea of the content their kids are being exposed to daily or the length of time they spend onscreen.

No doubt, most kids are subjected to scenes of violence, sex, drug use, and other inappropriate material. Kids who spend too much time on screens are at increased risk for suffering a variety of mental health problems, including depression, anxiety, stress, and poor self-image.

No research exists on the effects of screens specifically on kids who develop OCD. However, common sense and research suggests that allowing young children to be exposed to material beyond their emotional maturity likely contributes to feelings of instability.

TECHNICAL STUFF

Research on screen time and child development is difficult to conduct. The gold standard of research is a randomized control study. Imagine getting a large group of parents and children to agree to the following study: You will be randomly selected to one of three groups. Group one agrees to not use screens. Group two agrees to use screens daily for 3 hours each day. Group three is told to use screens for 10 hours a day. The study lasts for three months. Do you think participants would fully comply with these instructions? How would the study monitor compliance? Not easy to do.

Modeling misguided thinking

Parents want to teach their kids appropriate behavior. But in doing so, sometimes parents inadvertently teach their children that having bad thoughts means they're bad people. The story about Tomas that follows illustrates how such teaching can foster OCD thinking (see the section "Worsening OCD with Bad Thinking," later in this chapter).

Five-year-old **Tomas** loves to play with his Legos. He builds castles and towers. When Tomas's three-year-old sister Michelle knocks over his tower, Tomas pushes her and shouts, "Get out of my room, you creep; I hate you!" Tomas's father overhears the ruckus and yells, "You should *always* love your sister; God punishes kids who have thoughts like that!"

Tomas's father may have gone overboard and frightened his son. Though his intentions were honorable (wanting Tomas to love his sister), he used a scare tactic that could lead to OCD-like thinking. In particular, Tomas's dad suggested that merely having bad thoughts equates with being a bad person, a style of thinking quite common in OCD. Thinking is not the same as doing, but kids can be convinced that they're bad people if they have greedy, mean, or even illogical thoughts. What starts as a random thought can become an obsession.

Seeking perfection

Parents naturally want children to put their best effort into everything they do, but parents can scare their children by telling them they must do things perfectly or not at all. The saying, "If it's worth doing, it's worth doing right," can be pushed too far. Children who feel they must do everything perfectly sometimes stop trying altogether because they're afraid of making mistakes. On the other hand, other children respond by attempting to make everything they do perfect, which is, of course, impossible. (See the section "Needing everything perfect," later in this chapter, for more on the role of perfectionism in OCD.)

Overprotecting

Parents are right in thinking that it's their job to protect their children, but they may contribute to the development of OCD if they become *over*protective and never allow their children to goof up or assume any responsibility. Parents who fall into this trap end up sending a message to their kids that they're not capable of dealing with the world. These kids sometimes grow up believing that the world is a dangerous place and that they have little control.

When bad things happen

Bad things happen to children and their families. When these experiences occur, they can start a pattern of worry and fear. These initial fears can contribute to the development of OCD in children who are susceptible.

Illness

Children who suffer from a serious illness or have close family members who are sick often believe that the illness could have been prevented. For example, a child may be told that if he doesn't wash his hands, he'll get sick. He then actually does get very sick and believes that it's his fault because he didn't wash his hands.

Thereafter, he spends more and more time washing his hands. Or a girl whose grandmother gets cancer believes it happened because her grandmother didn't pray at night. She may start performing rituals to protect herself and other family members.

Accidents

Accidents happen every day. Children, their friends, or family members are often involved in car accidents. Children are exposed to other accidents by overhearing adult conversations or by watching media. Because accidents are frightening and difficult for children to understand, kids often invent ways to protect themselves by using magical chants, rituals, or avoidance. The story below about eight-year-old Austin illustrates how a ritual may emerge after an accident.

> **Austin** returns home from a visit at his cousin's house. On the way, his parents' car is rear-ended by a drunk driver. His brother is seriously injured and hospitalized. Luckily, no one else in the car is hurt. However, Austin is traumatized. Austin thinks he hears someone ask about the seat belts. Austin jumps to the conclusion that his brother did not correctly fasten his seat belt. In the ensuing weeks, Austin starts checking to see whether his belt is fastened "just right."

> At first, he buckles and unbuckles it several times before allowing his mother to pull out of the driveway. This activity gradually develops into a complex pattern — including locking and unlocking the car doors, positioning himself "just so" in the seat, and fastening and unfastening his seat belt until the click sounds "just right." This ritual must be performed every time he gets into the family car. His ritual starts consuming a lot of time, and then he starts other "protective" rituals. Austin develops a full-blown case of OCD.

Austin's story shows how easily children can develop OCD from their attempts to understand and cope with traumatic events. The symptoms sometimes start out making a little bit of sense (such as Austin carefully checking his seat belt) but evolve into activities that have little to do with anything that could realistically serve to protect.

Stress

When children are exposed to lots of stress, symptoms of OCD become worse. No study has directly linked a stressful event to the start of OCD; however, plenty of evidence suggests that stress leads to an increase in distorted thinking, which is characteristic of OCD.

Children may have a bad thought, such as wanting a younger sibling to be hurt. In rare cases, the sibling actually gets hurt sometime later. Children who experience bad thoughts that happen to come true may believe that their thoughts cause bad things to happen.

For example, a girl wishes that her father would stop yelling at her mother. Sometimes she has thoughts of hating her father when he yells. Later, her parents get a divorce, and her father moves out. She believes that her thoughts of hating her father and wishing that he'd stop yelling caused him to leave. Thinking that thoughts cause events to happen is typical of OCD thinking. For more on this, see the later section, "Worsening OCD with Bad Thinking."

Stress can also develop from giving children too much responsibility before they're developmentally ready. For example, an older child who has to assume care for younger siblings can become overwhelmed by the responsibility. The older child worries about somehow hurting the younger ones. The child in charge of his siblings develops an OCD style of thinking; see the "Being too responsible" section later in this chapter.

Trauma

Unfortunately, many children experience abuse or trauma. These events trigger worry and fear. Some children react with anger or depression. Others develop symptoms of OCD. For example, a boy who is at a bank with his father when it's robbed starts to worry about making sure the doors and windows at his house are locked. His daily checking routine starts each evening and involves both of his parents. He also frequently asks his parents to check throughout the house before he goes to bed.

Learning by seeing

Children learn from watching their parents. Thus, parents who exhibit OCD inadvertently can teach or model OCD to their children. The following example of a mother named Jane demonstrates how a parent with OCD can pass it along without intending to do so.

> **Jane** (a mother with OCD) worries about contamination. She obsesses about germs and the possibility of her or her family coming down with a serious illness. In order to protect everyone, Jane compulsively cleans the house with bleach for hours every day. She warns her children about all the dangers from germs. She makes her kids take baths every morning and before bed — as well as when they

return home from school or play outside. Her children listen and accept their mother's fears as being reasonable. Therefore, they begin to fear getting contaminated themselves.

Jane shows how a mother with OCD can model and teach her children to develop the disorder, quite possibly whether they have a genetic predisposition or not. However, not every child with a parent like Jane will develop OCD. Some kids may be more resistant or resilient, whether due to genes or some other unknown factor.

Developing OCD as an Adult

Sometimes adults develop OCD even though they did not suffer from it as children. Major life changes such as divorce, loss of loved ones, natural disasters, and significant financial setbacks, all can trigger the emergence of OCD in an adult. OCD symptoms can start gradually or have a sudden onset. Trauma would be particularly likely to cause a sudden onset of OCD. OCD is especially likely to occur in adults who tend to be anxious and/or have a genetic predisposition for developing OCD.

TRAUMA AND PTSD VERSUS OCD

Traumatic events frequently cause severe emotional pain. One of the more common reactions to severe trauma is known as post-traumatic stress disorder (or PTSD). PTSD involves recurrent thoughts or images of the event and avoidance of reminders of the trauma. For example, a soldier may have repeated images of a bomb exploding and avoid driving near construction sites and congested traffic because loud noises trigger the images.

Less often, trauma may trigger the onset of OCD. But distinguishing between OCD and PTSD can be tricky. If the obsessions and compulsions closely relate to the traumatic event in some way, then PTSD is usually diagnosed as the only emotional disorder. However, in the case of the soldier, if he obsessed about only cleanliness and avoided public restrooms, he would be deemed as suffering from OCD that was triggered by trauma. Finally, if the soldier had repeated images of the bomb exploding, avoided driving in noisy areas, and then began to obsess about cleanliness, he would be suffering from both PTSD and OCD.

Reinforcing OCD with Positives and Negatives

If left alone and untreated, OCD usually gets worse. One reason that OCD becomes more time-consuming and more distressing is because of what psychologists call reinforcement. Before I explain how reinforcement works specifically with OCD, here is the basic premise: *Reinforcement increases the likelihood of something occurring again.* Reinforcement can be positive, negative, or both negative and positive.

Supporting OCD with positive reinforcement

Most people don't go to work without getting a paycheck. The paycheck increases the likelihood of working and is, therefore, a positive reinforcement. Dogs are trained to associate getting a reward for sitting. Dogs will sit for their owners when they expect to get a treat. Even when they don't get a treat, they still have hope. Dog treats positively reward dog sitting.

TIP

Positive reinforcement can be found in encouraging words, a pat on the back, an ice cream cone, or a hug. Praise can also be a powerful form of positive reinforcement.

Friends and family can fall into a trap of positively reinforcing those with OCD. When people you care about suffer from obsessional worries such as the need for order and symmetry, it would be easy to overly compliment the tidiness of someone's home or office. Or, a child with contamination fears could be told that it's nice that they stay so clean. However, the even more powerful contributor to OCD is called negative reinforcement.

Supporting OCD with negative reinforcement

Negative reinforcement happens when a behavior gets rid of a distressing, unpleasant event or feeling. Like positive reinforcement, negative reinforcement increases the likelihood of a behavior occurring in the future. The behavior becomes more frequent because it *reduces* distress.

My dog Ollie is a master at negative reinforcement. Ollie loves to be petted. When Ollie wants a pat, he finds any human who's sitting down and purposely begins scratching that human's kneecap. The feeling is never pleasant, and sometimes it's downright painful. Ollie stops scratching as soon as he is petted. He knows that most people figure out quite quickly what he wants. So, people increase their petting because Ollie has negatively reinforced them for doing so.

Between sleeping in a sunny spot, occasionally stretching, eating, and going outside to . . . well, you know, Ollie spends his day going back and forth scratching people. Sometimes he doesn't even have to scratch them before they start petting him — he has trained them that well with negative reinforcement.

The negative reinforcement process is a little more complex when applied to OCD. Negative reinforcement comes into play when people with OCD experience an obsession and try to deal with it through either avoidance or a compulsion. The process goes like this:

1. **Obsession:** The OCD sufferer experiences an unpleasant, distressing, obsessive thought, urge, or image that creates anxiety.

2. **Avoidance or compulsion:** The sufferer attempts to cope with the obsession by avoiding it or engaging in a compulsion.

   - **Avoidance** is an attempt to suppress the obsession by avoiding potential causes, such as staying away from things that may be contaminated or not driving due to fear of hitting someone.

   - **Compulsions** are acts intended to neutralize the obsession, such as handwashing or frequently stopping the car to see whether someone was hurt.

   In both instances, the sufferer's anxiety is temporarily relieved.

3. **Negative Reinforcement:** Both avoidance and compulsions become more frequent because they succeed in temporarily reducing anxiety and distress. In other words, anxiety and distress are unpleasant. Negative reinforcement involves a behavior that succeeds in reducing this unpleasantness. People tend to do things far more often when they are negatively reinforced by having their distress reduced.

The temporary relief that people with OCD get when they try to avoid an obsession or act out a compulsion makes these strategies seem like they're working. So, people repeat them, and the cycle becomes more ingrained and compelling. The following example clarifies the concept.

Bert worries about dirt and germs. He particularly hates touching other people's hands. When someone attempts to shake hands with him, he imagines filthy bathrooms and disease-carrying germs. Along with the image, he feels a surge of anxiety. Whenever possible, Bert avoids shaking hands. When he successfully avoids a handshake, Bert feels a huge sense of relief (his anxiety goes down sharply). Therefore, not shaking hands is negatively reinforced.

If Bert is forced to shake hands, his anxiety and distress increase. He limply puts out his hand and withdraws it quickly. He then excuses himself and washes or disinfects his hands. After this act, he feels a bit better. So, the next time he feels distress, he's more likely to wash and disinfect his hands. Washing and disinfecting become more frequent because they've been negatively reinforced. Bert's hand-shaking aversion fit right in during the pandemic, however his obsession with cleanliness expands to almost any surfaces he comes into brief contact with. Bert's behaviors interfere with his work and his interactions with friends and family. Without treatment, his OCD is likely to intensify. Bert is a typical example of how OCD grows and intensifies over time.

Combining positive and negative reinforcement: A double whammy

People with OCD ask for reassurance as a way of getting both positive and negative reinforcement. Positive reinforcement comes from the care and understanding the person receives. Negative reinforcement happens because the reassurance temporarily removes the feelings of worry and distress.

So, what happens when something is both positively and negatively reinforced? In short, it becomes more frequent. People with OCD who ask for reassurance do so with increasing frequency as time goes on. Yet the more often they ask, the more insecure they feel. A few quick examples can help clarify how the reassurance cycle works.

Arthur has obsessive thoughts about having sex with children. He is appalled by those thoughts and has never even come close to acting them out. He goes to confession every day. On bad days he goes to more than one church so that he can confess more than once. He asks each priest for reassurance that he will not go to hell for having bad thoughts. Every priest has patiently answered that thoughts are not the same as acts. Arthur feels momentarily better after the confession. Though unintended, the care and concern of the priest both positively and negatively reinforce Arthur because his anxiety is temporarily decreased, and he enjoys receiving the concern.

Brenda believes that she has left the stove or other appliances on. She is often late for work because she returns home to check. She also calls her husband and asks him whether he thinks she may have left the stove on. Brenda's husband reassures her that he's sure she turned it off. Five minutes later, she may call him again and ask the same question. Sometimes she asks about the coffeepot. Brenda's husband loves his wife and puts up with frequent interruptions during his workday.

Colin lives alone. He is obsessed with order and cleanliness. His house is spotless. He arranges the food in his cupboards alphabetically. He spends hours each day arranging and rearranging his belongings. When something is amiss, he gets very upset. Colin seeks reassurance by calling his mother four or five times a day. He asks her whether she loves him and whether he is a good person. His mother worries about Colin but is always there for him.

Family members, counselors, and friends can unknowingly contribute to OCD by giving reassurance. See Chapters 21 and 22 for information about how to handle reassurance-seeking in children, family, or friends with OCD. That's one of the most important lessons to learn in order to help those you care about with OCD.

Worsening OCD with Bad Thinking

The thinking styles of those with OCD make OCD worse. These ways of thinking likely originate from early experiences and are perpetuated by continuing reinforcement, as discussed in earlier sections. As these ways of thinking become engrained, they deepen and intensify OCD. Even when peoples' OCD originates in adulthood, it is quite possible that they developed styles of thinking consistent with OCD during childhood. These styles of thinking likely increase the risk of acquiring OCD later in life.

Everyone's brain fills with weird thoughts, impulses, or urges once in a while. Having strange or scary thoughts is perfectly normal. For example:

>> You're walking down stairs carrying an infant, and you fear you might drop the baby.

>> Standing on a balcony, you have an impulse to jump.

>> You hear someone coughing, and you think you might get sick and die.

>> You feel like taking all of your clothes off in public.

>> You find a certain minister very attractive, so you must be a sinner.

Those thoughts can be pretty uncomfortable. But if you don't have OCD, you may dismiss them as odd or a bit disgusting. However, people with OCD misinterpret their thoughts as overly important or dangerous. They try to stop thinking the thoughts or do something to prevent the thoughts from occurring.

Various types of OCD thinking often work in concert with each other. Thus, most obsessions or compulsions involve more than one type of distorted thought. The story of Diane shows you how this collusion works.

Diane believes that in order to protect her children, she must repeat the number 3 all day long in her mind and do everything in sets of three. Thus, she washes the dishes three times and she flushes the toilets three times. As you can imagine, Diane has trouble getting things done.

Diane's story illustrates how many types of OCD thinking gang up to ruin her life. Although her obsessions and compulsions all revolve around the number 3, you can see how these thought distortions overlap. Diane's thinking includes:

>> Being too responsible

>> Needing to control thoughts

>> Exaggerating risk

>> Thinking magically and illogically

>> Viewing thoughts as real

But all is not lost for Diane or for you. Chapters 8 and 9 explain how to untangle OCD thinking. The next sections describe the most common OCD thinking errors.

Exaggerating risk

People with OCD tend to believe that bad things happen all the time and that bad things have horrible consequences. For example, no one likes to be around people who are coughing and sneezing and not covering their mouths. Have you ever been on an airplane seated next to someone with a bad cold? Yuck. OCD turns that unpleasant feeling into panic about getting sick. The OCD mind imagines that catching a virus will result in bronchitis, pneumonia, COVID, or even death. OCD thinking exaggerates the likelihood of catching something as well as the consequences of getting ill. Of course, serious pandemics change the risk of getting ill from airborne viruses, which may call for additional measures such as masks and vaccines.

The thinking of those with OCD tends to rate the likelihood of almost all types of obsessional fears actually occurring as much higher than logic would dictate. For example, a woman with scrupulosity OCD (see Chapters 2 and 15 for more information) has obsessions about screaming out profanities in church. She worries about doing so at each and every service. In actuality, she has never in her life even said an obscenity out loud in front of anyone. But when asked by her therapist, she rates the likelihood that someday she'll lose control in church at around 80 percent.

Not accepting uncertainty

Life does not come with guarantees. But those who suffer from OCD attempt to eliminate uncertainty of all kinds. Unfortunately, this creates greater misery than you might imagine. The following example of Ed shows how intolerance of uncertainty becomes a never-ending, nerve-wracking quest.

> **Ed** suffers from a type of OCD in which he greatly fears that he is a pedophile, one who sexually abuses children (see Chapters 2 and 15 for more information). He has never abused a child, and he really doesn't have sexual desires for children. However, he worries constantly about the possibility, no matter how remote, that he might one day actually attack a child sexually. His relatives are puzzled as to why he never attends their gatherings, but that's because children attend those events. He spends hours each day reading about pedophiles to assure himself that he isn't like them. This reading reduces his worries for a little while, but the uncertainty always returns. And, of course, the more time he spends reading about pedophilia, the more he thinks about it. He believes that he must stay away from children at all costs, at least until he's finally able to achieve 100-percent certainty that he is not a pedophile.

Ed's story shows how desperately those with OCD crave certainty. Unfortunately, living without some degree of uncertainty is impossible.

Needing everything perfect

OCD thinking drives its sufferers to seek perfection. Perfectionists believe that perfection is actually possible, and they should strive for it. Perfectionistic thinking dictates that everything should be arranged "just so" and completed without errors. This thinking often prevents people with OCD from finishing important work due to fear of making mistakes. Even miniscule mistakes are viewed with loathing and fear. If errors do occur, this thinking greatly magnifies their significance. You can probably see why perfectionism leads to avoidance and procrastination.

Controlling thoughts

Typically, people don't spend a whole lot of time thinking about their thinking. Once in a while, a strange or disturbing thought may pop into people's minds, and they usually dismiss the odd thought as unimportant. For example, Melinda may have the thought that she could let her car drift into an oncoming lane of traffic. But she quickly realizes that the thought is pretty silly and lets it go. Her attention returns to driving and listening to the radio.

However, those with OCD believe that thoughts are very important. They believe they should exert mental control by not allowing disturbing thoughts to occur in the first place. They think that controlling one's thoughts is both possible and essential. If Sam, who has OCD, has a thought about driving into an oncoming lane of traffic, he believes that having that thought is a sign of poor mental health or even insanity. He worries that one day the thought may compel him to actually turn into oncoming traffic. Ironically, Sam finds himself focusing on his fearful thought for a long time.

Being too responsible

Those with OCD believe that they must be vigilant and do everything possible to protect others from harm. And if a bad outcome does occur, they think they probably could and should have done something to prevent it. Sometimes this thinking gets pretty bent out of shape. The story of Ellen demonstrates this inflated sense of responsibility run amok.

> **Ellen** believes that she must never fall ill out of concern for making others around her sick. She rarely goes out during the cold season, takes extra vitamins and zinc tablets (hoping they will prevent illness), and washes her hands three times an hour. She believes that her compulsions protect those around her from contracting any germs, which she feels she carries even if she isn't sick. If one of her family members catches a cold, she obsesses over what she did to cause the illness. She firmly believes that there must have been something she could have done to prevent the cold.

Like many who have OCD, Ellen starts with an idea that sounds almost reasonable — she wants to avoid making others sick. But the OCD throws the sense of responsibility into hyper-drive. She enormously inflates the extent to which she influences events and blames herself for things she has little or no control over.

Viewing thoughts as real

The OCD mind tends to view thoughts way too seriously — so much so that it blurs the distinction between thoughts and actions. This distinction can be blurred in three ways:

>> **Bad thoughts = bad deeds.** This way of blurring thoughts and actions involves thinking that having a bad thought is the same thing as actually carrying out a bad deed. Thus, someone who has a thought of robbing a bank may conclude that they are as immoral as if they'd actually robbed the bank.

>> **Thoughts are always true.** For example, if someone with OCD has a thought that the wallpaper is contaminated, they conclude that it must actually *be* contaminated.

>> **Thoughts cause events.** Another way of thinking about thoughts as real is by making the assumption that thoughts can actually *cause* events in the world to occur. Thus, some people with OCD think that if they experience a thought about a loved one dying, the thought itself may cause the person to die.

Thinking magically and illogically

OCD thinking usually has a magical, illogical quality to it. Thus, those with OCD often imbue numbers with magical properties. For example, some numbers are thought to be either safe or dangerous, good or bad. Some with OCD feel a compulsion to repeat actions a certain number of times in order to prevent a catastrophe from occurring.

Superstitions lack logic as well. In OCD, superstitions can look particularly bizarre. For example, someone with superstitious OCD (see Chapters 2 and 17 for more information) may feel driven to wear certain colors in order to feel safe from harm. Someone else may avoid driving on streets that start with the letter C out of a conviction that C is an unlucky letter.

REMEMBER

Lots of people have a few superstitious beliefs and even a little magical thinking — especially kids. It's not OCD thinking until the beliefs start interfering with a person's life. So, if you don't like the number 13 or the color black, so what? But if you spend hours each day consumed with thoughts about numbers and colors, you may have a problem.

2

Starting Down the Treatment Path

Chapter **6**

Overcoming OCD Obstacles to Change

The process of change often stirs up deep-seated, almost primal fear. Change for anyone can be uncomfortable. Fear of change leads many to live with the devil they know rather than the one they don't. Other times people say and believe that they want to change, but they end up engaging in self-defeating behaviors without even knowing why.

The nature of OCD makes change even more challenging for those entangled in its throes, and resistance is more multifaceted. This chapter helps you understand the nature and frequency of resisting effective treatment for OCD. It lays out precisely how people defeat themselves before they even start. Then it discusses why engaging in such resistance is so understandable. Most importantly, this chapter shows you what can be done to turn from self-defeat to self-success.

Realizing Resistance Is Futile

People who try to overcome OCD rarely succeed without first putting up a really good fight, against themselves. As odd as it may seem, their first instinct is often to resist necessary change and remain stuck exactly where they are.

Does this mean that people *want* to hold onto their problems such as OCD? That's not the case. Nobody actually wants to have OCD. Why would they? OCD consumes large chunks of time, causes extreme distress, and creates misery both for those affected and those who care about them.

People resist and avoid treatment of their OCD for various reasons. These roadblocks to change fall into three major categories:

>> Specific fears and myths about OCD treatment

>> Self-handicapping and fear of shame

>> Self-beliefs that make change seem out of reach

Each of these three change-blockers are examined and tips and hints for dealing with those beliefs are spelled out in the following sections.

Fearing treatment

Unless they have gone to school to study psychology, most people don't understand mental-health issues particularly well. Because OCD comes in highly varied forms (see Chapters 2 and 3 for information about the types of OCD and its relatives), it is even less understood than other mental-health problems, such as depression or anxiety. And lack of knowledge provides fertile ground for fears and myths to grow like weeds.

The following sections discuss some of the common fears and myths sufferers experience related to OCD and its treatment. Often, they're the reasons people avoid or stop seeking treatment.

Going crazy

Some people are afraid that not being allowed to perform the compulsions that define their disorder may literally drive them crazy. This fear stems from the fact that compulsions often feel *absolutely necessary* to the person who performs them. OCD sufferers have described the desire to act on a compulsion as being as strong as the need to breathe.

The distress that OCD brings is very frightening, and carrying out compulsions provides a temporary sense of reduction in anxiety or distress. Thus, for a little while, it feels better to

>> Arrange items perfectly in the closet for someone with symmetry concerns

>> Check the locks 25 times for someone with checking and doubting worries

>> Stop the car to check whether someone has been hit for someone with hit-and-run OCD

>> Wash hands repeatedly for someone with contamination worries

I've never seen or heard of anyone going crazy by not carrying out a compulsion, but it's an understandable and legitimate fear, nonetheless. Getting over this fear means learning to trust in the advice you're given and slowly acting on that trust.

Resisting risk

People with OCD hate nothing more than uncertainty and risk. Many OCD thoughts and behaviors are specifically designed to insulate against risk of any kind. And the OCD mind continuously conjures up all kinds of possible dangers and potential disasters.

ERP FOR OCD

Estimates vary widely, but it appears that at least 25 to 50 percent of people who are offered treatment for their OCD either refuse treatment entirely, drop out early, or fail to comply with treatment fully. Although many people refuse treatments such as medication, refusal may also come in relation to a specific type of treatment. This issue is particularly common with what's known as *exposure and response prevention* (ERP) treatment (see Chapter 10 for more information about ERP). But refusal is quite unfortunate, because ERP may be the most effective treatment currently available for OCD.

Briefly, ERP involves asking people to expose themselves to the very things that tend to trigger their obsessions and compulsions. While doing so, they must work very hard to resist engaging in the compulsions that they feel desperate to perform. For example, people with fears of contamination may be asked to touch doorknobs, dirt, and motor oil while their therapists instruct them to avoid washing their hands for a period of time. As you may imagine, ERP is not an especially easy or comfortable procedure, especially if you have OCD. So, it isn't surprising that many people who might benefit from ERP refuse to carry it out.

Although ERP *may* be the most effective treatment for OCD, the edge it holds over other approaches is modest. Alternatives do exist that are quite effective and that may arouse less fear (see especially Chapters 8, 9, and 11 for information on cognitive-behavioral therapy, metacognitive therapy, mindfulness, and medications).

Treatments for OCD work (see Chapters 8 through 18 for lots of information about the types of treatment for OCD and its subtypes). In fact, they work very well — especially when people can be persuaded to stick with their treatment.

That's why some people with OCD check things over and over again, just to be sure. Some repeatedly wash their hands to be absolutely certain of eliminating all germs. Still others engage in various rituals designed to protect the ones they love, all in the name of reducing risk.

REMEMBER

Life comes with a degree of uncertainty, and when all is said and done, nothing can truly eliminate all risk. Review Chapters 8 and 9 for ideas on coping with risk.

Being wary of inconsistency

Psychologists have known for a long time that people try to remain largely consistent in the behaviors, beliefs, and attitudes they exhibit. Being consistent simplifies life and makes everything feel a little more predictable. You may not like your OCD thoughts or behaviors, but at least they're familiar and predictable. Fear of inconsistency and the discomfort that accompanies breaking old routines and replacing them with new ones may keep you from following through on treatment that demands change.

REMEMBER

At first, shaking old habits creates an uncomfortable shift from what you've come to know. Embracing new patterns of thoughts isn't easy, but sticking with treatment is crucial for success. With time and practice, you and your world will settle into a new consistency. Life will seem no less predictable than before treatment if you have a little patience.

Missing OCD

People with OCD come to believe that their thoughts or behaviors keep bad things from happening. Because they've become so accustomed to using compulsions to manage their obsessions, they often worry that eliminating their OCD will leave them without any tools for coping with distress.

REMEMBER

If you have this concern, realize that out of all the patients I've successfully treated for OCD, no one has ever begged to have their OCD back! I suspect such an outcome would be very rare, but if you were indeed to discover yourself missing your OCD, you could always go back to it if you wanted to (which you won't).

Getting sick or worse

People starting OCD treatment worry that they might really get sick and die if they move ahead with treatment. For example, those who consider ERP treatment (see the previous sidebar and Chapter 10), frequently fear that exposure of certain types may result in death. Someone with contamination concerns is almost certain to greatly fear exposure to dirt and surfaces that other people have touched.

The risk of getting sick cannot be 100 percent eliminated. That's because a very small degree of risk does indeed exist with exposure treatment. It's conceivable, though exquisitely unlikely, that you could pick up a virus, get sick, and even die from touching a doorknob. Mind you, I've never heard of anyone undergoing ERP and dying in this manner, but *anything* is possible. Part of overcoming OCD involves finding ways to overcome the exaggerated fears of uncertainty and risk that accompany it. These fears can be overcome by taking a slow, gradual approach — but you can never fully eliminate risk.

Hurting someone else

People with a type of OCD known as doubting and checking OCD sometimes fear hurting others. They develop elaborate ways of ensuring that they won't carry out these feared acts, especially against a loved one. They truly fear that terrible things will happen if they don't listen to what their OCD tells them to do. Parents often have fears of hurting their children. The following story about Valerie shows how one mother resists treatment for her OCD due to fear that her obsessional worries may come true.

> **Valerie**, a mother with OCD, believes she needs to count each step she takes up to the number six, over and over, or her children will get seriously injured.
> Throughout the day, she spends so much time counting that she can't get the basic chores of everyday living completed. She loves her children and doesn't want to chance hurting them. She feels terrified when a therapist tells her that in order to treat her problems she needs to stop counting. She worries that in spite of what the therapist says, there may be truth to her obsession and her kids might get hurt. No wonder following the therapist's advice is so hard to do.
>
> Valerie's OCD controls her mind. She leaves therapy because of her intense fears. Her therapist may have pushed her a little too far too quickly. However, six months later, she returns to therapy and works out a plan with her therapist to take a more gradual approach.

Valerie's story is not uncommon. Many OCD obsessions seem quite real to the person who has them. That's what makes fighting them so difficult.

Another common OCD fear is the fear of losing control and hurting or abusing someone as a result. Once again, this fear is exaggerated, as those with this type of OCD concern are actually at *lower* risk of harming others than most people. But in order to deal with this OCD-related fear, one must once again be willing to deal with a very small degree of uncertainty. Building up sufficient trust to work on this issue takes time.

A skilled therapist will take whatever time you need to gain courage to fight your OCD. It may take multiple sessions before you feel comfortable enough to describe exactly what you are thinking and feeling. For treatment to work, you must eventually learn to trust your therapist to be a safe guide through your journey to recovery.

Doing things against your will

People with OCD worry that their mental-health professional will make them do things that they don't want to do. However, no competent, ethical therapist will ever insist that you engage in anything that you say you simply cannot do. Therapists may try to help you see the advantages in following a treatment plan, but they will not force you to do so.

Being unable to stand the treatment

Some people are so afraid that the distress associated with OCD treatment may overwhelm them that they can't even contemplate treatment. If you fear discomfort greatly, you may benefit from reading Chapter 8 to gear yourself up to seek treatment.

Thinking therapy doesn't work

Some people have heard that therapy is ineffective, expensive, and takes an extraordinary amount of time to work. In reality, OCD treatments of various types do work, and they usually improve symptoms significantly in months rather than years (though treatment for complicated OCD and OCD along with other problems can take much longer).

The outcomes for cognitive behavioral therapy, metacognitive therapy, mindfulness, ERP, and medication are reviewed in Chapters 8, 9, 10, and 11, respectively. These treatments are considered very successful. Just one catch . . . you have to show up and participate actively in the treatments for them to work.

Handicapping against treatment success

Many of those with OCD fear working hard on their issues, so they engage in *self-handicapping* instead. What is self-handicapping? Essentially, it amounts to anything you do to limit yourself or your efforts in ways that provide an excuse for not making progress. It's like engaging in a wrestling match with one arm tied behind your back. If you lose the match, you can always say, "But I had one arm tied behind my back!"

You may wonder why anyone would do this. The answer is actually quite simple: Self-handicapping avoids a loss of face and the resulting shame you might otherwise feel if you were to work very hard and still fail. It also allows you to save face if you succeed for a little while, but then fail later.

No one likes feeling ashamed. Yet those with OCD often feel ashamed of their symptoms and fear seeking treatment because they fear being judged negatively. They think the therapist will see them as crazy; after all, some of the symptoms of OCD can look very strange indeed. But therapists are very good at being non-judgmental. They don't see you as a defective human being just because of your OCD. On the contrary, they know that OCD is a complicated problem, and almost everyone engages in behavior that's a little OCD-like from time to time.

So, what does self-handicapping look like? It comes in a fascinating array of colors, shapes, and sizes. In the following sections, I discuss some of the ways people self-handicap their efforts. Head to the later section "Overcoming Resistance and Changing for the Better" to find out how you can recognize and deal with your own self-handicapping behaviors.

Waiting until you're "ready"

By delaying therapy until you feel really ready, you avoid failure by never really starting. In other words, you're waiting for the *perfect* time. The problem, of course, is that the perfect time doesn't exist — except for the time you actually begin therapy.

Reducing effort

If you don't try very hard, you're giving yourself a built-in excuse for failure: "Well, I would have done rather well if I had actually made the effort." Missing sessions and showing up late can be ways of reducing effort. This self-handicapping strategy fits the earlier example of tying one hand behind your back while wrestling.

Raising the bar

Sometimes people self-handicap by declaring that they can succeed only if they're 100 percent perfect in their attempts to change. Anything less is unacceptable. Thus, attaining a 65 percent reduction in OCD symptoms does not represent success. Although this strategy avoids declaring success, it indirectly avoids failure. People who raise the bar in this way know that failing to achieve perfection isn't really failing because no one can be perfect anyway.

Giving up early

Some folks will make a run at improving their lot, but abandon the effort prematurely. Thus, they may try a few sessions of therapy, but quit well before treatment has had a chance to succeed. At the first moment that therapy gets difficult or feels scary, they jump ship. That's because doing so avoids the chance of failure.

Seeing yourself as hopeless

If you're already hopeless, it's pretty hard to fail, isn't it? Hopelessness is a little like the "reducing effort" form of self-handicapping, but taken to the extreme. If you're hopeless, why even bother to try?

Blaming others

One way to limit yourself is to totally blame others for your problems. If you blame your parents, your therapist, or even your friends for not doing enough for you, then you don't have to put forth your own efforts to change. If you don't make an effort, you effectively prevent failure (unfortunately, you prevent success as well).

Reporting symptoms dishonestly

Sometimes those with OCD feel such shame about their symptoms that they lie or fail to tell their therapists the nature of their problems. In fact, I believe that OCD is an underreported epidemic because so many people are intensely embarrassed and ashamed of their symptoms.

Criticizing yourself harshly

Harsh self-criticism robs you of motivation and, thus, reduces your ability to keep putting forth effort. People engage in harsh criticism because they think that by doing so, they'll beat everyone else to the punch. But like all self-handicapping strategies, it simply prevents success.

Arguing with the therapist

One way people avoid dealing with their problems is by going into therapy and then constantly disagreeing with the therapist. Thus, the focus of the discussion is about how wrong the therapist is rather than on the work that's necessary in order to get better. Others avoid working by questioning the competence or skills of the therapist or dismissing therapy as nonsense.

Although arguing for the purpose of avoiding treatment is never a good idea, sometimes disagreeing with a therapist is actually very appropriate. Some practitioners are not well-trained or may not be a good match for you. If this is true in your case, you need to change therapists. See Chapter 7 for more information about getting professional help and knowing whether you've found a good match.

Passive acceptance

While arguing excessively with your therapist isn't a good idea, passive acceptance isn't good either. Some people enter therapy and sit quietly waiting for the therapist to change them. That doesn't work. Getting better takes active involvement and cooperation.

Presenting distractions

Most people with OCD find it difficult to talk about their symptoms. A common way to avoid dealing with difficult subjects is through distraction. Clients want to talk about another problem at work or a difficult relationship. Sometimes their pressing concerns are really just ways of staying away from doing the hard work of therapy.

Waiting for the guarantee

Some people with OCD want an absolute guarantee that if they're going to make the effort to try a difficult treatment like ERP, it will work. Of course, no such guarantee is possible. The outcome data is highly promising, but no one can provide absolute assurance that it will work.

Denying improvement

Another way to self-handicap and avoid failure is to deny success. Some clients improve a great deal on a wide variety of indicators (such as psychological tests) of their OCD severity. Yet they insist that they're doing no better. Denying improvement provides a buffer — just in case things take a turn for the worse. However, denying real improvements when they occur can also rob you of the motivation needed for continuing with difficult treatments.

Putting too much blame on biology

Chapter 4 points out that the brain is heavily involved in OCD. Problems with the way the brain functions clearly contribute to the development of the disorder. But other factors also enter in. And as discussed in Chapter 4, when you change your thinking and your behavior, studies have shown you can literally affect the way your brain functions, for the better. But if you completely chalk up your OCD to a brain disease, you may be less willing to engage in some of these other effective, albeit a little challenging, strategies. You probably just want to take medication. Although medicines do play a role in treating OCD, you can limit your success by not considering the adjuncts or alternatives.

Believing the worst about yourself

All people hold certain beliefs about themselves. Some of these beliefs are positive, and others may hold you back. Negative beliefs such as seeing yourself as inadequate, dependent, undeserving, and/or blameworthy, can negatively impact your ability to deal with OCD. The following sections explain the most common types of self-beliefs that can get in the way of dealing with your OCD.

Believing you are inadequate

OCD can make people lose confidence in their ability to handle the everyday stresses in the world. No wonder many who suffer from OCD start to feel that they can't solve their problems. Feelings of inadequacy go hand in hand with OCD. The belief that you can't do something (like change or get better) stops you from trying.

Inadequacy often leads to dependency. Because people with OCD feel that they're inadequate, they frequently seek some outside help. They often become dependent on friends or partners, asking for excessive reassurance. Unfortunately, getting reassurance may give temporary relief, but doubt quickly returns (see Chapter 5 for more on the dangers of reassurance).

Believing you are guilty

Some people with OCD believe they're 100 percent to blame for having the disorder. Feeling guilty about something takes a lot of mental energy. And that energy is needed for the work of getting better. If people with OCD feel guilty, they may also feel that somehow they deserve to suffer, and therefore, they deserve the pain of OCD.

Guilt focuses on the past. In order to get better, you need to move past the guilt and go forward. If you feel guilty and ashamed about having OCD, ponder these questions:

>> Do I remember ever having wanted to get OCD?

>> Does feeling guilty about my OCD help me get better?

>> If I had friends with OCD, would I tell them they were to blame for having it?

>> Is it possible that if I stop feeling guilty about having OCD, I might actually have more energy to devote toward recovery?

>> Is it possible that my OCD is largely a result of genetics, my early development, and other experiences (such as stress and trauma) I encountered over the years?

Use your answers to these questions to help you find self-acceptance. When you can accept yourself where you are right now, you will find it much easier to move forward.

Believing you are undeserving

Those who believe that they're undeserving don't feel that they're worthy of getting better. Typically, they received those messages in childhood. They feel uncomfortable when others are kind to them. They often wallow in their own misery sincerely convinced that happiness is meant for others and that they don't deserve the relief that treatment can bring.

Friends and family may find that those who feel undeserving can be rather frustrating because they resist help. Such friends and family may want to read Chapter 22 for ideas about how to help without making themselves miserable in the process.

Believing you are a victim

As discussed in Chapter 5, OCD is sometimes triggered or worsened by traumatic events. When terrible things happen to people, their views of the world and themselves change. More often than not, they shift from viewing themselves as independent, competent, and capable to dependent, incompetent, and incapable. This is a completely natural and understandable reaction to the horrible event. Victims often focus on unfairness and injustice. They feel angry about what's happened, but fail to see their responsibility for taking positive action in order to recover. Victims tend to believe that their fate and emotional well-being are largely controlled by outside forces.

At the same time, some who suffer from OCD unrelated to trauma also feel like victims of their OCD. Their reactions are also understandable because OCD is a terrible affliction. However, in order to progress, victims must learn to let go of these views of themselves and shift to the perspective of those who've found ways to cope. Those who cope have also had something bad happen to them, but they've managed to focus on what they can do to recover. Theirs is a more active, involved stance.

Overcoming Resistance and Changing for the Better

The preceding sections help you understand that resistance to treatment is both common and understandable. At the same time, fighting or refusing treatment doesn't help you overcome OCD. Realizing that you did nothing to ask for your

OCD is important. And as much as you may resist treatment, you probably hate having OCD just as much.

The way out of this mess is to stop blaming yourself and stop seeing yourself as a victim. You just need to take responsibility for doing something about your problem.

Embracing the process of change

Change of almost any type frequently requires multiple attempts. Psychologists and researchers, Drs. James Prochaska, John Norcross, and Carlo DiClemente have studied the process of change and discovered that it typically involves six phases — whether you're talking about OCD, stopping smoking, losing weight, or overcoming depression. Understanding these phases and how they work can help you stay on the right path. The phases are

1. **Precontemplation:** In this phase, people haven't even started to ponder doing anything about their problem. Sometimes in this stage people deny that they have a problem at all. The good news here is that if you have OCD and you're reading this book, you've no doubt moved past this stage.

2. **Contemplation:** This phase is where people start giving serious thought to doing something about their problem. Sometimes they feel that their problem is a little overwhelming, so they remain on the sidelines for a while until they can see a light at the end of the tunnel that doesn't look like an oncoming train. This chapter is designed to help you with this phase.

3. **Preparation:** At this point, people usually feel there is something they can do to get better. So, they design a plan for how they can attack their problem. Chapters 8, 9, 10, and 11 help you with ideas for this stage and the next one — taking action.

4. **Action:** This is where the rubber meets the road. In this phase, people carry out the plan that they've designed.

5. **Maintenance:** This phase is one that people often don't think about ahead of time. It's when you've gotten better, but then discover that maintaining those gains requires a little more effort than you thought it would. You, however, will be ready because you will be prepared for this phase beforehand. Chapter 12 gives you lots of information about avoiding relapse and maintaining your gains.

6. **Termination:** Some people manage to reach a phase where their change is so complete and ingrained that they no longer have to put much effort into holding onto their gains. Not everyone reaches this phase, and it isn't realistic for most of those who have OCD to expect a virtually complete cure with no

further effort required. However, people with OCD can improve greatly and, with continued maintenance strategies, manage to live very fulfilling lives that are far less weighed down with OCD than when they had not yet contemplated change.

You may think that these phases occur sequentially, one through six. And sometimes they do. However, it's more common to jump around these stages a number of times. For example, some people leap into action without having made much of a plan. Then when the action fails, they bounce back to the precontemplation phase and don't consider changing for a while.

Jenny's story is a typical example of someone who vacillates from one phase of change to another. Though it takes her several years to successfully tackle her OCD, she eventually makes great strides.

Jenny, an X-ray technician working for a major hospital, has frequent obsessions regarding the patients she works with. Her obsessions occur throughout the day. She fears that she is somehow sending high levels of radiation to her patients despite her strict adherence to safety protocols. When she looks at her patients, she sees horrible images of blood flowing out through their eyes, noses, and mouths. They appear hairless, and their skin melts away from the instant effects of radiation poisoning.

These images haunt her daily and continue throughout the evenings after work. She develops several odd compulsions to help ward off danger. These compulsions start with muttered prayers for safety when she begins her procedure with patients. However, over time, her mutterings become louder and longer. Patients begin to complain about their weird X-ray tech to the office staff, who report these incidents to her supervisor.

Jenny's supervisor invites her to meet to discuss her strange behavior. Jenny's work, other than her odd behavior, is exemplary, so the supervisor advises Jenny to seek help. At this point, Jenny is in the precontemplation stage.

However, after her conversation with her supervisor, she moves to the preparation stage by entering treatment. She immediately finds a therapist and starts exposure and response prevention (ERP) therapy. She tries very hard to stay the course. She attempts to stop her prayers and chants prior to performing an X-ray.

Unfortunately, after two sessions, Jenny's OCD overwhelms her, and she gives up, quits therapy, and returns once again to the precontemplation phase. Jenny's supervisor recommends that Jenny try a different treatment approach that may feel less intense and threatening.

Jenny ultimately selects a therapist trained in cognitive therapy because it sounds a little easier. She also talks to her physician about medication (see Chapter 11).

A few months later, Jenny's symptoms improve greatly. At this point, she's in the maintenance phase.

A year later, she experiences a relapse, and her symptoms return completely. She needs to regroup and moves into the contemplation phase. Finally, she selects mindfulness (see Chapter 9) and a little ERP (see Chapter 10). These strategies work very well for her. In the ensuing four years, she experiences minimal trouble with her OCD, although she needs to remain vigilant and continues in the maintenance phase.

Jenny's story shows you that change isn't always smooth, even, and easy. Most people make progress and have slip-ups. But each time Jenny struggled, she gained something from the process.

REMEMBER

People who succeed at improving their OCD (or anything else) take a number of runs at their problems. Just because you've made a few attempts only to slide back does *not* mean that you won't ultimately succeed. The fact is, each time you make a solid attempt, you discover things that will help you in your next go-round.

Defeating self-handicapping

Self-handicapping occurs whenever you do anything that interferes with making progress. People with OCD are especially vulnerable to the self-handicapping trap because the treatments can be so challenging. If you have OCD and are starting treatment, monitor your behavior for any signs of self-handicapping. When you see self-handicapping occurring, try to respond to it by recognizing how self-defeating this behavior can be. Talk back to the self-handicapping part of your OCD mind.

In the following example, Art had started treatment for his OCD six weeks earlier and struggled to stay on track. Art's story shows how self-handicapping can interfere with treatment until you start attacking it.

> **Art** suffers from what's sometimes called *hit-and-run OCD* (see Chapters 2 and 14 for more information). Whenever he drives, it isn't long before he feels some type of bump in the road — usually from a pothole, running over a speed bump, an out-of-balance tire, or going over a rock. When he feels the bump, he instantly imagines that he's run over a person. His body floods with adrenaline and fear as his heart races and his shirt becomes soaked with sweat.
>
> He pulls over to the side of the road and looks back. At that moment, he's quite certain that he will find a body. He never does. Sometimes Art inspects his car looking for signs of blood or dents from the impact. He also returns to the scene multiple times just to be sure that nothing has happened. Needless to say, it takes Art an awfully long time to get where he's going.

At his wife's insistence, Art seeks therapy for his problem. Art encounters a lot of difficulty getting started with his treatment. Therefore, his therapist suggests that he monitor his self-handicapping, recognize it for what it is, and respond to it. Table 6-1 shows what Art came up with.

TABLE 6-1 **Art's Monitoring of Self-Handicapping**

Day	Self-Handicapping	Response
Monday	I didn't read the material my psychologist suggested.	When I don't do these things, I'm handicapping myself. OK, this reading will take 15 minutes; I'm not going to let my OCD mind defeat me!
Tuesday	I was 20 minutes late for my appointment.	Sure, I was busy, but in truth, I think I was self-handicapping again. At least I caught you in action, OCD mind.
Wednesday	Today, I stopped my car and looked for a body on the road. My therapist has asked me to not do that. Maybe I'm hopeless.	I'm defeating myself again. I knew I didn't have to cave in. But I also don't have to see myself as hopeless. Next time, I'll be on the lookout for this.
Thursday	I had a partial success today in that I resisted going back to the scene, but I did look into my rearview mirror. I must not be doing any of this right.	I am self-handicapping when I view actual progress as a failure. I need to pat myself on the back whenever I take a step in the right direction.
Friday	I had a thought that this treatment is too difficult. Why should I do all this when I've read that OCD is all biological anyway? Maybe I should just take some medication and be done with it.	My therapist talked with me about medication, and he pointed out that it is an option, but this treatment will probably work better in the long run. I'm just handicapping myself when I see it as entirely biological.
Saturday	I've gone two days now without stopping my car. I understand this approach now, so I think I can quit therapy.	Wow, that's a great way to snatch defeat from the jaws of victory. I have so many other issues, and I'm pretty sure there's more to be done with my hit-and-run OCD. I'm just kidding myself by thinking it's gone just because I've done well for two days.
Sunday	Today I found myself getting really mad at my mother. She's the cause of my OCD — what with the way she used to clean the house all the time and warn us constantly about every imaginable danger. When I learned to drive, all she would do is yell at me.	OK, perhaps she did contribute to my OCD. But if I focus only on blaming her, I won't get anywhere myself. I need to let my anger go.

My Reflections: I can see that my OCD mind has lots of ways of handicapping my efforts. I'm going to have to be very vigilant and recognize when I'm starting to defeat myself. I can win this war, but only if I stay alert.

Art's story illustrates how easy it is to self-handicap. When you start your treatment for OCD, be on the lookout for things like missing appointments, blaming others, not wanting to carry out assignments between sessions, and so on. Also try tracking your self-handicapping on a "Monitoring Self-Handicapping" form.

Here's how to go about monitoring and responding to your self-handicapping tendencies:

1. In either a notebook or on your device write down the date that you are monitoring your self-handicapping.

2. To the right of that, indicate what behaviors or thoughts you've had that indicate some type of self-handicapping.

3. Respond to your self-handicapping by talking back to that part of your OCD mind. Formulate a reason to not engage in that type of self-handicapping.

4. After you've recorded your self-handicapping for at least a week, write down what you've discovered from the exercise.

TIP

Although you don't have to explicitly label your self-handicapping, you may find it useful to review the list of ways people engage in self-handicapping. Refer to the earlier section, "Handicapping against treatment success."

Dismantling change-blocking beliefs

Recognizing that you may be holding onto negative beliefs about yourself (such as feeling guilty, inadequate, undeserving, or a victim) is the first step toward pushing them out of your way. The second step involves analyzing those beliefs in order to help you see how badly they interfere with your desire to change.

For that step, I recommend that you carry out a cost/benefit analysis. A cost/benefit analysis is a simple, but highly effective, technique. It helps you focus on the problem and develop a sensible alternative. Although most beliefs at least *seem* to confer a few benefits or advantages, close scrutiny usually reveals that those advantages are far outweighed by the costs.

Here's an example of how Roberto carries out a cost/benefit analysis of his success-busting belief about himself:

> **Roberto** is an engineer in his late twenties. Other than work, he lives a very solitary life. He has always felt different from others and avoided making friends because he assumes others won't like him. Roberto suffers from *obsessive superstitions.* He feels driven to engage in rituals throughout the day. In the morning, he reads from the Bible. No problem, right? Well, Roberto reads every other word from

specific passages. He has to repeat this ritual three times before he gets out of bed. This ritual is repeated prior to meals and in the evening before retiring. Altogether, he spends about an hour and a half every day on this task.

But that's not all. Roberto also has a routine of praying for 30 minutes in his church every morning before work. He never misses a day. That's because he is obsessed with the idea that he is evil and perverted. He believes that he will go to hell if he does not complete these rituals compulsively. Between reading and praying, he has no time to connect with others or engage in enjoyable activities.

His family is quite concerned and wants Roberto to seek help. His pastor explains to Roberto that he likely has OCD and needs therapy. However, Roberto does not believe he can change his behavior, because he is not up to the enormity of the task. Roberto feels overwhelmed and incapable of making changes. However, the therapist that Roberto's pastor recommended suggests that Roberto might be engaged in self-defeating beliefs, specifically, the thought that he is inadequate.

Roberto contemplates taking a shot at his OCD. He realizes that his success-busting belief of inadequacy stands in his way. So, following his therapist's advice, he carries out a cost/benefit analysis of this belief, as shown in Table 6-2.

TABLE 6-2

Cost/Benefit Analysis of Roberto's Inadequacy Belief

Goal, problematic thought, belief, or decision: I believe I am inadequate.	
Benefits	Costs
If I feel inadequate, I don't have to work hard to make changes.	If I feel inadequate, I may not have to work at making changes, but I won't make any changes!
Maybe I can get my mother to help me with this problem if I feel inadequate to do it myself.	Feeling inadequate invites my mother to keep controlling my life. She makes me feel even more stupid when she takes over.
I won't have to tackle my problem and then fail.	If I continue feeling inadequate, I won't make changes.
	By holding onto my belief in my inadequacy, I ruin any chance I have of meeting someone.
	Believing in my inadequacy feels awful.

My Reflections: Now I can see how much my belief in inadequacy has been hurting me. I need to be on the lookout for that belief.

After Roberto reviews his cost/benefit analysis of his success–busting belief, he decides to act as if he were actually adequate. He realizes that staying stuck will enable his OCD to keep him down. He looks forward to his next appointment with his psychologist and feels ready to face his OCD.

Here's how to design a cost/benefit analysis of your problematic beliefs:

1. Either in a notebook or on your device, write down a success-busting belief that you think applies to you.

2. Underneath the heading "Benefits," write all the imaginable advantages or ways in which your belief feels useful to you.

3. Under "Costs," write down all the ways that your belief may be holding you back, costing you, or causing you harm.

4. Beneath your table, write "My Reflections" and summarize what you've discovered from your cost/benefit analysis.

TIP

You can use a cost/benefit analysis to change a belief, make a decision, rethink your perspective, decide about goals, and motivate your efforts. It helps you move past contemplating changes and actually start moving forward.

If you discover that your cost/benefit analysis results in more benefits or advantages for retaining your core belief about yourself, you will likely profit from professional help.

Taking one step at a time

You may think that you're sick of your OCD, and you want to change it and change it now. Great! But, be careful. Successful change requires careful contemplation, planning, and work. Thinking you can just jump right into eliminating your OCD sets you up to have unrealistic expectations. Those expectations can cause you to crash quite suddenly if and when your attempts falter.

Try a slow and steady strategy for tackling OCD. For example, if you're trying ERP therapy (see Chapter 10) to help rid you of your fears of contamination, starting out by rubbing the inside of a dumpster with your hand probably isn't a good idea. But you might be able to tackle touching a doorknob.

The same advice holds for how you approach this book. You can be sure that almost anything anyone would want to know about OCD is covered in these pages. But you don't have to read every single chapter, and you certainly don't need to carry out every single exercise. Furthermore, you should take it at your own pace.

REMEMBER

Resistance to change is not productive or useful. Taking reasonable risks and accepting occasional setbacks in your therapy will keep you on track to overcoming OCD.

Chapter **7**

Getting Help for OCD

Many people who have obsessive-compulsive disorder (OCD) never seek help for their problem. Those who suffer often fail to get help because they feel ashamed of their obsessions and compulsions. Unlike the worries associated with anxiety or the sadness that comes with depression, the thoughts and behaviors of OCD can appear quite bizarre to others. People with OCD fear that their disorder will make them look crazy, so they work hard to hide their symptoms. But OCD can worsen over time if treatment is not received.

This chapter tells you about the kinds of help available for treating OCD. If your symptoms are quite mild, you may want to try self-help for your OCD. However, most people with OCD benefit more if they also receive some type of professional help. In any case, educating yourself about OCD should be part of your treatment plan.

The cast of characters in the mental-health field who are available can seem overwhelming. No worries, this chapter introduces them all. More importantly, read about how to find the right person and what to expect when you make an appointment. Finally, I'll give you a guide to help evaluate whether your choice is a good fit for you.

Going After the Types of Help You Need

If your brakes fail, you take your car in to a garage and let the mechanic do the repair job. If you have an ear infection, you go to a medical provider and get some antibiotics. You can pretty much leave the fixing to the experts. You have to cooperate, that is, pay the bill or take the pill, but little personal effort is required.

Taking on OCD is different, however. When you fight OCD, you have to go into the boxing ring yourself and engage in the battle. You may have someone in your corner coaching you, but you're the one who has to throw the punches and bob and weave to avoid getting hit.

If you or someone you care about has OCD, you probably wish the solution could be quick and easy. Unfortunately, there are no quick fixes for OCD. But don't despair, highly effective treatments are available.

WARNING

OCD can be severe and is sometimes accompanied by depression (see Chapter 3). If you have thoughts of hopelessness or suicidal thoughts, please seek immediate help from a mental health professional. Furthermore, if OCD is making it nearly impossible to get to work, sleep, eat, or get along with others, you should get professional help without delay.

Educating yourself about OCD

Self-help is a necessary part of any successful OCD treatment, and a huge chunk of that self-help is becoming educated about OCD causes and treatments. You may seek professional help in addition to self-help for guidance, support, and motivation (see Chapter 6 on overcoming obstacles and resistance to change), or you may be ready to jump-start treatment on your own. Either way, you need to actively participate in your treatment program, and self-help motivates you to do so.

You can help yourself in two ways — by finding out all you can about OCD and by getting support from family, friends, and others. This section discusses the educational aspect of self-help. (Skip ahead to the next section for more on enlisting support.)

Obtaining information about what you're up against prepares you for the battle ahead. Prior to the Super Bowl, the coaches try to find out all they can about the opposing team so they're prepared to make the right moves at the right time. In the same way, educating yourself about OCD can help you come up with a winning game plan.

Reading through this book gives you a solid foundation about the types of OCD, the possible causes of OCD, the research-backed treatments of OCD, and where to find help. In addition, you can find examples throughout that may help you understand your own issues.

Most people learn best by repetition. I know that I frequently return to trusted sources when I am puzzled by some aspect in my own life. You should feel free to skim *OCD For Dummies* and then go back and reread for greater understanding.

In addition to this book, I recommend reading material offered by The International OCD Foundation. This foundation is a non-profit organization that provides support and information to those with OCD, their families, and professionals working with OCD. Their website, `iocdf.org`, contains information about conferences, training, and specific topics pertaining to OCD.

TIP

You also can learn about OCD from watching movies and series that feature OCD characters. Some are quite accurate; others not so much. I have found that some trivialize or romanticize the suffering that many people with OCD experience. Having OCD is not a comedy. So, enjoy the show, but take in the information as a grain of salt, because the show's real intent is usually to entertain, not inform.

WARNING

Of course, other great books and resources are available for learning about and helping with OCD. However, be careful. Look at the author's credentials. Just because an author has some initials after their name doesn't necessarily mean that they have training in a particular field. You can have a PhD in chemistry and write a book about OCD, but it's not likely to be very accurate. In addition, be wary of those promising quick fixes. OCD is a highly treatable disorder, but it does take expertise, time, and patience.

Getting support from family, friends, and others

People with OCD are isolated. Obsessions and compulsions take up time and energy. Many people with OCD can barely make it through the day, let alone have time to socialize. Yet, getting support can be an integral part of getting better. One OCD treatment in particular, exposure and response prevention (ERP — see Chapter 10), may involve getting together with a buddy or partner to carry out some of the assignments. Social support can come in the form of the following:

>> **Friends and family:** If you have an understanding family or friends, they may be willing to pitch in and help. First, they'll need to become educated about the ins and outs of OCD — this book can be a great start for them. After they're educated, they can serve as assistants to using ERP. Typically, their

assistance should be guided by a professional whom you are seeing for your OCD. Friends and family can also serve as gentle coaches, giving you needed encouragement (see Chapter 22 for more information about the role played by family and friends).

>> **Online support:** Online chat rooms, forums, and other support groups related to OCD allow you to be anonymous, and many people benefit from sharing with others online. The good online groups abide by codes of conduct — offensive, inappropriate, and unrelated comments are discouraged. Some of these groups even have moderators who edit and delete prohibited messages. Other groups provide a specific community with related news, updates, and a chance to talk with others through e-mails only. A few groups even involve professionals who volunteer their time to the online community.

>> **Support groups:** Groups for people with OCD can provide compassionate support. Some groups involve a mental-health professional who leads the discussion, provides education, and offers suggestions. Other groups consist of people with OCD and function mainly as places to talk about experiences, solve problems, and offer empathy.

Be careful about who you share personal information with and don't buy into what anyone trying to sell you quick-cure products may tell you.

Choosing a professional to help you

Not every mental-health professional is well acquainted with OCD. That's because at one time, OCD was thought to be extremely difficult to treat and quite rare. Now we know that these ideas are not true at all. OCD is both treatable and fairly common. The bottom line is that you need to ask your mental-health professional about their experience and training with OCD. A qualified person will have received training and education about OCD and treated OCD fairly frequently.

Anyone you choose should be familiar with the major therapeutic approaches to OCD, such as cognitive-behavioral therapy (CBT), metacognitive therapy, mindfulness, a specific type of CBT known as exposure and response prevention (ERP), and medications (see Chapters 8, 9, 10, and 11, respectively).

Picking the right professional

You may have to seek services from more than one professional. Although all of them should be familiar with the treatment approaches to OCD, not everyone administers all OCD treatments. For example, you could obtain ERP training from a psychologist and medication from a psychiatrist. Here are the types of professionals who sometimes work with OCD sufferers:

- » **Coaches:** Coaches or life coaches are fairly new in the area of mental- health treatment. Some coaches have good skills (and are also trained counselors or psychologists). However, at this time no licensing requirements exist for this class of professionals. And coaching doesn't have a lot of science backing it up. Coaching can be great for setting goals and increasing motivation in your personal or business life, but I recommend sticking to a licensed practitioner for OCD.

- » **Counselors:** Counselors have graduate training in counseling, education, theology, or psychology. They obtain a master's degree and are licensed to practice in their state of residence. The backgrounds of counselors vary widely, and you need to check on the specific training of the counselor whom you choose. Many counselors are very well trained and have expertise in treating OCD.

- » **Psychiatrists:** Psychiatrists attend medical school and obtain an MD degree. They follow the attainment of this degree with additional training in the diagnosis and treatment of emotional disorders as well as other disorders that involve the brain and behavior. Psychiatrists are experts in prescribing medications for OCD. Most psychiatric practices emphasize biological treatments for emotional disorders and do not typically engage in psychotherapy treatments for OCD, such as ERP, mindfulness, and CBT.

- » **Psychoanalysts:** A psychoanalyst usually starts out as a psychiatrist, psychologist, or other therapist and gets additional training. This approach looks at deep-seated childhood issues. Treatment usually requires several sessions a week for many years, and no research that I know of has been conducted on its use with OCD. Effective OCD treatment targets symptoms directly and usually brings at least some relief within a few months or less. Psychoanalysis is not usually a good fit for someone with OCD.

- » **Psychologists:** This group of professionals is most likely to have extensive training in the various psychotherapies specific to OCD. Psychologists have doctoral degrees (PhD or PsyD) in psychology and are licensed by the state in which they practice. The psychotherapies they deliver have been scientifically proven to be effective. Although most psychologists do not prescribe medication for OCD, some states now allow prescription privileges for psychologists who obtain additional training in that area.

- » **Social workers:** Social workers attend graduate school and obtain a master's degree in social work. Many social workers also obtain supervision and training in psychotherapy, including techniques for treating OCD. They are licensed by the state in which they practice. Social workers also have training and expertise in case management and helping people obtain needed social or governmental services.

You may hear the word *therapist* or *psychotherapist* used to describe a mental-health professional. "Therapist" is a general word used to describe someone who does therapy. Sometimes the word "psychotherapist" is used to describe a person who does psychotherapy. A therapist may be a social worker, counselor, or psychologist.

Although most professionals obtain licenses through state boards, territories and the military also grant some licenses.

The International OCD Foundation offers an intensive training course for licensed mental health professionals. In addition to in-person training, supervision by seasoned professionals after the coursework is required. This training leads to a certification by the foundation. You can find therapists in your area with this certificate at `iocdf.org`.

Avoiding the wrong pseudo-professional

Lots of people hang shingles on their door proclaiming their expertise in various healing arts. They provide a range of services, such as chiropractic healing, massage, and acupuncture. A few of these approaches work for pain or other disorders, but they have not demonstrated effectiveness for OCD.

In addition, some individuals have strings of letters after their names (designating something, but I have no idea what) and may not have a license to practice anything. They may advertise services such as:

>> Ear candling

>> Herbs and supplements

>> Listening to special sounds while lying on a vibrating table

>> Past-life regression

I live in New Mexico — trust me, I see lots of interesting alternative health practices. By the way, I heard of one guy who listed CCG after his name. What the heck is that I asked? Certified Crystal Gazer.

Asking the important questions

When you decide to call the office of a professional, you'll probably want to know some things before making your first appointment. Some of these questions can be answered by the office manager or secretary if there is one. These questions include the following:

>> **How soon can I be seen?** If the answer is in several months, you may want to keep checking around. Recently, there has been a shortage of trained mental health professionals; you may have to wait longer than you want. In the meanwhile, take the opportunity to read over the material in this book. It will help prepare you for therapy.

>> **What are the fees, and do you take my insurance plan?** Not all practitioners accept all insurance plans, and some do not accept any. You need to know the fee schedule upfront.

>> **What are your practice hours?** If you require evening or weekend appointments, you need to see whether these are available.

>> **Do you practice telehealth?** Some people find telehealth convenient and easily accessible. Others need face to face in order to establish rapport. The option can be very appealing depending on your individual circumstances.

>> **Does this person hold a license to practice in this state?** If not, I recommend you seek services elsewhere. You can verify this information on the internet in most cases (usually through your state licensing board).

TIP

With all the complex ins and outs of insurance these days be sure to call your health insurance plan — assuming you can get through to a real, live person! Ask about how many sessions your policy allows, how frequently those sessions can occur, and at what rate your policy will reimburse for OCD treatment. If your provider does not accept insurance, inquire as to whether your insurance carrier will consider reimbursing you for sessions with a receipt from the provider.

TIP

You may also want to consider the convenience of the professional's office in relation to where you live. However, convenience is relatively less important than the person's experience and skill in working with OCD.

You'll want to ask the mental-health professional a few questions directly. These only require about five or ten minutes of time, and most professionals will be willing to answer them on the phone prior to you making your first appointment. These questions include the following:

>> **Do you ever consider administering treatment outside of your office for OCD?** Although most professionals do not conduct treatment outside of their offices for most problems, OCD treatment sometimes calls for flexibility.

>> **Do you teach your OCD clients how to administer ERP for themselves?** A good therapist not only guides you through ERP, but also teaches you how to apply it for yourself. See Chapter 10 for information about ERP.

>> **Do you treat and/or evaluate OCD?** Not everyone does, so be sure to ask. You may not know for sure whether you have OCD, but if you suspect that you do, you need a good evaluation.

>> **Do you treat OCD regularly?** You want to hear that the professional either regularly treats OCD or will get supervision from someone who does.

>> **Do you use scientifically validated therapies for OCD?** You certainly want a treatment that has been proven effective in the treatment of OCD. The professional should mention at least one of the following therapies: CBT, ERP, metacognitive therapy, mindfulness, or medications.

>> **Is your treatment for OCD confined to single, one-hour sessions each week?** Sometimes effective OCD treatment calls for more frequent and longer sessions. These may or may not be covered by your insurance, so you may want to ask about that as well. Your provider may be able to facilitate obtaining coverage for OCD treatment that exceeds usual policy coverage. That's because the treatments that really work for OCD often require more than one standard, 50-minute session per week.

If you receive the answers you hoped to hear, ask yourself how talking with that person felt. Were you comfortable? Did you feel rushed? Did the person sound interested in treating your problem? If your answers are positive, make an appointment! If you talk to someone who doesn't have a lot of experience with OCD, ask for a recommendation; many professionals who don't treat OCD themselves know of others who do.

BILLIONS OF BUCKS COULDN'T SAVE HOWARD HUGHES

Billionaire Howard Hughes, famous airplane designer, pilot, movie maker, and womanizer, lived from 1905 to 1976. It is well-known that he also happened to suffer from OCD. He had various symptoms, including intense fears of contamination along with elaborate rituals for handling all sorts of objects. His symptoms worsened over time, and he disappeared from public view in his later years. In those last years, he spent his days and nights lying naked in bed in darkened hotel rooms — as a way of creating what he considered to be a germ-free zone. He even burned his clothes if someone near him was stricken ill.

Unfortunately, little was known about the treatment of OCD in Howard Hughes's day. It wasn't until the 1970s that ERP was studied and found to be an effective treatment for OCD. Furthermore, effective medication options for OCD weren't available. Today, Howard Hughes could be treated with a good expectation of success. You can, too, and you don't even need billions of dollars.

What to Expect in Therapy

When the door closes and the first session begins, feeling a bit nervous is normal. Whether you're going to a psychologist, psychiatrist, social worker, or counselor, generally the initial session is one in which you are asked a lot of questions. The questions are the start of the assessment process. Your therapist is trying to understand you and your symptoms in order to come up with a treatment plan. Therapists have different approaches, but generally the following areas are covered in the first session:

» **Problems:** What are your current symptoms? How severe are they? How often do they occur? Do certain situations make them worse? Do you avoid people, places, or situations? How healthy are your current relationships? Do your obsessions or compulsions interfere with your life? How are your moods? How do you handle anger? How do you sleep? Has your appetite changed lately? Do you have trouble making decisions or concentrating? Do you ever have trouble thinking clearly?

» **Daily responsibilities:** Do you work in or out of the home? How are you handling your responsibilities? Have there been any recent changes in your job, family, or finances? Do you have trouble following through on important tasks?

» **Safety:** Have you ever thought about hurting yourself? Have you ever attempted suicide? Do you feel hopeless? Have you ever worried about hurting anyone else? Have there been times in your life when you have lost control and hurt someone?

» **History:** When did you first notice these problems? Have there been times when the symptoms have decreased or increased? Have you had other emotional problems in the past? Have members of your family had emotional or behavioral problems?

» **History of treatment:** Have you ever seen a therapist before? What was your experience like? Did you learn anything useful? What did you like about therapy? Do you have any complaints about your past therapy?

» **Health:** Are you healthy? Have you ever had significant health problems? Serious injuries? Are you taking any medications? Have you ever taken medication for an emotional problem in the past? If so, was it effective? Do you smoke or drink? How much and how often? Do you use any other drugs?

» **Trauma:** Have you ever been abused? Are you afraid of someone hurting you? Have you ever been exposed to traumatic events? Has anyone close to you experienced trauma?

» **Anything else:** Is there anything else that you would like to mention during this session?

Don't expect the first session to be primarily focused on the symptoms of OCD. That's because critical areas like safety, health, and functioning must be considered before treating OCD. For example, if you're feeling suicidal, that danger must be addressed immediately. Or there could be significant substance abuse that may have to be dealt with before OCD treatment can be effective. Furthermore, your therapist may discover that you're not actually suffering from OCD, but something else entirely — or that you have OCD in addition to one or more other problems.

The first session is also a time for you to assess how comfortable you are talking about your problems. Ask yourself whether you were able to communicate your concerns and leave the session with hope.

Keeping your therapy private

Maybe you've heard the saying, "What happens in Vegas, stays in Vegas." The implication is that whatever you choose to do in Las Vegas, no one else ever has to know about it. The therapeutic relationship is like this saying in that what you say in therapy, stays in therapy.

The relationship that you have with your therapist is unique because of the practice of confidentiality — the promise that what you say will not be disclosed to others. Without that promise (backed by law), therapy would not feel safe, nor would it be very effective. There are only a few exceptions to this confidentiality rule, such as:

>> **Abuse:** If you tell your therapist that you are abusing someone, your therapist may have to inform authorities. That does not mean to say that if you lose your temper and scream at your kids or partner your therapist will report you. Abuse is usually reported when it is physical, serious, chronic, and dangerous to children, disabled individuals, or the elderly.

>> **Dangerousness:** If your therapist feels that you pose an imminent danger to yourself or others, authorities may have to be informed. Again, that means that the therapist believes you may have access to a lethal weapon and/or that you intend to seriously harm someone. It does not mean that when you tell your therapist, "I'm so angry I could strangle him," that they will call the police.

TIP

Having intense worry that you may hurt someone else (but finding the thought abhorrent) is not usually considered a sign of dangerousness. In fact, it's more likely a sign of a particular type of OCD (see Chapter 2 and 15). Those people are generally at lower risk than most people of actually hurting someone, so your therapist won't be calling authorities if that's the case for you.

Finally, your therapist could be subpoenaed if you are involved in litigation. This issue should be discussed prior to beginning therapy if it is potentially relevant to you. Exceptions such as these are rather rare, and you should be sure to talk about them in detail with your therapist if you have any concerns. Overall, you can rest assured that what you say in therapy will remain in confidence with your therapist.

Digging deep into an OCD diagnosis

Sometimes diagnosing OCD can be pretty difficult. After the first interview, the doctor or therapist will often use a more formal checklist, test, or interview to better understand your symptoms. *The Yale-Brown Obsessive Compulsive Scale* (Y-BOCS) is the most commonly used interview to nail down the specifics of OCD. The Y-BOCS asks about obsessions and compulsions that have to do with contamination fears, hoarding, religion, symmetry, sexual obsessions, aggressive obsessions, worries about illness, superstitious thoughts, rituals, and checking (of locks, appliances, and so on). Several forms of Y-BOCS are used, including a clinician interview, a self-report, and a children's form.

Not all practitioners use this instrument, but your therapist is likely to ask many questions specific to a wide variety of OCD types. Your therapist will also want to know about the triggers that set your OCD off. Be patient; the evaluation and assessment process can take up to two or three sessions. But that time will pay off by allowing your therapist to know what symptoms to target and in what order.

Speaking the truth to your therapist

Lots of people believe that psychologists, psychiatrists, or other mental health professionals have special powers and can read the minds of the people they treat. Oh, if only it were true. The job sure would be a lot easier. Although training and experience provide mental health professionals with the ability to understand, diagnose, and treat emotional disorders — and they are usually pretty good at understanding their clients — they certainly can be fooled.

Most people who step into a therapist's office want to be helped. But sometimes they're embarrassed to discuss their deepest fears, worries, weaknesses, or thoughts. It's human nature to try and present a good front. And the thoughts and worries that the OCD brain gives you can feel disturbing.

It's perfectly normal to lie to a health-care professional. Normal? Right. In fact, research studies throughout many years have found that the majority of patients lie to their health-care (and mental healthcare) providers. Studies range from a low of 40 percent to a high of just over 90 percent. Common lies, or shall I say exaggerations of the truth, include the following:

>> Severity of symptoms (usually minimized)

>> How horrible they feel

>> Compliance with homework/treatment

>> Exercise

>> Diet

>> Medication compliance

>> Alcohol or drug use

>> Temper outbursts or mean behavior

>> Sexual acts, desires, or fantasies

>> Agreement with therapist

>> Self-harm or suicidal thoughts

>> Relationship problems with others

>> Excuses for missing appointments

Experienced health-care providers understand their patients' reluctance to be perfectly honest. And they feel empathy for a human need for approval. People don't want to display their weakness or weirdness. Those are perfectly natural desires. Nonetheless, dig down deep and open up with your mental health professional. Believe it or not, there are very few symptoms that professionals experienced in treating OCD haven't heard. As you read other chapters in this book, you may see that at least a number of your symptoms show up. It may help to know you're not the only person in the world to experience troubles like yours.

REMEMBER

The more open you can be with your mental (or physical) health-care provider, the more your provider will be able to come up with a solid treatment plan. Health-care providers are still not able to read minds!

Evaluating your therapist

After you've been to two or three sessions, the evaluation phase is usually complete. Soon thereafter, you need to start an evaluation of your own. Does your therapist seem like a good fit for you? Does there seem to be a reasonable game plan for your therapy?

The relationship between you and your therapist matters. Considerable research supports the idea that the quality of that relationship contributes a lot to the amount of progress you're likely to make. So, what makes a good relationship with a therapist? Here are some questions to ask yourself:

>> **Do I feel comfortable telling my therapist almost anything?** If the answer is no, that's something you should discuss. If you still feel uncomfortable after that discussion, you may not have the right therapist. On the other hand, if your own shame is what keeps you from discussing your thoughts or feelings with your therapist, that difficulty can also be discussed.

>> **Do I feel judged or criticized?** Good therapists are experts at not judging or criticizing their clients. Your therapist may not think what you're doing is a great idea (such as checking the stove 40 times each hour), but you shouldn't feel put down for that. If you do feel criticized or judged, that's something to discuss.

>> **Does my therapist seem to really listen?** If your therapist is playing on the phone or answering texts during your session, that's really not a good sign! But seriously, you need to feel truly heard. Signs of being listened to include eye contact, head nods, expressions of concern or empathy, and being provided with brief summaries of what you've said.

>> **Does my therapist speak to me in language I can understand?** Occasionally therapists use professional jargon. However, most of them try to communicate clearly and only use technical words when they must. You should feel comfortable asking for clarification of any idea or word your therapist uses.

>> **How do I feel talking with my therapist?** You should feel that your therapist cares about you and wants to help. Therapy is a professional relationship and not the same as a friendship. However, like a friend, a therapist should be reasonably warm and understanding.

REMEMBER

The treatment of OCD will likely involve times of discomfort and some struggle. Having the support of a therapist who has a good connection with you is important. But you also need a good game plan.

Reviewing the game plan

Therapy for OCD involves more than a good relationship, as important as that is. In addition, your therapist needs to help you devise a set of goals and come up with a plan to reach them. By the third or fourth session, you should know whether you have OCD. You should also know whether you have problems above and beyond OCD.

You and your therapist should discuss a plan to address the problems. Your therapist should be using one or more of the therapies discussed in Chapters 8, 9, 10, and 11. You should have some idea of which problems are to be tackled, in what order, and with what strategies. If you're unclear about the game plan, ask. Both of you should have an idea of what progress will look like as well.

REMEMBER

Occasionally, therapists and clients find that they are not a good match. For example, you may feel you're not being heard or supported, and your attempts to discuss the issue don't improve things. Or you may find that your therapist's training in OCD is lacking and goals are not made clear to you. Or maybe your therapist looks exactly like your ex-spouse or mother — possibly taking your attention away from a collaborative relationship. In any event, if you feel things aren't working, first discuss the issue with your therapist. If that doesn't work, look for a new therapist. Or ask for a referral.

3

Overcoming OCD

Chapter **8**

Cleaning Up OCD Thinking

Cognitive behavioral therapy (CBT) is based on the relationship between your thoughts and the way you feel. The premise is that the way you interpret situations (what you think) greatly influences your emotional response (what you feel). Hundreds of studies have shown that learning to change the way you think can improve the way you feel.

If you have OCD, you more than likely tend to misinterpret aspects of your reality in various ways. This leads to a sort of misalignment between how you feel about what's going on around you and the actual reality of the situation.

Researchers have identified a number of ways that people with OCD tend to interpret or think about situations related to their OCD that are particularly problematic. This chapter presents seven ways that OCD sufferers misinterpret events and provides various CBT-based methods for changing them. Modifying these misinterpretations allows you to develop more balanced ways of thinking that reduce your OCD and the distress that goes along with it.

Realigning Interpretations with Reality

Although people with OCD interpret many events in their lives rationally in the same way that most people do, they interpret *portions* of their lives in highly distorted ways. The distorted interpretations primarily occur in response to events that have something to do with *that person's* OCD. So, someone with contamination OCD perceives a dirty towel as dangerous, but probably does not obsess about running people over on the way to work. And someone with symmetry OCD looks at disorder with shock and distress, but isn't likely to worry about touching doorknobs.

Seeing common types of OCD distortions

These seven ways of misinterpreting reality show you how the thinking of those with OCD is distorted. Regardless of the specific type of OCD one has, these misinterpretations are particularly common:

>> Doubting

>> Exaggerating risk

>> Viewing thoughts as real

>> Confusing facts and feelings

>> Needing perfection

>> Needing to control thoughts

>> Being excessively responsible

See Chapter 5 for more information about how these types of thinking interact with and aggravate OCD. Although a few of these types of distorted perceptions show up in other emotional disorders as well, they appear especially troublesome for those with OCD.

Using CBT to correct distorted thinking

CBT applies techniques that aim to improve well-being by bringing about specific changes in the way you think, which leads to changes in the way you feel and behave. CBT, when applied to these distorted OCD interpretations, helps you more accurately align your feelings with reality.

CBT: CHANGING THOUGHTS VERSUS CHANGING BEHAVIORS

The first highly successful treatment for OCD was developed in the late 1960s and was a specific cognitive behavioral technique called exposure and response prevention (ERP). See Chapter 10 for more information about ERP. Subsequent research over several decades has consistently demonstrated that ERP works very well. There's just one problem — many people refuse ERP and/or drop out of the treatment before they complete it.

Why do people drop out of or even refuse ERP altogether? Well, it's icky, yucky, and sometimes downright disgusting. For example, people with worries about dirt and germs may find themselves instructed by their therapists to touch dirt, doorknobs, toilet seats, urine, and maybe even the inside of a dumpster. People who fear hurting somebody may be asked to talk about stabbing loved ones, pick up knives, and carry babies they fear they may harm. As you can imagine, not exactly everybody is willing to do those things — even with the guidance of a trusted, competent therapist.

Because of these concerns, behavioral scientists have searched for other ways to treat OCD. Research findings support the idea that cognitive-behavioral therapy (CBT) techniques primarily aimed at changing thinking are effective for OCD, and for some may be as effective as the specific CBT strategy known as ERP. CBT thinking techniques are often combined with ERP as well.

This section describes and discusses seven ways of misinterpreting reality commonly associated with OCD (see the preceding section for a list). In addition, it shows you how CBT can be used to realign distorted thinking.

Defeating unreasonable doubts

The doubts that plague those with OCD are not based on reality, direct evidence, or the actual here and now, but rather on imagined scenarios that are concocted in the sufferer's mind. What all these OCD doubts have in common is that they're not tied to experience and information from the body's senses — that is, sight, touch, sound, smell, and taste. For example, the obsession about whether one closed the windows in the house before leaving is not connected to not having felt the windows actually click shut. Similarly, those imagined microbes emanating from the microwave cannot be seen, felt, or touched.

People with OCD accept a reasonable degree of uncertainty and doubt in some areas of their lives. For example, they may assume that the sun will rise and set each day, even knowing there could be a slight possibility that it won't. But when the OCD mind takes control over a particular topic or concern (for example, contamination, harming others, and so forth) doubt permeates, creating a haze that makes seeing reality almost impossible. Even though they usually know their thoughts are going against their own common sense and gut feelings, OCD sufferers repeatedly lose out to the "what if" mentality. In other words, they distrust their own senses and perceptions. So, they ask themselves:

>> What if I don't scrub the counters with bleach?

>> What if I left the windows unlocked?

>> What if I lose control and shove that person I am walking behind?

>> What if I take that knife out and stab my dog?

>> What if that microwave is emitting radioactive microbes?

Obsessive thoughts that cause distress usually are based on a premise that something really bad may happen. Doubt lurks behind almost all obsessions. *Maybe, just maybe* the obsession will come true if action is not taken to prevent it.

Distinguishing doubts from what's real

Most true dangers have elements that can be directly sensed. Natural gas comes with an added smell of rotten eggs to serve as a warning. And if something is burning on your stove, you can see or smell smoke coming from the kitchen.

Of course, some dangers are not easily detectable by the average person's senses. In many of these cases, warning signs are posted, such as, "Danger: High Voltage," "Danger: Radioactive Materials," or "Warning: Non-Potable Water." Or a loud siren may be sounded to warn of tornadoes in the area. Those warning signs are put there by people who are knowledgeable about the risks and whose senses (often aided by scientific instruments) enable them to assess specific risks that others might not be aware of. The signs themselves, though, are directly observable by *your* senses.

Even less obvious dangers, such as the risk associated with some germs, can usually be assessed by logical means. For example, during the recent pandemic, people could gauge the dangerousness of situations by accessing public information about local infection rates and then taking reasonable precautions.

The OCD mind creates warning signs based entirely on exaggerated, made-up, fanciful material. The story of doubt becomes grabbing and compelling because it can't be disconfirmed absolutely. But as the story departs from that which can be confirmed by your senses, it also drifts far from any likely reality.

Dismissing unrealistic doubts

The first step toward changing the way you think is becoming aware of the basis for your thoughts. If you're plagued by OCD doubts, ask yourself the following questions to help you realize that these doubts are not realistic:

>> Are your doubts based on direct information from your senses (sight, sound, smell, taste, or touch)?

>> Does your doubt seem to have a life of its own and keep coming back, even without new evidence to support it?

>> Is there anything about your doubt that other people would see as illogical?

>> Is there anything that would convince you that your doubt is likely false?

Realistic doubts are based on evidence from the senses; they don't keep returning without new supporting evidence; other people see them as reasonable; and they can be disproved or proved. Realistic doubts keep you safe from danger, but OCD doubts only keep you upset.

WARNING

Unreliable news sources can also encourage you to feel doubt. Try to check out those doubts by doing research using multiple sources of information including authorities on the subject.

The following story about Pam and Debbie shows you how realistic doubts and OCD doubts are as different as night and day.

> **Pam** and **Debbie** are sales representatives for a large pharmaceutical company. Their jobs require weekly travel. A few months earlier, they both came down with a case of food poisoning after eating hamburgers in a messy airport restaurant. Pam happens to have OCD, and Debbie does not. Since the illness, Pam's OCD goes into hyper-drive whenever she travels. She no longer eats at restaurants, opting to carry her own food wherever she goes.
>
> At a sales conference, Pam and Debbie are seated at the same table for a company luncheon. They reminisce about their previous bad experience at the restaurant together. Debbie tells Pam that she had a few qualms and doubts for a little while about eating in airport restaurants, and tends to avoid ordering rare hamburgers now; plus, she checks the place out for general cleanliness.
>
> Pam says, "That doesn't do it for me. I haven't gone into a restaurant ever since that happened." She then pulls out her can of liquid meal replacement for her lunch while she wipes the table top with a bleach towelette.
>
> Debbie asks, "Are you on a diet?"

Pam says, "No, but this place is crawling with germs. You never know what the waiters have touched. Lots of times they don't even wash their hands after going to the bathroom."

Debbie responds, "It looks pristine and clean to me. What are you talking about?"

"You can't see the microbes on the glasses, but I know they're there. You should know, too; we both got sick that way once. Some waiters carry hepatitis C. Do you know how horrible that is? You can catch it from unclean plates. That's not going to happen to me — ever!"

An important point to take away from Pam and Debbie's story is that sometimes OCD fears do come true. However, Debbie's doubts are realistic and based on evidence from her senses. She now takes precautions to avoid undercooked meat and messy-looking restaurants. Pam, on the other hand, has interpreted events related to food and restaurants with extreme, non–reality-based doubts and a refusal to accept any uncertainty. She avoids all restaurants and imagines microbes and diseases that cannot be seen.

How can you tell the difference between the two types of doubt? Filtering doubts through the series of questions from earlier in this section can help you determine whether your doubts are reasonable or not. Here's the result of asking these questions about Debbie's and Pam's doubts in Table 8-1.

The answers to the questions in Table 8-1 illustrate how OCD doubts are not based on reality that is observable. And when doubts are not based on solid evidence and logic, the quest to disconfirm them never ends — because they simply cannot be totally disconfirmed. In fact, if you try to disprove OCD doubts, they only intensify because they can't be absolutely proven as false.

REMEMBER

The OCD mind directs you to eliminate *all* doubts and uncertainty, especially in areas related to your OCD (such as contamination, imagined catastrophes, harming others, and symmetry). But doubt and uncertainty can *never* be fully eliminated and must be accepted as an inherent part of life.

Ending exaggerating risk

When thinking about their OCD-related concerns, OCD sufferers inflate the risks. And should any of those worries actually come true, the OCD mind substantially exaggerates the degree of suffering that is likely to result. This way of interpreting the world keeps anxiety and distress levels high.

Most people without OCD know that touching a doorknob could conceivably allow a cold virus to infect them. However, they proceed to touch many doorknobs each day knowing that the actual risk they incur each time is rather small. And they know that catching a cold is hardly catastrophic. Touching doorknobs took on more risk at the beginning of the worldwide pandemic; however, researchers soon found that the virus was primarily airborne and that the likelihood of catching COVID from surfaces was very low.

TABLE 8-1

Distinguishing Debbie's Doubts from Pam's

Question	Debbie	Pam
Are your doubts based on direct information from your senses (sight, sound, smell, taste, or touch)?	Yes. She ate an undercooked, bad hamburger in a messy restaurant.	Yes. She ate an undercooked hamburger in a messy restaurant. But now her fears are not based on her senses. She cannot see the microbes she imagines and cannot tell whether her waiters have diseases.
Does your doubt seem to have a life of its own and keep coming back even without new evidence to support it?	No. Debbie has an occasional qualm, but those have gotten much better with time.	Yes. The more Pam thinks about her doubts, the more they seem to grow. She does more and more things to avoid possible contamination.
Is there anything about your doubt that other people would see as illogical?	No. It is reasonable to avoid unclean restaurants and undercooked meat.	Yes. Most people know that eating in restaurants carries a slight risk, but they don't make assumptions about unseen microbes and diseases.
Is there anything that would convince you that your doubt is likely false?	Debbie uses evidence about how restaurants look and cook their meat. She only had food poisoning once in her life and knows it could happen again, but probably not for a long time.	Because she can't see the imagined microbes and diseases, *nothing* can convince Pam that restaurants are essentially safe.

However, for someone with OCD contamination obsessions, each and every doorknob is crawling with millions of highly contagious viruses of all kinds — COVID, flu, HIV, colds, tuberculosis, SARS, you name it. A touch of a doorknob sets off emergency warning sirens in the OCD mind. These sirens urge the person to take immediate action to eliminate the viruses and avoid illness. Even the possibility of a cold becomes greatly feared because there's at least *some* chance that a cold could turn into pneumonia and ultimately result in death.

DOUBTING THOMAS

The term *doubting Thomas* refers to a skeptic — one who is not easily convinced. The expression "doubting Thomas" comes from the biblical account of a disciple of Jesus. After Jesus was crucified, Thomas did not believe that Jesus had risen from the dead. Although other disciples told Thomas that Jesus had appeared to them, he wanted evidence. The following week, Jesus appeared to Thomas and allowed him to touch his wounds. After that, Thomas became a believer. He was able to see and touch Jesus. People with OCD have doubts as well. However, they don't look to real evidence to check out their doubts.

Religious practices are largely based on faith rather than direct evidence from one's senses. Faith is known to be extremely helpful for billions of people worldwide. However, faith and OCD don't mix. OCD does not enhance people's lives. So, if you want to act on faith, do it with respect to spirituality, not to deal with obsessions and compulsions.

One way to deal with the tendency of OCD to exaggerate risks is to check the evidence and logic of one's obsessive fears. You may find that this helps you reevaluate the exaggerated risks that your OCD mind is fooling you with. Working with a therapist can greatly facilitate this process. Consider answering these questions:

>> Do I have any direct evidence that is contrary to my fears?

>> Do I have any direct evidence to confirm my fears?

>> How often have my fears of this risk come true (versus not coming true) in the past?

>> Is there anything about the risks I'm imagining that other people would likely see as illogical?

The following story of Blair illustrates how OCD can exaggerate risks and how her therapist helps her.

Blair is a 39-year-old CPA. For years, she has struggled with OCD that's focused on contamination and germs. Blair worries about contamination that may emanate from health-care facilities. There is a clinic near her workplace, and she walks several blocks out of her way in order to avoid coming close to the clinic.

Her therapist asks her to estimate the probability that serious, potentially lethal contaminates could be picked up simply by walking near the clinic. She tells him the risk is about 10 percent — not exactly a certainty, but rather troubling for the likelihood of contracting a serious, life-threatening infection. Her therapist guides her to a reexamination of her estimated risks. He asks her to search for any evidence or logic she can think of that might change her estimated risks. She comes up with the following evidence and logic:

>> If the real risk was 10 percent, that would mean that a full 10 percent of those who walk by the clinic would die. Hard to imagine that someone wouldn't have noticed that.

>> If walking by a clinic incurs a 10 percent risk, then working there would probably kill off half of the employees within a short time. Blair assumes that's not happening.

>> Blair figures that she's probably walked by hundreds, if not thousands, of doctors' offices, hospitals, and clinics without even realizing it. If her estimate was real, she'd be dead by now.

Blair's new evidence allows her to re-estimate her risks as far less than 1 percent. She is more ready to try her therapist's next suggestion of walking by feared places like health clinics (ERP therapy; see Chapter 10 for more information).

WARNING

After you have scrutinized your OCD mind's ways of misinterpreting risk, re-rate that risk once, and only once, for any given thought. *Do not* keep returning to this exercise. If you do, the technique can actually become a compulsion that you are using to reassure yourself (see Chapter 5 for the problem with reassurance with OCD). Used once, and only once, for any particular OCD thought, this strategy can help you see that risks are much smaller than you think and allow you to work on accepting a certain amount of uncertainty in your life.

Rethinking the idea that thoughts have real power

If you have OCD, you may give thoughts far more importance than they merit. Just because you think something weird, strange, immoral, or cruel, does not mean that you are bad, crazy, or mean. *All* people have weird thoughts once in a while. That's perfectly normal. When that happens to most people, the thoughts are quickly dismissed or forgotten. Not so in OCD. The OCD mind takes thoughts way too seriously, thereby causing anxiety, guilt, shame, and revulsion.

Just because you think something doesn't make it true. Imagine that you have an obnoxious manager at work. After a frustrating day, you think, "I wish I could wave a magic wand and make him disappear."

Pretend that the offensive manager just happens to run away to Tahiti with his secretary the very next day (leaving his job, wife, and children). You celebrate, throw a party. But someone with OCD may think that the thought of wanting someone to disappear caused the occurrence. The OCD mind may say, "I had a bad thought; therefore, I am a horrible person. My thought caused my manager to run away. I have ruined the lives of his poor wife and seven children."

An obsession is an unwanted, intrusive thought. Everyone has obsessive thoughts once in a while. Say you don't have OCD and you think, "Wow, it's really hot in my office today. I feel like taking off all my clothes!" Do you worry that you might start stripping? Probably not. In fact, you may not think about the thought at all and go get yourself a cold drink instead.

But if you have OCD and you have the same thought, your OCD mind may say something like this: "Oh, my, I am really a weirdo. I wonder how many other people in the office know what I'm thinking? People must think I'm loony. What if I can't control myself, and I actually rip off my clothes? How can I stop myself? I better start counting the ceiling tiles to distract myself from that horrible thought. I'm starting to sweat. People will know. I better go home. I hope I can make it to the car without losing it completely."

TIP

If your OCD mind tricks you into thinking that thoughts are very important, try this experiment to help you understand that thoughts don't equal action:

1. Put a glass of water next to this book on a table.

2. Stare at the water.

3. Now say to yourself, "I think I am going to spill the water on top of this book with my thoughts alone."

4. Say it again.

5. Think really hard.

6. Did you spill the water?

I'm betting that most readers did not spill the water. You can't make things happen just by thinking them. And if you did spill the water just by thinking about it, a visit to Las Vegas may be in order.

TIP

Think up some other experiments to help you remember that bad thoughts are not the same as bad actions — that thinking about something does not cause it to happen. Be creative. If you're working with a therapist, this may be a very good activity to bring up in a session. Here are a few examples of other experiments designed to show you that thoughts don't cause events:

>> **Take out a ten-dollar bill and stare at it.** Try to turn it into a 100-dollar bill. Command it to change. (**Note:** It doesn't count if an unexpected check shows up in your mailbox in a few days — that's just a random happening).

>> **Stare at your car and command it to change color.** If it's white, try turning it to black. Good luck. How did that work out for you?. Consider starting an auto painting business if you succeed.

>> **Stare at the speed-limit signs on your daily commute and command them to raise the limit so you can speed your way along.** By the way, don't start speeding until they actually change.

Decoupling facts and feelings

Feelings serve many purposes. For example, feelings may give you joy and pleasure or they may warn you of impending danger. But when OCD kicks in, feelings lead you astray. That's because OCD causes the brain to turn on the burglar alarm when there's no actual sign of a break-in (see Chapter 4 for the biological explanation of this process).

People with OCD are flooded with feelings of dread and doom when no logical cause for alarm exists. However, the OCD mind tells them that there must be a real reason for these feelings. And if the feelings are true, whatever meaning you associate with those feelings must be true, too. For example:

>> I feel ashamed, so I must be a sinner.

>> I feel dirty, so I must be contaminated.

>> I feel dizzy, so I must have a brain tumor.

>> I feel guilty, so I must have done something wrong.

>> I feel out of sorts, so I must be coming down with something.

>> I feel scared, so there must be real danger.

Feelings like the ones listed can be very powerful. Anxious, negative feelings are merely an indication that your brain's alarm system has been set off — but just like a home burglar alarm system, lots of false alarms can occur. Winds, a neighbor's cat, your teenage son sneaking in late at night, and an electrical short can also start the sirens blaring.

To get a grip on your feelings, start reminding yourself that feeling bad doesn't mean you *are* bad or that something bad is going on. When your brain's alarm system goes off, resist the urge to scream, run, or hide. Hold off on making a judgment and carefully check for evidence. If you can't find clear signs based on what you can see, hear, smell, taste, or feel, consider assuming the alarm was false. With lots of practice, you can stop your brain from setting off so many false alarms.

Overcoming the need for perfection

Perfection permeates the OCD mind by telling you that mistakes are horrible and must be avoided at all costs. Perfectionism leads to procrastination and avoidance because perfection is impossible to obtain. For example, a student may write and rewrite a paper and never turn it in because she knows it must contain errors. Although many people without OCD struggle with perfectionism from time to time, OCD ups the ante. How can you ever be 100 percent sure that

» You will never say anything that could offend anyone, ever?

» The books are lined up precisely and perfectly?

» The kitchen counters have absolutely no microbes or germs of any kind?

» The tone of voice and words in your prayer are exactly what God demands of you?

If these kinds of concerns plague you, you may want to ask yourself these questions:

» Does my perfectionism benefit my life?

» Does my perfectionism hurt me in any way?

» If a friend of mine had such perfectionistic thoughts, what would I tell him?

» What would my life be like if I allowed for a little more leniency in the way I judge myself?

TIP

Most perfectionists have far more compassion and understanding for the flaws and foibles of others than they have for themselves. Learning to judge yourself by the same standards you set for your friends may help you let go of the excessively harsh standards you set for yourself.

Sidestepping obsessive thoughts

One of the hallmarks of OCD is that the thoughts, urges, and impulses known as obsessions become extremely upsetting and unwanted. Therefore, most people with OCD feel driven to rid themselves of their obsessions. The problem with that strategy is that it flat-out doesn't work. Not only that, trying to suppress thoughts actually intensifies them. And as the thoughts intensify, so does the distress.

In the story that follows, Marty is plagued by the obsession that his shameful thoughts might lead to horrible actions. Marty believes that his thoughts have special powers (see the earlier section, "Rethinking the idea that thoughts have real power"), so this belief causes him to work very hard at ridding himself of these appalling thoughts. The story shows you what happens as he tries to suppress his thoughts.

> **Marty** works at an electronics store at the mall. He has obsessions about the possibility that he could lose control and fondle women inappropriately when they walk into his store — abhorrent, dirty thoughts. Whenever Marty has those thoughts, he believes he might lose control and actually abuse women.
>
> From that premise, it's pretty easy to understand why Marty desperately tries to suppress all such thinking. However, the more he tries not to have the thoughts, the more they grow. He finds that day after day, he spends more time trying to "not think" about these things. He sings to himself; he tries to repeat phrases such as "clean thoughts/clean mind;" and he repeatedly counts the inventory even though that task is only required once each month. His co-workers start noticing that he seems distracted all the time.

Attempting to suppress thoughts causes them to increase for a pretty simple reason. When you try to avoid thinking about something, you have to constantly search your mind for any sign of the thoughts that you're trying to avoid. The act of being on the lookout for the unwanted thoughts actually causes them to pop up to the surface more easily.

TIP

If you find yourself trying to control your OCD obsessional thoughts, try this experiment. You will see how trying to suppress thoughts usually just adds to your difficulties:

1. Pick one obsessional thought that you wish you didn't have. Write that thought down in your OCD notebook.

2. Spend one day trying as hard as you can not to have the thought at all. At the end of the day, estimate how many times the thought managed to break through your defenses and pop into your mind and write it down. Also rate and record how disturbing the thought felt from 0 (not at all) to 10 (highly disturbing).

3. Spend the next day allowing the obsessional thought to do whatever it wants — pop into your mind or not. Again, write down your estimate of how many times the thought came into your mind and how disturbing it felt on a scale of 0 to 10.

4. Continue alternating days for at least six days (three suppressing days with three days of no attempt at suppressing).

5. Write down your conclusions and reflections about what attempting to suppress your thoughts does to you.

You're likely to discover that the harder you work to stop thinking about your obsessions, the more they increase and disturb you. If you find that thought control really works for you, go for it. I suspect that it won't. If it does seem to work, most likely the effect will be temporary and partial. Consider working with a therapist if you discover that you're continuing to struggle with attempts to control your thoughts.

Letting go of feeling excessively responsible

People with OCD often believe that their thoughts, urges, or images, as well as their actions, cause harm to others or to themselves. They spend lots of time worrying about whether they may have done, said, or thought something that may possibly hurt someone. They dwell on the slightest possibility of causing such harm. Whenever an event has a bad outcome, they feel totally, morally responsible, even though they had little or no influence on the event and did not want it to happen.

One way to challenge your beliefs about being excessively responsible is to develop a picture of how responsible you really are by using a pie chart. The pie chart is a graph that illustrates all the factors that generate a particular outcome. The process goes like this:

1. Estimate the percentage of the bad outcome for which you believe you're personally responsible.

2. List any other factors that could conceivably have contributed to the event. Assign percentages indicating the extent to which these other factors may also be responsible.

3. Make a pie chart to graph the percentages from Steps 1 and 2 accordingly.

4. Examine the resulting chart to assess your relative responsibility for the outcome.

5. Develop a statement that affirms the fact that you are not solely responsible and repeat it to yourself often.

The following example of Raul illustrates this process.

Raul works as a physical therapist at an assisted living facility. He obsesses about hurting the residents. He imagines pushing frail, elderly people down the stairs, dumping them from their wheelchairs, or suffocating them. Of course, he has never hurt any of his patients and finds the idea totally repugnant, but he has repeated urges, images, and thoughts. When any of the residents becomes ill or dies, Raul believes that he is fully responsible for the outcome. He thinks he surely could have done something to prevent the illness or death. He obsesses over whether he failed to wash his hands or maintain perfect care, or whether his thoughts alone caused the patient's condition. He is disgusted with himself and believes that someday he will be punished for his horrible obsessions.

Following the death of one of his elderly patients, Raul's distress is so great that he admits to his therapist how he believes he caused the death. His therapist, Dr. James, asks him to estimate exactly to what extent he owns personal responsibility for the patient's death. Raul responds, "100 percent." This is illustrated by the pie chart in Figure 8-1.

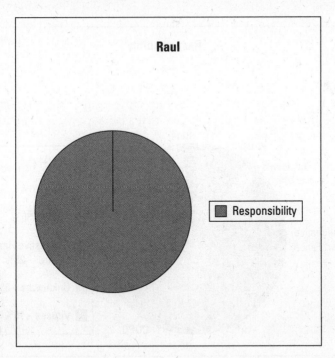

Raul

■ Responsibility

FIGURE 8-1:
Raul believes that he is 100 percent responsible for the death of a patient.

Dr. James draws a circle on the white board in his office. He labels it "Responsibility for Patient's Death" and writes Raul's name on it. He then turns to Raul and asks, "Are there *any* other possible factors that could have caused the death of this patient?"

Raul responds, "Well she was in her late 90s, and she started with a bad cold. Then she caught that flu that's been going around."

"So Raul," Dr. James expands, "her age may have been a factor, she had the flu, and she was already pretty frail. Let's add these to the pie chart. Were there any other things that may have contributed?"

Raul goes on to say, "Well, she did have advanced chronic obstructive pulmonary disease (COPD), which greatly increases the chances of dying from almost any-thing. And she'd had congestive heart failure for six years."

Their conversation ultimately produces a wide variety of potential contributors to the patient's death. At the end of the session, Raul and Dr. James conclude that he probably did not have much to do with the death of the 98-year-old woman. The pie chart they develop is shown in Figure 8-2.

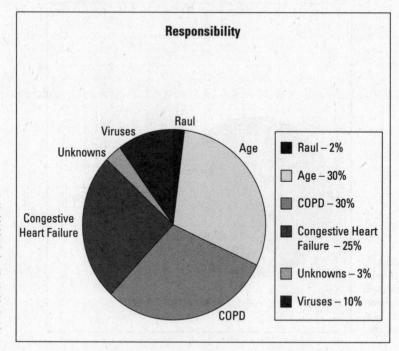

FIGURE 8-2: Raul's pie chart indicates that Raul's responsibility for the patient's death is insignificant compared to the other contributing factors.

Raul remains concerned about his obsessions. Dr. James doesn't really buy that Raul owns even 2 percent of the responsibility for the patient's death. However, Raul still clings to feelings of guilt and shame. He dwells on the slight possibility that his 2 percent contribution may have been the tipping point. Thus, Dr. James tells Raul that continued work on his excessive responsibility OCD is necessary.

This exercise helps Raul understand that his obsessive urges and impulses don't really have the power to hurt others. He still feels somewhat responsible, but using the pie chart technique helps him talk back to his OCD. He learns to say, "Just because I feel overly responsible, doesn't mean that I am. No one's care can be perfect, and even if it were, people would still die."

REMEMBER

The pie chart technique helps people realize that many factors are involved in outcomes. Usually no one person or one reason can be held 100 percent responsible when something bad happens.

Pushing Out OCD Thinking with New Narratives

Mysteries, horror, and science fiction capture the minds and emotions of audiences all over the world. The audience is immersed in a story that may be highly unlikely or even illogical, but it appears possible because the audience suspends judgment and logic for a few hours. When the movie or book reaches a conclusion, the audience returns to reality.

OCD grabs your mind and emotions in much the same manner, but the story or movie never ends. Logic and reality remain suspended. Endless skewed narratives (obsessive thoughts) that misinterpret reality exhaustively plague the OCD mind.

It's as though those with OCD have a fiction writer living in their heads churning out compelling narratives, or stories, one after the other. The OCD mind sees just enough elements of *possibility* to make the story *seem* totally believable. The best way to shut these OCD-fueled stories down is to rewrite your mind's narratives and give them a good dose of reality. This involves a three-step process:

1. Making up OCD-like stories

2. Writing your own OCD narratives

3. Assessing and rewriting your OCD narratives

But before you start writing fictitious OCD stories, it's a good idea to see what a typical OCD story looks like. Consider the story of Pam, from the earlier section, "Dismissing unrealistic doubts." Pam has doubts about the safety of food, the cleanliness of restaurants, and the possibility of contracting diseases from waiters. Her OCD story contains many OCD misinterpretations. Her therapist suggests that she write out her complete OCD narrative. Here's what she comes up with.

> Germs are everywhere. I keep thinking about filth. You never know who might be sick or have open sores. If a waiter with hepatitis has a cut and then touches my plate, I could easily get hepatitis. If I get hepatitis, I could pass it on to my family before I even know I'm sick. I saw a waiter smoking a cigarette outside in the parking lot. The parking lot is full of germs from rotting food and animal droppings. The waiters can pick up dirt and feces on their shoes, and then contaminate their hands when they tie their shoes. Then they touch everything on the table. I'm not certain that all the glasses, plates, and utensils are sterilized after each meal. I look at the plates and feel disgusted; if I feel disgusted, I'm pretty sure that means they must be contaminated. Walking into a restaurant feels like walking into a cesspool. I was lucky to just get food poisoning. If I eat in a restaurant again, I could get something much worse. So, it makes sense to carry my own food in sterilized plastic bags. If I have to go to a restaurant for work, I just don't eat. As soon as I'm out of there, I shower for at least 30 minutes, and then I sanitize my clothes.

Pam's OCD narrative has many elements that seem reasonable. Germs *are* everywhere, miniscule amounts of feces *are* found in food, parking lots *are* dirty, and hepatitis *is* occasionally transmitted by food handlers. What makes this an OCD story is that Pam has no direct evidence to confirm or disconfirm her concerns about all these contaminants making their way to her dinner plate. Her OCD story illustrates the following OCD misinterpretations:

>> Confusing facts and feelings

>> Doubting her own senses' ability to detect cleanliness and safety

>> Inflating the importance of her thoughts

>> Overestimating the risk of getting sick

>> Seeking unobtainable perfectionism (perfect cleanliness)

Due to the type of OCD misinterpretations she uses, her story spins entirely out of her OCD mind. You see how to write out your personal OCD stories and assess them for misinterpretations in the later sections of this chapter. But first, indulge in a little fantasy.

Creating made-up, OCD-like stories

In order to prepare you for dealing with your personal OCD stories, you may find it helpful to create OCD-like stories about things that *you normally don't worry about at all*. Doing so allows you to see how similar these completely made-up stories are to those your OCD mind has already created. You can see that there is absolutely no end to such stories and remind yourself that your personal OCD stories are merely fictitious creations of your OCD mind.

These fictitious stories are actually sort of fun to write. But the point of writing them is to remind yourself that these fanciful stories are exactly like the OCD stories that run through your mind and scare you all the time. Try viewing your OCD stories as creative, emotionally interesting, and even a little entertaining. Follow this process to author your own work of OCD fiction:

1. **Think about some mundane, everyday event that causes you no particular worry or distress.**

   Examples include walking along a sidewalk, searching for a book on the library's shelves, going to the mall, or sitting in your hot tub. Just be sure to choose something that you do with no trouble and that's unrelated to the actual OCD stories that currently run through your mind.

2. **Include details concerning everything that could conceivably go wrong in your story.** This can include contamination, death, illness, harm to others, imperfections, and so on.

3. **Read your made-up story and notice how similar it is to the ones that really do scare you.** Compare it to the stories that run through the movie theater in your mind on a daily basis.

4. **Practice watching how creative the OCD mind can be.** Consider writing two or three of these stories each day for a while.

5. **Consider becoming a Hollywood horror-movie author.** (Just kidding.)

I'm pretty sure you'll discover that it isn't difficult to imagine many conceivable scenarios of danger. For example, how worried are you right now, *this very moment*, that your house may ignite into a ball of fire? Probably not very (at least until I brought up the possibility).

Now turn on the OCD fiction writer and watch how the story unfolds:

Maybe the electrician who installed the wiring in your home office was a drug abuser who was high that day and crossed a few wires. It's also possible that moisture has accumulated behind the walls and some connections are about to short out. Maybe your neighbors haven't cleaned their fireplace chimney and an ember could spark, fly out, and land on your roof. And the U.S. Navy just shot a satellite out of the sky. You can imagine a big chunk falling onto your house, setting it ablaze. It's been a while since you cleaned out the dryer vent. What if the cat tips over a lamp while you're out, and it ignites the curtains? Are you absolutely, positively certain that you turned off the stove?

The point is that the above scenario is remotely possible. But the OCD story is not based on anything that is happening right now. Of course, you should take reasonable precautions to keep your house safe. But the OCD fiction writer keeps these thoughts churning despite the lack of any objective supporting evidence. And OCD doubt would not be assuaged by cleaning out the dryer vent — *there's always something else* that could be done to prevent fire. In actuality, the list is potentially endless. You could no doubt spend every waking moment of each and every day trying to eliminate risks of fire and still not succeed 100 percent.

WARNING

There is a slight chance that writing fictitious OCD stories could cause you to develop a few new worries. If you find that to be the case for you, please stop this process and seek professional consultation. If your OCD is fairly severe (that is, quite worrisome and disruptive to your life), you should seek such consultation before attempting any of the exercises in this book on your own at all.

Writing down your OCD narratives

In order to change the endings to the OCD stories that run continuously through your mind, you need to write them out. Take some time to start writing your personal stories, the ones that actually run through your mind and worry you from day to day. Be sure to tell the whole story (or as they say in New Mexico, "the whole enchilada"), including all your doubts, distorted interpretations, beliefs, reasoning, images, and worries — everything your mind tells you about your obsessions and compulsions. Here's how:

>> **Write a complete narrative about every OCD fear or worry that bothers you.**

You don't have to do all of these stories at once — you may need several writing sessions to complete the task. Write them down one at a time. Go back to your story a number of times and add details as they occur to you.

>> **Be sure to include all thoughts, images, and urges that run through your head as they relate to the OCD story.**

>> **Write down what makes you believe in your OCD story — your reasoning process (regardless of whether it seems logical).**

>> **Don't forget to include your fears of what may happen if you fail to obey your OCD and take actions to avoid bad outcomes.**

>> **Include any people or characters that may be involved in your story.**
   Often stories revolve around harm to others.

Review your story fairly often and embellish it further if additional details come to mind. Don't worry; there is a plan to help you change your story. In the next section, you find out how to write alternative, non-OCD stories to live by. But for now, you need to be aware of the existing stories and hear what they're telling you.

Assessing and rewriting OCD narratives

After you've written out your OCD story, you're ready to rewrite it with a different outcome. There are two steps to rewriting your OCD story:

1. Assessing your story

2. Creating a balanced story

Assessing your OCD narrative

In order to assess your OCD narrative, you need to determine what types of OCD misinterpretations (such as exaggerating risks, doubts, confusing facts, and feelings, and so forth) your personal OCD story contains. Then you'll have the information you need to write an alternative, balanced story. Here are questions that can help you analyze the elements of your narratives:

>> Does your OCD story involve doubt? If so, is your doubt based on direct evidence?

>> Would other people agree with your story or find it illogical?

>> How great is the risk of your OCD story happening? Are you exaggerating the risk?

>> Are you viewing your thoughts as having special powers or as being real?

>> Are you confusing your feelings with facts?

>> Are you too worried about being perfect?

>> Are you trying to control your thoughts?

>> Are you being overly responsible and believing that you should be able to protect yourself and others from harm?

Write out the answers and take some time to reflect upon them. The answers alone will not greatly impact your OCD, but they will prepare you to write a new, more balanced story.

To give you a better idea of how this step works, take a look at Tracy's story.

Tracy is a 45-year-old elementary school teacher with contamination fears. Her story provides an opportunity for you to practice analyzing OCD stories for OCD misinterpretations. Then you'll be ready to analyze your own OCD stories and, finally, rewrite them.

The modern world is full of radiation and unknown dangers from cellphone towers and other signals in the air. Whenever I spot a tower, I feel nervous, and my entire body tingles. I am pretty sure it's due to the signals bombarding my body and disrupting nerve cells. The danger lurks everywhere. Thousands of satellites beam signals all over the planet. So, I've lined my car roof with aluminum foil. I also had contractors place rolls of foil across my entire attic. But I still worry. I wear hats lined with foil everywhere for a little extra protection.

I try to explain these problems to my family, but they think I'm crazy. I tell them the things they should do to protect themselves. I'd just die if they got cancer when I could have prevented it. Sometimes, I try hard not to think about these dangers because the thoughts just upset me. But the thoughts keep coming back. Maybe my brain has become contaminated, and that's preventing me from being able to control my thoughts.

Now let's take a look at Tracy's story and analyze it for OCD misinterpretations. Is her story based on faulty logic or thinking? By applying the eight questions noted earlier, you can see evidence of faulty thinking.

» **Does her OCD story involve doubt? If so, is her doubt based on direct evidence?**

Tracy's story is full of OCD doubt and not based on any clear evidence. Perhaps someday science will figure out whether the types of signals Tracy worries about pose any real risk, but until that day, no justification exists for her actions.

» **Would other people agree with her story or find it illogical?**

Everyone that Tracy has shared her story with finds it quite unlikely.

» **How great is the risk of Tracy's OCD story happening? Is she exaggerating the risk?**

As is typical with OCD, Tracy is profoundly exaggerating risks.

>> **Is Tracy viewing her thoughts as having special powers or as being real?**

She believes that merely because she has these thoughts, they must be real.

>> **Is Tracy confusing her feelings with facts?**

Yes. She feels tingling in her body, which is probably due to anxiety. She then assumes that the tingling represents proof of damage to her body.

>> **Is Tracy too worried about being perfect?**

Tracy's story does not show evidence that she is too much of a perfectionist.

>> **Is Tracy trying to control her thoughts?**

Yes, but like most people, she finds that attempts to control her thoughts just make the situation worse.

>> **Is Tracy being overly responsible and believing that she should be able to protect herself and others from harm?**

Yes, Tracy is assuming that she can do things to prevent cancer from occurring in her family by getting them to take the same actions she has — that is, by creating barriers to block signals and radiation.

By answering the preceding questions, you can see the types of OCD misinterpretations Tracy has been making. You can assess your own OCD stories the same way.

Creating a balanced narrative

Now it's time to start writing an alternative, non-OCD story. This story will stand in sharp contrast to your OCD story. Your new story needs to take the opposite view. Consider how someone who doesn't have OCD might tell the story. You probably won't believe in this new story right away — that's expected. However, with time and practice, you will make slow but sure progress toward buying into your new story.

TIP

Writing and rewriting your OCD stories will likely be much easier to do with the collaborative help of a therapist. If your OCD is fairly severe, please realize that while these exercises are likely to help you, you'll also need to do many of the other strategies presented throughout this book. I strongly suggest professional help.

Here's how to proceed:

>> **Take your time.** Don't expect to write your new story in one sitting.

>> **Include at least as many details in your non-OCD story as you have in your OCD story.** Add even more details over time.

>> **Make sure your story is based only on evidence that you can see, touch, taste, feel, or hear.**

>> **Act as if you believe your story.** Read it and imagine it to be true several times each day. Continue this process for a number of weeks.

>> **Don't pull out your story to deal with distress that arises when your OCD story becomes active.** Instead, read your new story repeatedly when you're feeling okay.

>> **As you practice your story, start rating how much you believe in your balanced, non-OCD story.** Also rate your belief in your OCD story and see whether it starts to slowly decline.

Following is Tracy's new, non-OCD story. (See "Assessing your OCD narrative" for the OCD version.) Because Tracy's OCD is pretty severe, she enlists the help of a therapist to complete this exercise.

> I realize that no one is on a mission to contaminate the world. Overall, most cancer rates have actually declined a little in the past decade. Telephone companies certainly don't want to kill their customers off. Real people work for those companies, and those people care about their own families and probably other people as well. My house and my car are safe, nice places to be. I enjoy spending time driving as well as having friends over to my home. I like going to other people's homes. Their homes are as safe as they need to be. Cellphone towers help people stay in touch with each other. Satellites allow us to predict the weather, stream movies, and enjoy modern life.

Tracy reads and imagines scenes from her story regularly. She remembers not to pull it out in order to deal with her OCD story when it pops up. With lots of support and practice, she discovers that her OCD story feels less and less believable. Her new story slowly becomes more comfortable. She finds that living her life as if the new story were true feels much better.

Chapter **9**

Meta-Mindfulness for OCD

large part of OCD suffering occurs inside the head. People with OCD monitor their thoughts for signs of danger, uncertainty, shameful images, or potential disorder. They dwell on these thoughts and fixate on possible threats. It's no surprise that some treatment strategies involve re-examining the thoughts that occur in the OCD brain.

This chapter takes a look at two of those treatments — one, fairly new and the other ancient. Metacognitive therapy is a strategy that helps those with OCD take a step back and look at thinking styles and beliefs. Mindfulness takes on OCD by helping those who suffer fully accept the present moment.

TECHNICAL STUFF

Cognitive behavioral therapy (CBT) and exposure and response prevention (ERP) are both well-researched effective treatments for OCD. However, almost a third of those who start these therapies drop out early or refuse treatment. And many more show some progress but still have residual symptoms. That is one reason that metacognitive and mindfulness strategies are often used successfully alone or in conjunction with CBT or ERP.

Thinking Erroneously

Metacognitive therapy addresses broad beliefs about thinking. In contrast to CBT's focus on individual distorted beliefs (see Chapter 8), metacognitive therapy takes a wider lens and focuses on what individuals believe about their obsessions and compulsions. The metacognitive model looks at how strongly individuals believe in the power of obsessional thinking and the negative consequences of not performing compulsions.

Three beliefs about obsessions have commonly been found in people with OCD. When someone with OCD has an intrusive thought (obsession), these beliefs increase the perception of dangerousness or importance of the obsession. Generally called the fusion beliefs, they are as follows:

>> **Thought Action Fusion:** Bad thoughts always lead to bad behavior. For example, "I have an obsession that I am sexually attracted to my priest; therefore, I will be unable to stop myself from acting out sexually."

>> **Thought Event Fusion:** Thinking about something will cause it to happen. For example, if I have an obsessive thought of pushing an elderly person off the sidewalk into the street, I believe it will definitely happen now or sometime in the future.

>> **Thought Object Fusion:** Bad, evil, or inappropriate thoughts can be transferred to objects. For example, "My thoughts can contaminate an object, which will then be dangerous to me or others."

A metacognitive approach to these fusion beliefs is to understand the fallacy of these beliefs and begin to respond to obsessional thinking more objectively. Obsessions are not all-powerful predictions of the future, but simply mental events. In addition to dealing with obsessions in a different way, metacognitive therapy helps to challenge the false belief that compulsions (rituals) must be performed or something terrible will happen.

TECHNICAL STUFF

Differences between therapeutic approaches such as CBT, mindfulness, and metacognitive therapy can seem quite subtle. And they are. Most effective therapies share much in common and differ in almost imperceptible ways. Metacognitive therapy has more of a philosophical bent than some of the other therapies, but don't worry about understanding the nuances.

Separating Your Thoughts from You

The concept of mindfulness means attending to the present moment with openness and without judgment. Achieving mindfulness can seem very challenging when your mind is busily bubbling with obsessions and compulsions. You may wonder how you can be accepting of the present moment when the present moment feels so distressful and uncomfortable.

TECHNICAL STUFF

Practicing mindfulness involves adopting a set of attitudes and is a good precursor to meditation. Research supports the use of meditation and mindfulness as adjuncts to cognitive-behavioral therapy (CBT). Mindfulness has been increasingly incorporated into CBT. Exciting research on mindfulness-based techniques has shown significant promise. In fact, CBT that includes a mindfulness component has demonstrated actual, positive changes in brain areas thought to be involved with OCD.

REMEMBER

To achieve mindfulness, you must be able to recognize that the thoughts you think and who you are as a person are not one and the same.

People with all types of emotional disorders universally fall into a trap set by their minds. And in truth, people who do not suffer from clear-cut emotional maladies sometimes fall into this same trap. The nature of this trap is that the mind tells you to take the thoughts it generates very seriously. The mind further dictates that you should believe that you and your thoughts are synonymous — one and the same.

But you need to realize that these directives from your mind are erroneous illusions. And believing in these illusions can lead you down a very rocky path indeed. The only way to avoid this trap is to find a way to step back and observe your OCD mind at work.

Here's an exercise to help you see what I'm getting at called "Discovering the Observant You versus Your OCD Thoughts."

1. **Sit down and make yourself comfortable.**

2. **Close your eyes and wait for a thought to pop into your mind** — any thought at all. Your thought could be about

   - How you're feeling (relaxed, anxious, sad, whatever)

   - The temperature in the room

   - What this exercise has to do with OCD

- What you want to cook for dinner

- Wondering when a darn thought is finally going to pop into your mind — yes, that's a thought, too!

You may have to wait a few seconds or perhaps a few minutes, but it won't take too long for some sort of thought to cross your mind. After all, the mind is a master at generating thoughts one right after another.

REMEMBER

Obsessions are thoughts, too. If an obsession is the first thing to pop into your mind, consider it a thought.

3. **Now, ask yourself this question about your thought: Who noticed the thought?**

The answer to that question is that there is an observant part of you that can see your thoughts separately from the part of you that generates your thoughts. Thus, *you* are not your thoughts. With time and practice, you can separate yourself from your thoughts — especially your OCD-related thoughts. Start listening for those OCD thoughts. Typical examples include the following:

>> I can't stand not being certain that things will be okay.

>> I could die from touching doorknobs.

>> I could never use a public restroom.

>> Elevator buttons are dangerous collectors of germs.

>> Restaurants are full of contaminants that could kill me.

Chapter 8 tells you how to rethink the content of your thoughts — by examining the evidence, rewriting OCD stories, looking for OCD misinterpretations, and so on. Now try your hand at viewing your OCD thoughts as simply random, meaningless output from your OCD mind. These thoughts can be interesting to observe, but they shouldn't be taken too seriously.

Some simple mental exercises can help you put your thoughts into the proper perspective and let them go effortlessly. To that end, try the following:

>> Close your eyes and imagine writing your OCD thought on a leaf. Then toss the leaf into a stream. Watch the leaf swirl in the eddies of the water as it slowly heads downstream.

>> Close your eyes and imagine you have a magic laser that writes your thoughts onto a cloud high in the sky. Just watch the cloud slowly drift.

>> Repeatedly remind yourself that "thoughts are merely thoughts, nothing more." Repeat this phrase over and over, but don't let it become a new compulsion for dealing with your obsessive thoughts!

The point of treating your thoughts this way is that slowly, but surely, you can relate to them differently. You can call upon the observant part of you to help you step back from your thoughts. Think of your thoughts as analogous to having your hand smashed up against your face, blocking your vision. The observant you can help you take the hand away, allowing you to see (think) more clearly.

BUILDING BRIDGES FROM BUDDHISM TO WESTERN PSYCHOLOGY

Dr. B. Alan Wallace of the Santa Barbara Institute for Consciousness Studies and Dr. Shauna L. Shapiro of Santa Clara University discussed their views on and approach to integrating Buddhist philosophy and mental-health practices in the journal, *American Psychologist*. In contrast to traditional psychology that often focuses on what is wrong with people, Buddhist philosophy is concerned with achieving states of balanced well-being. Wallace and Shapiro believe that good mental health consists of mental balance in four areas. Achieving this balance could help relieve OCD symptoms. The four areas are

- **Conative Balance:** Conative behavior means purposeful and goal-directed. A person must have willful intentions and carry them out. These intentions must be realistic and consistent with the well-being of oneself and others. For example, with OCD, there must be an intention or willingness to face fear and some discomfort in order to benefit from treatment.

- **Attentional Balance:** Attentional balance refers to the ability to attend to and focus voluntarily. Lack of attentional control is a problem for those who suffer with OCD. They can be distracted by their obsessions and unable to concentrate on what is important. The development of voluntary and sustained attention allows a person with OCD to practice mindfulness instead of dwelling on obsessional thoughts.

- **Cognitive Balance:** Maintaining cognitive balance means having a clear mind that is open to experiences and not distorted by thoughts or emotions. A person with cognitive balance is grounded in reality. For OCD sufferers, this means identifying OCD distortions that cloud their thinking (see Chapter 8).

- **Affective Balance:** Affective refers to one's emotions. People with affective balance experience a full range of emotions and respond to reality with appropriate emotional expressions. They are empathic, compassionate, and joyful as appropriate, based on reality, as opposed to those with OCD who tend to become overly fearful and anxious because of their OCD beliefs.

Acquiring the Attitudes of Mindfulness

Mindfulness consists of a set of adoptable attitudes, which are described in this section. When you embrace these attitudes, you can start ever-so-slowly to form a new perspective on life that can help you manage your OCD mind instead of allowing it to manage you. These ways of thinking can also prepare you for mindful meditation. These attitudes are

>> Making time

>> Having patience

>> Letting go

>> Learning acceptance

>> Suspending judgment

>> Living in the now

Making time to be mindful

Adopting mindful attitudes and becoming skilled at mindfulness require you to open up some space and time in your life. Simply put, to change, you have to want to change, and you have to make time to change.

I can almost hear you saying, "Okay, but I'm awfully busy. Exactly how much time will I need to put in on this?" That question actually comes from the OCD part of your mind, which doesn't want you to spend time on things that will take you away from your OCD!

In actuality, you don't need to practice mindfulness for any absolute amount of time. If you're feeling really pressed, try giving mindfulness ten formal minutes a day. As you get used to it, and it begins to feel more natural, you'll probably find it easier to devote an increasing amount of time to it. Try to work up to 30 to 45 minutes a day.

REMEMBER

If you're thinking, "Gasp, I could never devote 45 minutes a day to something like this," don't forget that less time can be helpful, too. You can always try being mindful for a couple of minutes ten times a day or develop some similar strategy. The more time you spend on being mindful, the less time you will be devoting to your OCD. Most people find that if they can reduce their OCD by 50 percent or more, a big chunk of time is freed up that was unavailable to them before.

Pursuing patience

Humans tend to be a rather impatient lot. But impatience can derail the most determined efforts to change. For example, dieters give up on dieting because they don't see results quickly enough — even though studies indicate that the more slowly you lose weight, the better you'll do in the long run. In the same way, impatience causes people to stop physical training when they can't observe results after a few weeks.

You simply cannot rush the process of adopting mindful attitudes. Consider running a long-distance race using the wrong motivation. Somewhere along the way, after running for what seems like an eternity, you realize you have not yet reached the finish line. To prod yourself to do better and run faster, you start smacking yourself on the head. I hope you can see the futility in this approach. It is only by accepting where you're at now that you can move forward.

OCD often devours hours of time and mental energy every day, so it's very understandable that you want quick relief. Be patient. Don't expect immediate balance and absolute well-being after a few days of practicing mindfulness.

Letting go of striving for striving's sake

In the Western world, and especially in the United States, people tend to emphasize hard work and striving for a purpose. The message is usually that if you aren't where you want to be in life, all you have to do is work harder, and you'll get there. Still not getting the results you want? Work even harder. Whew! I'm tired just from thinking about it! What about working *smarter* with mindfulness?

Adapting a mindful attitude may feel very strange indeed if you, like most people, belong to the "work hard and then work some more" school of thinking. Mindfulness just doesn't happen that way. Rather, unlike almost everything else you do, mindfulness comes from letting go of working harder. In a sense, you want to strive to not strive. You *allow* mindfulness to come in while allowing yourself to let go of striving for striving's sake.

You could easily conclude that I am suggesting that hard work is a bad thing. But that's not the case at all. For example, the treatment of OCD usually involves hard, difficult work. Most people will need to participate in some type of psychotherapy in order to get better. That means going to sessions, talking about difficult topics, and even doing things that may be really hard (see Chapters 8 and 10 for more information). But my experience with people is that when they work too hard at therapy and become, well, obsessive, then progress can be slowed.

Discovering acceptance

Most clients start therapy wanting to change something about themselves or their world. They come for help because they're uncomfortable and feeling great distress. They want something different in their lives. They want to feel better. Although therapy helps them feel better, it cannot eliminate all the bad stuff they will encounter the rest of their lives.

Certainly, if you suffer from OCD, you want change — change from suffering and change from feeling overtaken and overwhelmed. What if I tell you that the only way out of suffering is to accept that you will suffer? But the pain of your suffering will impact you far less when you practice acceptance.

Life is difficult. If you live a long life, you will necessarily experience pain, loss, and sadness. All humans do! But you may wonder, why do some people fall apart when bad things happen while others march on or even benefit from hardship?

Lots of factors play a role in how people respond to life's bumps in the road. People are made stronger by having supportive family and friends, enjoying productive work, and being strong mentally and physically. But something else protects against misfortune. People who are shocked and surprised when the inevitable obstacle shows up have a harder time handling it than do people who acknowledge and anticipate distress. Knowing and *accepting* that some moments in life are going to be uncomfortable, and even expecting those moments, make those difficult moments less, well, difficult.

REMEMBER

Acceptance means cultivating a willingness to experience life as it comes your way. Allow bad feelings in when they arrive and *actually embrace* them. The more you fight, the bigger the battle. That is the paradox of acceptance. Thus, acceptance is neither pessimistic nor optimistic. Acceptance is *realistic*.

Okay, enough of the philosophical chatter. Here, in a nutshell, is what acceptance has to do with you and your OCD: When you struggle against your own thinking, your mind bubbles over with even more obsessive thoughts. This means the more you can't stand to have an obsessive thought, the more likely that obsessive thought is to materialize.

Here's an exercise to make the point clearer. Think of a pink elephant. Bright pink, big, and fat. Concentrate. Picture that big, fat, pink elephant in your mind. Now, stop. Stop thinking about that pink elephant. Think about paying your bills or something. Seriously, I mean it! Whatever you do, don't think about that elephant. Don't let any thought of pink elephants enter your mind for the rest of the day. Tell yourself that the absolute worst thing you can do is think about pink elephants.

Did it work? Did you succeed in having absolutely no thoughts about that pink elephant? Probably not. That's because it is pretty hard to stop yourself from thinking. Active attempts to suppress thoughts usually boomerang.

By contrast, when you accept your thoughts for what they are — just thoughts — they lose some of their stranglehold over your OCD mind and dissipate more quickly. See, you've probably already stopped thinking about that pink elephant. Oh, sorry.

TIP

Mind you, acquiring acceptance takes time. Most humans will never be fully and readily accepting of whatever happens to them 100 percent of the time. For example, if you suffer a serious loss, you can't simply accept the loss and instantly move on. That's not fair. Rather, it's important to accept the grief into your life. Feel it, observe it, and don't try to push it away. This approach will gradually guide you toward a healthy resolution of the loss. If you try to simply squelch difficult thoughts and feelings (whether related to loss or OCD), they will hang around far longer. Acceptance acknowledges the loss, the grief, and the lessening of the pain over time.

Suspending judgment about emotions

The vast majority of OCD thoughts that produce difficult emotions, such as anxiety, distress, sadness, stress, and controllable urges, include making strong judgments about the thought or events. The powerful emotions brought on by these judgments frequently trigger troubling episodes of OCD. The process is cyclical and looks something like this:

1. A thought enters your awareness, or an event occurs.

2. You make an OCD-biased judgment about the thought or event.

3. Your judgment of the thought or event triggers an emotion.

4. You make an OCD-biased judgment about the emotion.

5. Your judgment of the emotion triggers OCD behavior.

6. As it says on the shampoo bottle, lather, rinse, and repeat. . . .

With practice, you can learn to release judgments and harsh evaluations of yourself and the world. Here are a few common OCD-related judgments and evaluations of the self and the world that you may want to watch for so that you can defend yourself against them:

>> I am a defective person who must always be on the lookout. Otherwise, I am bound to seriously harm or kill someone.

>> I could never forgive myself if I failed to keep my kitchen 100 percent clean and someone in my family came down with food poisoning.

>> If I mess up in any way at all, I am a truly horrible person.

>> No sane person would ever have thoughts like mine. I'm a disaster!

So how do you defend yourself against these kinds of judgments and evaluations? As an alternative, try realizing that all humans are an incredibly mixed bag of actions that can be judged positively or negatively. I'm not saying that people are not responsible for intentional, immoral, illegal, and unkind actions. However, devoting much of your time to negatively judging yourself or others only makes you miserable and provides further fuel for your OCD mind. Stuff happens! When it does, remember that emotions are neither right nor wrong — they just are.

REMEMBER

Please realize that suspending judgment and acquiring self-acceptance is an ever-evolving process. As with all mindful attitudes, you'll never achieve perfection with it. But that's okay, because considerable research has shown that people who struggle for perfection wind up feeling much worse than those who can accept themselves as they are.

TIP

Try to avoid judging your attempts at becoming nonjudgmental! Of course you will make many slips along the way. Just remember that no one is keeping score — other than the OCD part of your mind.

Living in the now

Everyone tends to worry now and then about things that haven't happened, and in many cases never will. For those with OCD, this kind of worrying is persistent, with one thought leading to another. What if I lose my job? What if that table is contaminated? What if I can't control myself? Or you may feel guilty or depressed about what has happened in the past. Why did I say or do that? I wish I could go back in my life and do something better with my relationships. If only my childhood had been better.

Even though I write lots of books on how to think better, I'm not always a master of my thoughts. Much of the time when I'm thinking, I'm not focused on the here and now. Instead, I'm somewhere else in time, often in the future (worried about what might happen). Sometimes I'm in the past — for example, giving myself grief for backing into the side of the garage and knocking off the passenger side mirror. But I am almost always able to bring myself around and become aware that I am *living* in the here and now and stop time-traveling in my thoughts.

If you suffer with OCD, thinking about the future can feel like being in the future. This can lead to experiencing the emotion of dread toward the future, even though the event has not and may not occur. So, if today is sunny and warm, yet you are focused on tomorrow's forecast of cold and rain, you miss the joy of the good day that *is* and experience the dread of the rainy day that may or may not actually occur. After all, the TV weather people are not infallible!

The following example is taken from my own experience and illustrates what focusing on anticipated dread versus present moments does:

Friday mornings I travel down the road to a small gym near home. There, I'm met by my personal torturer, uh, I mean personal *trainer*. All the way there in the car I'm thinking about how early it is and how I didn't have enough coffee. My mind is spinning and spewing negative thoughts. I begin to conjecture. What if

- She makes me go up on weights this time?
- She makes me stand on one leg and twist into a pretzel?
- I fall over, and everyone laughs?
- I have to jump rope for three minutes and can only do two?
- I stop breathing and die?

Still, when I arrive at the gym, I drag myself out of the car, continuing to dread what is coming next.

My trainer greets me, smiling. "Hi, I've been taking some great continuing education classes. I've got some new routines that involve abs, core strength, triceps, and biceps. Oh, yeah, and the gluteus, too!"

Oh, goodie, I think.

But then something happens. As I give myself to the magic of rigorous, physical exercise, within just a couple of minutes, the dreadful thoughts disappear. Attention focuses purely on how to balance, coordinate, and sustain the muscles necessary to complete each set. The "now" I am experiencing is really not that bad, and its aim is to keep me healthy. The mind calms. After the workout, smiles and happy moods prevail. See you next week!

This example from my own life shows you how absurdly self-defeating thoughts about the future are typically poor predictors of actual experience (like those faulty weather reporters). The OCD mind is particularly good at this kind of catastrophic thinking about the future.

However, the mind becomes still when you fully engage with the present moment and live in the now. When you pay attention — full attention — to what is in front of you rather than what is behind you or ahead of you, your mind fully engages in the now.

Minding Meditation

Acquiring mindful attitudes (see the preceding sections) greatly enhances your ability to engage in what's known as meditation. Both being mindful and practicing meditation can help relieve your OCD.

OCD involves intolerance of distress, discomfort, urges, and uncertainty. Meditation teaches you to tolerate these frustrations. Meditation also increases your concentration and helps OCD sufferers view intrusive thoughts as less important.

The really great thing about meditation is that it's not especially complicated or expensive — you don't even need formal lessons or classes, although many people find them helpful. You can get started just by setting aside a few minutes each day.

There are many types of meditation. You may be instructed to focus on a candle or pay attention to each breath. Some forms of meditation ask you to concentrate on your body as you walk. Yoga and Tai Chi are considered types of meditation.

Which form of meditation is the best one for OCD? No one knows, and I rather suspect almost any one of them will work as well as any other. Although large, controlled studies on meditation for OCD are lacking, future studies will most likely demonstrate that meditation works for OCD. The next two sections show you the basics of two easy-to-learn forms of meditation.

WARNING

One type of meditation uses mantras (a word, phrase, or meaningless sound that you repeat over and over in order to focus and block out thoughts). You can use this approach to meditation, but if you do, be sure *not* to use it in direct response to an obsession. If you do, you run some risk of the mantra becoming a type of compulsion — in other words, something you feel compelled to do in order to reduce the distress brought on by your obsession. Definitely not something I recommend for those with OCD.

WARNING

When something seems too good to be true, it usually is. Some scammers purport that they have special techniques and powers. If you are asked to pay a significant amount of money for meditation training, beware of con artists. Meditation is not a path to instant success or happiness. Meditation practice takes time and patience and usually doesn't cost much more than your time and effort.

Breathing meditation

Breathing meditation is a common type of meditation. Do this one while sitting down in the following manner:

>> **Find some place pleasant where you will be undisturbed.** This place can be inside or outside. Quiet is nice, too, but less important than finding a place where you won't be interrupted.

>> **Find something to sit on.** Many people choose to purchase formal mats and pillows called *zabutans* and *zafus* for their meditation. But you can also use a chair or couch.

>> **Experiment with a sitting position.** You can assume any of quite a few different postures while meditating — nothing is especially magical about any of them. Try to maintain the posture you choose for a period of time. Practice remaining still. Not many people find this easy to do, but you'll get better with practice. Physical training and/or yoga are great for strengthening your body so that you can remain still for increasing amounts of time.

>> **Invite all feelings in, including discomfort.** Yep, that's right. Notice little feelings of unease, discomfort, anxiety, obsessions, and urges. Sit with them a while. Stay connected with these feelings and try not to judge them. You'll see over time that you can tolerate these feelings longer and longer if you don't evaluate them as "horrible" or "awful."

>> **Allow whatever thoughts you have to go through your mind — including your obsessions.** Some people think meditation involves blocking thoughts out. But meditation actually teaches you to relate to your thoughts differently — dispassionately observing them rather than taking them so seriously. So, if you hear an obsession or other negative thought calling, just notice the thought. Allow it to pass, as eventually it will.

>> **Don't hold onto positive thoughts.** Everyone enjoys positive thoughts, but this instruction involves just noticing your positive thoughts. They, too, will pass, and that's okay.

>> **Focus on your breathing.** Notice the air as it passes through your nose and down into your lungs. Take slow, deep breaths. Allow the tension in your muscles to release. Let go of any tightness you sense. Scan your entire body and allow it to relax. Let your eyes and face soften. If you choose to count your breaths, that's fine. Breath in on one, out on two, in on three, out on four. You can count to ten and then start over or keep on going. There is no right or wrong in meditation.

>> **Be kind and accepting of yourself.** Realize that no one finds meditation immediately rewarding and beneficial. If you struggle with meditation, give it more time. You can take a class later if it continues to be difficult. Results come slowly. But studies show it has benefits well beyond OCD. Improvements may occur in blood pressure, chronic pain, anxiety, and general health.

TIP

Engaging in regular meditation enhances the mindful attitudes discussed in the previous sections. And mindful attitudes aid your efforts with meditation.

WARNING

In a few cases, people find that meditation triggers especially troubling feelings, such as anxiety or panic. Although meditative practices call for allowing and noticing difficult feelings, don't let things get out of hand. If you find the approach too disturbing, stop immediately! You still may want to learn meditation, but in these cases, you should get assistance from a mental-health professional, who is also trained in meditation. This distressing reaction is less common with walking meditation, described next.

Walking meditation

Consider observing people scurrying about on a busy sidewalk or in a shopping mall. Notice how they rush to and fro. Take a glance at their faces and bodies — furrowed brows, tense foreheads, and arms swinging wildly. Many folks rush through their days, never noticing their own keyed-up states.

Mindful walking meditation can help you let go and refocus. Walking meditation is probably one of the easiest meditation methods around, so it's often a good way to start. And the great thing is that you can do it almost anywhere. Here's how walking meditation works:

1. **Pause for a moment before you start and take a deep breath.** Focus on the air as it flows through your nose and lungs.

2. **Start walking.** The pace doesn't matter much, but don't rush.

3. **Focus on the sensations in your body as you walk.** Pay attention to your leg muscles, feet, thighs, ankles, calves, and the rhythmic swinging of your arms.

   If thoughts, obsessions, or bad feelings intrude, allow some space for them. Notice those thoughts and feelings, but do not judge them. When you can, shift your focus back to the sensations in your body.

4. **Concentrate on your feet for a while.** Focus on how they strike the ground as your heel hits first, your foot rolls, and you use your toes and the ball of your foot to push off. Just notice these sensations.

   Again, thoughts, obsessions, and bad feelings are welcome. Do not judge them.

5. **Focus again on the flow of air as you breathe.** Inhale slowly and exhale as you notice the rhythm of your breath.

6. **Focus on any sights, smells, or sounds that you encounter on your walk.** Do this without judgment or evaluation.

7. **Shift your focus back to the muscles in your body and the rhythm of your walking.**

   If any of your obsessions come in, allow and notice them, but resist acting on them. You can tell yourself that when the walking meditation is over, you can engage in a compulsion if you feel you must — but continue the walking for at least 15 minutes.

That's it. Consider practicing walking meditation every day for 15 or 20 minutes. The exercise from the walking can't hurt, and the meditation is likely to help you.

TIP

Meditation apps may be a useful way for some people to start meditating. They provide structure and guided practice. However, start with a free trial, and see what you think before you purchase an app. Realize that research is somewhat limited regarding the effectiveness of these apps.

REMEMBER

There is no absolute, correct way to do breathing or walking meditation. You can experiment with varying what you decide to focus on, but generally you want to concentrate on bodily sensations and your breath. Finally, with meditation, you do not want to block out thoughts, including obsessions. Rather, you want to relate differently to them by allowing them to come in and pass through as they will.

Chapter **10**

Tackling OCD Behavior with ERP

O ver the years of my career, I've worked with many clients with OCD. Far too many of these clients previously received years of treatment, including various medications, all types of psychotherapy, and even electroconvulsive shock therapy yet continued to suffer. Sometimes OCD had not been correctly assessed and diagnosed. Other times the diagnosis was on target, but the therapies and medications were ill-chosen. A few of these cases had even been described as hopeless, and family members had been told to expect a lifetime of serious disability, if not institutionalization. I'm happy to report that with the right diagnosis and treatment, most people with OCD can get better, often much better.

Fortunately, in recent years the outlook for OCD clients has been improving. Many more mental-health professionals are aware of how to recognize OCD and accurately diagnose it, as well as which treatments work and which ones don't. Of the available treatments for OCD, the specific type of cognitive-behavioral therapy (CBT) called exposure and response prevention (ERP) stands as the most widely researched and accepted treatment strategy.

This chapter explains what ERP is, why it works, and how to implement this strategy. Unless your OCD is very mild, you will want to collaborate with a professional in using ERP. In fact, it may be best to consult with a therapist before using ERP at least once even if your case is mild. This chapter lays out the essentials and can help prepare you to work with your therapist. See Chapter 7 for information about seeking the services of a professional with appropriate training in ERP.

Exposing the Basics and Benefits of ERP

Don't panic! The "exposure" part of ERP doesn't mean you take off your clothes and walk around in public nude — that's *not* what ERP is about! But exposure *is* involved. ERP is pretty straightforward and can be broken out into two parts:

>> **Exposure:** The exposure part of ERP involves putting yourself in contact with the situations, cues, events, and triggers that lead to your *obsessional fears* (frequently recurring thoughts, images, or urges that are unwanted and cause considerable distress). For example, if you fear touching numerous everyday objects like telephones, doorknobs, and kitchen counters, you're asked to gradually start touching these feared surfaces.

As you make contact with these triggers, you're asked to pay close attention to how you feel, which will likely involve some distress. However, that distress will diminish as you continue making contact. In fact, you will be expected to repeatedly come in contact with these triggers and cues until your distress *does* diminish. It may take a while for you to feel better, but you will.

>> **Response prevention:** The response prevention part of ERP simply refers to resisting the urge to engage in or carry out your usual *compulsions* (behaviors or mental acts that you use to reduce the distress caused by an obsession) in response to the discomfort you feel from making contact with the triggers. In the preceding example, after touching objects, you're likely to want to wash your hands (a compulsion), but while practicing ERP, you're instructed to work very hard to avoid handwashing at least for a while.

The description of ERP initially may sound like, "Just stop having your obsessions and compulsions!" That reaction is perfectly understandable. But I'm guessing that if you could, you would have already stopped your OCD.

So how is ERP more than an instruction to "just stop"? Well, with ERP you are carefully guided to systematically — slowly, but surely — make contact with your problematic triggers while gradually building up your ability to resist engaging in your compulsions.

It seems that psychologists are pretty much addicted to acronyms, but they don't particularly agree on which ones to use. Exposure and response prevention is sometimes referred to as ERP, but you may also see acronyms such as E&RP, EX/RP, and ERPT used to refer to the same thing. Occasionally, you may see the terms behavior therapy (BT) or cognitive-behavioral therapy (CBT) used to refer to ERP, but those are actually much more general types of therapy that may or may not include ERP.

Understanding why and how ERP works

People learn best through repeated, direct experience and practice. The more times you do something, the more ingrained the learning becomes. Your OCD is well practiced and deeply ingrained. ERP helps you unlearn your OCD behaviors by reconditioning your responses to your obsessions. You can start with the least problematic trigger and progress to the most challenging one or start with the trigger that interferes most in your life. It's totally up to you.

Ringing in change with ERP

In the late 1890s, a Russian scientist by the name of Ivan Pavlov conducted experiments that demonstrated a learning principle that helps explain how ERP works. Pavlov noticed that dogs begin to salivate upon seeing the person who normally feeds them. He then decided to see if he could teach the dogs to associate the same response with the sound of a bell (something that dogs would normally never salivate in response to). He rang a bell and closely followed the sound with giving the dogs food. Soon the dogs began to drool merely in response to the bell — even without receiving food. Even more importantly, he discovered that this response could be *unlearned* (essentially, that the association could be broken) by repeatedly sounding the bell over and over again without following the sound with food.

Humans also have used dinner bells for centuries to announce that dinner is ready. The users of dinner bells find that they, like Pavlov's dogs, begin to salivate in response to the bell — and sometimes even bells other than dinner bells. But if someone continuously rang bells with no food to follow, humans also unlearn the response.

The first principle of why ERP works is based on this same idea. The triggers, cues, situations, and events (what shrinks call *stimuli*) that set off your obsessions and compulsions have a powerful negative emotional charge — in other words, you associate them with great distress. So, if touching a doorknob triggers an obsession about contamination, you feel freaked out. Just looking at a doorknob may even make you feel upset.

However, if you make repeated, prolonged contact with doorknobs, you can actually unlearn this association. The association is broken or unlearned because the anticipated horrible outcome doesn't occur. In other words, you hold onto the doorknob until your freaked-out feelings diminish, and they will with enough time and repetition.

It may take you a while to believe that nothing bad will happen during exposure to fearful, distressing stimuli — which is why many, if not most, people need some assistance in going through ERP.

For a few people with mild OCD primarily involving obsessions, exposure is the only treatment necessary. Gradual, repeated exposures decrease their obsessions to the point that they feel good enough and leave treatment.

Reconditioning behavior with ERP

For those people who have both obsessions and compulsions (the vast majority of those with OCD), an additional principle explains why ERP works. That principle is known as *reinforcement.* Reinforcement refers to the fact that people tend to do more of almost anything that makes them feel better (see Chapter 5 for a more detailed explanation of both positive and negative reinforcement). Thus, if what you do results in either pleasurable feelings or marked reductions in anxiety or distress, you have a strong incentive to keep doing more of what leads you to these feelings.

Compulsions are powerfully reinforced because they *temporarily* make you feel better. ERP therapy instructs you not to carry out your compulsions so that your brain won't remain stuck in the OCD loop of an obsession causing distress and a compulsion reducing that distress, which reinforces the cycle.

See Chapter 4 for a description of how the brains of those with OCD differ a little from the brains of those without OCD. In OCD, certain brain areas are enlarged, and others show increased activity. Particularly exciting research shows that ERP (as well as medications) can restore these alterations to normal. Remind yourself repeatedly that with each ERP trial, you are literally rewiring and normalizing the way your brain works. That's actually the best incentive for undergoing ERP.

Seeing the upsides and downsides of ERP

ERP has been extensively studied as a treatment for OCD since the 1970s. These studies have consistently demonstrated that ERP is highly effective as a treatment for OCD, as long as the patient stays the course.

The major downside of ERP (and it's significant) is that it has a moderately high dropout and/or refusal rate. Some people just won't consider doing ERP, and others drop out after they start. Combining cognitive therapy or medication with ERP appears to reduce the rate of refusal, but it's unclear whether fewer people ultimately drop out of such combined treatments. More studies are needed on this issue.

However, the positives of ERP, when you follow through, are many. Here are the major findings at this time:

>> ERP appears to be at least as effective as medication and may be even more so, although the literature on this issue is mixed. A combination of ERP and medication does not lead to dramatic improvements over either one alone but is generally recommended for those with severe cases.

>> The effectiveness of ERP appears to be similar to that of other CBT techniques for OCD (see Chapter 8 and 9), but comparisons of those techniques have not been studied as extensively. Furthermore, most studies of CBT for OCD to date have included at least some component of ERP. And ERP usually has a few elements of CBT. Therefore, the jury is still out regarding the overall comparable effectiveness of CBT alone for OCD or, for that matter, ERP with no other elements of CBT.

>> ERP can be done in a therapist's office or in a patient's home environment. I often conducted exposure therapy outside the office or in the waiting room, depending on the issue. There's no hard and fast rule on the location.

>> ERP usually works better when guidance is provided by a trained professional. However, self-directed ERP seems to work fairly well for some people, especially those with mild cases.

>> ERP works better than psychological treatments aimed only at anxiety reduction (like progressive muscle relaxation and deep-breathing techniques).

>> ERP works over the long term, and those who practice it appear to resist relapse for a number of years (if not longer). By contrast, medication alone leads to rapid relapse if discontinued.

>> Understanding the basics of ERP and practicing it with a therapist often encourages clients to become their own ERP therapists in everyday life.

Exploring an alternative when ERP isn't appropriate

Real-life exposure generally works best whenever carrying it out is practical. However, a lot of people with OCD experience obsessive thoughts or images having to do with worries about engaging in violent, inappropriate, dangerous, or immoral behaviors. For example, some people with OCD obsess about shouting obscenities out loud and compulsively chant to prevent them from losing control. ERP would not have those people shout obscenities at a religious service.

Obviously, exposure is inappropriate when obsessions have to do with horrible or socially inappropriate things, such as murder, rape, or doing something indecent in public. However, another approach to exposure *can* be used for these kinds of problems. This alternative is called *imaginal exposure.*

TIP

A very small percentage of those with OCD report experiencing obsessive thoughts without any compulsive mental or behavioral actions. Some of these people may have horrible images of hurting someone else without any compulsive actions to keep them from doing so. Imaginal exposure also can work for this issue when regular exposure would be impractical.

Imaginal exposure strategies include the following:

>> **Scripts:** With this approach, you write out a vivid story about your obsessions. For example, you might write out a scene involving catching a terrible disease from eating contaminated food. Or, if your OCD theme is about harming other people, your script might include detailed descriptions of you losing control and doing what you fear, such as stabbing all your family members to death. The scripts are usually one to five minutes in length. Scripts should be listened to or read multiple times. If you use a script, be sure that you keep it secure.

>> **Video:** Sometimes you can find a scene closely related to your OCD theme from a horror movie that you can play repeatedly.

>> **Virtual Reality (VR):** Computers can generate environments that mimic obsessional concerns. VR can be applied to a variety of situations, especially shame-based obsessions, which would not be appropriate for real life exposure. One small study used VR as exposure to filthy bathrooms. Participants were asked to "touch" toilets and walls of progressively filthier stalls. Practical application of VR in clinical practice has been hampered by cost and the availability of specific technologies, but it has great potential.

WARNING

If your obsessions are highly disturbing and include themes about harming yourself or others, engaging in violence, or doing illegal activities, I strongly recommend that you consult a therapist. Although those with OCD are at lower risk than most people for actually engaging in such behavior, you need a mental-health professional to assess your risks and provide an actual diagnosis.

Working through ERP Therapy

Setting up and working through ERP involves a series of five steps. Although you can read most of this book in any order you want, if you're ready to consider ERP start with Step 1 and proceed through Step 5. Most people find going through ERP is easier when working with a therapist.

1. Find your OCD theme.

2. List your OCD triggers, their Ugh Factor Ratings, and choose the trigger you want to start with.

3. Identify and prevent the compulsive response.

4. Warm up to ERP.

5. Work through your triggers by doing ERP.

Step 1: Determining your OCD theme

Although obsessions and compulsions vary widely from one person to another, in almost all cases, OCD consists of one or more unifying themes or subjects. These themes are often referred to as OCD types (see Chapter 2 for more specific information). The most frequent themes are fears and worries about:

>> Contamination

>> Doing something inappropriate (usually sexual or aggressive)

>> Doubts, fears, and uncertainties

>> Physical health

>> Superstitions and rituals

>> Sinning

>> Symmetry and order

The first step in ERP is to determine the main theme or type of *your* OCD. That isn't difficult to do. Simply review the list above and/or look through Chapter 2 and find the types of OCD concerns that give you the most trouble. You may identify more than one.

Step 2: Making a list and choosing your challenge

When you know the theme or themes surrounding your obsessional thoughts and worries, the next step is to look for all the triggers, actions, events, cues, and situations (also known as stimuli) that set your whole OCD cycle off. These triggers include a variety of situations that you probably avoid much of the time right now. For instance, if your obsessional theme is contamination, you may stay away from public bathrooms or avoid touching doorknobs, dirt, kitchen counters, or phones. Or if lack of symmetry is your theme, then keeping your belongings in a particular order prevents you from encountering a trigger. A *trigger* is something that sets off your desire to use a compulsion (like washing your hands or arranging your cupboards) if you come across it.

TIP

The nature of a given person's OCD may involve triggers that don't lend themselves to standard ERP in real-life situations. For example, someone who fears exposure to radioactive material would not be encouraged to actually take a field trip to the national labs at Los Alamos, New Mexico, and walk into a room labeled: "Warning! Highly Radioactive Material Inside!" If your OCD involves impractical triggers like this example, see the earlier section, "Exploring an alternative when ERP isn't appropriate."

After you've made your list of problematic OCD triggers, actions, cues, events, and situations, rate each one for the amount of difficulty it would cause you if you were to make contact with it. I like to whimsically call these *Ugh Factor Ratings*. I use Ugh Factor Ratings because the word "Ugh" captures the essence of distress and upset.

TECHNICAL
STUFF

The technical term that most psychologists use is Subjective Units of Distress or SUDS. Only psychologists would come up with an acronym like SUDS. These ratings are personal and arbitrary — basically, good guesses. SUDS sounds important, but it just means a good guesstimate.

Here are the steps to follow for listing and rating your OCD triggers.

1. **Make a list of about 10 to 20 distressing situations — the events, cues, actions, and triggers for your OCD.**

   All items in your list should relate to your particular OCD theme, such as contamination. Make a separate list for each theme or type of OCD you struggle with. As you create your list, consider the following guidelines:

   - Include situations that you normally completely avoid, but that would upset you if you were to encounter them. Thus, if you never go into public restrooms (and you fear doing so), that would go on your list.

   - Try to include items on your list that vary in the difficulty they would cause you if you were to make contact with them. Have several relatively easy items, a few that would cause you moderate distress, and some that would be very difficult.

   - Unless you're working with a professional therapist, do not include items that someone without OCD would probably be unwilling to do. For example, most people would be pretty reluctant to touch the inside of a dumpster or the inside of a public toilet.

2. **Go through your list and give each item an Ugh Factor Rating on a 0–100-point scale of difficulty.**

On this scale, a 0 indicates that you would anticipate no distress whatsoever, and a 100 indicates that nothing imaginable could cause more distress. Thus, a 25 would cause you mild distress, a 50 would start feeling intense, and a 75 would set off strong negative feelings.

Gil's story illustrates the process of making a list of OCD triggers related to contamination fears and assigning an Ugh Factor Rating to each item on the list.

Gil is a 19-year-old college student majoring in physics. Since he was about 10 years old, Gil has worried about germs and becoming ill, and he fears exposure to all kinds of possible environmental toxins. Through an ad in the school newspaper, he discovers that the student mental-health clinic on his campus happens to have a clinic for treating OCD. Gil recognizes himself in the ad's description of OCD and makes an appointment at the clinic. A therapist interviews him carefully, gives him some questionnaires about OCD, and concludes that Gil indeed has OCD.

The therapist then suggests that Gil list his problematic OCD triggers (events, situations, and cues). He recommends that Gil rate each item on his list in terms of the Ugh Factor. Table 10-1 shows Gil's list and associated Ugh Factor Ratings.

Gil's therapist is pleased with his list and Ugh Factor Ratings. However, the therapist notices that no items are in the range between 30 and 50. Because that's quite a jump, they work together to come up with two items that Gil forgot — specifically, shaking hands (40) and checking out at the grocery store (45).

Gil's list is typical of someone with the OCD theme of contamination. Now he's ready to use his list and ratings to create an exposure plan.

TIP

Each person's list will differ both in content and Ugh Factor Ratings. For example, one person with contamination fears may not feel any distress at all in touching doorknobs while someone else may dread doing so. Someone who has doubt about safety could be worried about locking doors and windows; another person might have a need to keep turning on and off lights. A person whose OCD compels them to keep things in a specific order may be obsessed about uneven, tangled fringes on a carpet and another with keeping items in specific places around the home. Compiling your list and rating each item is likely to take you a little time and creativity. Don't rush the process.

WARNING

Developing and rating your list can cause anxiety. In a way, that's good because the process actually represents the beginning of the exposure task — just writing down the items and rating them is a type of exposure. However, if you experience overwhelming anxiety, get professional assistance.

TABLE 10-1   ## Gil's OCD Trigger List and Ugh Factor Ratings

OCD Trigger	Ugh Factor Rating (On a Scale of 0–100)
Touching doorknobs	70
Walking on lawns (fear of exposure to toxins)	30
Touching classroom desks	50
Using public toilets	80
Eating at a public restaurant	65
Eating at the school cafeteria	75
Picking up the mail	25
Touching money	50
Touching the door to a health clinic	80
Touching motor oil	50
Touching handrails	55
Pressing elevator buttons	55
Using a public phone	60
Visiting a hospital room	90
Being close to someone who is sick or disabled	95
Driving by a homeless person	30

Step 3: Identifying and preventing the response to compulsions

When you look at your list, your first reaction will likely be "Ugh." That's perfectly normal. Ask yourself what you would normally feel compelled to do when you see the items on your list. Most people feel compelled to engage in a compulsion when an obsessive worry is activated. Compulsions come in two forms:

>> **Actions:** Examples include washing your hands, spraying disinfectants, touching or moving in a certain way, or arranging things in a certain order.

>> **Mental acts:** Examples include counting, praying, chanting, or having certain good thoughts.

Compulsions may seem logically connected to the OCD triggers, as in the case of wanting to wash your hands after touching something you see as contaminated, or they may have no clear logical connection to the trigger at all — they may simply feel like the right thing to do in order to alleviate your discomfort. Thus, after touching a doorknob you may feel compelled to think certain "clean thoughts" over and over as a way of neutralizing your obsessional fears — that may not be logical, but somehow it makes you feel better.

WARNING

Sometimes compulsive behavior makes perfect sense. For example, during the pandemic, people were advised to wash hands frequently, wear masks, and avoid crowded indoor areas. These behaviors were not technically compulsions because they followed public health recommendations. See Chapter 13 for more information on how people with OCD fared during the pandemic.

In either case, compulsions bring a sense of temporary relief and are, therefore, very rewarding. Some people with OCD describe the compulsive act as somehow protecting them or their loved ones from danger. Others say that performing a compulsion neutralizes the obsession.

Very good reasons exist for preventing your compulsions. They include the following:

>> In the long run, the feelings of relief are short-lived, but compulsions usually take more and more of your time.

>> Compulsions prevent you from discovering that obsessions are merely obsessive and rarely, if ever, come true.

>> Compulsions can involve other people and make you feel foolish.

>> Compulsions ultimately make OCD worse.

>> Compulsions often hurt your self-esteem. They don't mean you are crazy, but they can sure make you feel that way.

Developing an awareness of the compulsions that your OCD mind urges you to do is essential. After making your list, note any and all actions (whether mental or physical) that you feel compelled to do when encountering any of those OCD triggers. This is your compulsion list — a list of the things you want to work very hard not to do.

In Gil's case (see the preceding sections), after going over his OCD trigger list, he realizes that he has a variety of compulsions, including

>> Counting backward from 100 to 0 slowly

>> Disinfecting what he's touched

>> Repeating the phrase "I'm clean" seven times

>> Showering four or five times each day

>> Washing his hands

Your list of compulsions may be quite short, such as only needing to say a certain prayer or wanting to wash your hands, or you may have a lengthy list of compulsions that you turn to. Jot down any and all compulsions that you notice yourself tempted to do in order to feel better. Keep your list handy — you may find that you discover new compulsions popping up. If you do, add them to your list.

REMEMBER

The "RP" in ERP stands for *response prevention*. The response are the compulsions that follow the obsessions. Preventing refers to not engaging in a compulsion.

Step 4: Preparing to engage in ERP

For many people, starting ERP feels like standing at the end of the highest diving board before taking the plunge (of course, if you're an Olympic diving champion, this is not a good metaphor). Nevertheless, here are a couple of tips for boosting your courage before you make the dive. You can think of these as warm-up exercises. They're not as intense as the real thing that comes next, but they're a great start.

>> **Take a few deep breaths and delay your compulsive act.** Put it off for 15 minutes; then, later, put it off for 30 minutes. Even later, go for an entire hour. Pay attention to how you feel during your delay time.

ARE TOXINS OCD OR REAL?

Global warming, greenhouse gases, pesticides, Escherichia coli (E. coli) in the food supply, air pollution — all represent legitimate concerns. People get sick and die from environmental contaminants. So, when do normal concerns about toxins cross the line into OCD? You probably don't want to hear this, but there is *no absolute, definitive line*. Perhaps some people viewed Al Gore as a little OCD when he began to rail against the dangers of global warming. Others thought he was a visionary, and today most of the scientific community sees him as the latter.

Al Gore's interest in the environment was passionate, welcomed, and under his deliberate control — all signs that he wasn't suffering from OCD. If your concerns are based on clear warning signs or a body of consistent, scientific evidence, they probably don't constitute OCD. On the other hand, if your concerns feel out of your control, highly disturbing, life disrupting, and intrusive, they are more likely to be indicative of OCD.

» **Do something different — alter your compulsions in some way.** If you usually have to count to 10 six times, count to 10 five times. Or perform your compulsion at top speed one time and at slow speed the next. Clean with a different hand if cleaning is your problem. Wash your hands in cold water or with just a trickle coming from the faucet. In other words, the more you change up your compulsion, the better. Again, pay attention to how you feel. These altered compulsions aren't likely to feel as satisfying to you, but they prepare you for living without compulsions altogether.

» **Remind yourself that you are not your OCD.** You will get better. You've started to reprogram and rewire the OCD part of your brain.

Step 5: Moving through your triggers with ERP

Take a look at your OCD trigger list as well as your list of usual compulsions. Set aside a couple of hours because ERP takes some time to work. That doesn't mean you'll hold onto a doorknob for two hours straight. Rather, you will touch a doorknob while not using any compulsions. Then you'll keep touching the doorknob frequently, but not constantly.

Realize that ERP is hard work, and that you need to be prepared to feel some discomfort. However, you're quite likely to find that you can tolerate that discomfort. Exposure is sort of like jumping into a cool swimming pool on a hot day — it feels freezing at first, but you get used to it. Acclimating to exposure takes a lot longer than getting used to the temperature of a pool, but you get the point.

REMEMBER

You'll find that the discomfort involved with ERP is well worth the effort because your symptoms will decrease greatly — and in some cases, a nearly complete cure is possible.

Here's how you proceed with your trigger list of subsequent compulsions:

1. **Pick a trigger from your list.**

   Some therapists recommend starting on a particular trigger that has an Ugh Factor Rating of at least 50. You can do that, but I suggest for the first exposure you start low and slow, especially if you're doing this on your own.

2. **Write the label for the trigger you're working on in the "Checking Your ERP Progress" form.**

   Refer to Table 10-2 to see Gil's progress form for an example. Any piece of paper or file on your device will do.

3. **Activate the trigger.**

   In other words, make contact with the OCD trigger. The nature of your contact very much depends upon the nature of the specific trigger. Thus, if your trigger involves having a shameful thought, deliberately think that thought. Go ahead and think it. Now, think it again. If your trigger involves eating a certain food or shaking someone's hand, obvious time limits will be necessary. Frequent, repeated contact is what usually matters most. If you're uncertain how to proceed, consult a professional.

4. **Record your Ugh Factor Rating (refer to Table 10-1) when you first make contact with your trigger. Stay in close contact with the trigger for about ten minutes or so.**

   Refrain from resorting to a compulsion.

REMEMBER

5. **Re-rate your Ugh Factor Rating about every ten minutes.**

   This rating may increase for a while but stay in contact with your trigger anyway.

6. **Remain in close contact with your trigger until your Ugh Factor Rating decreases.**

   Don't be rigid about the amount of the drop — any truly significant improvement in your feelings can suffice if the ERP has gone on for over an hour.

REMEMBER

The more distress or higher Ugh factor you allow yourself to experience, the greater the progress you'll make. Some people choose to dive off the high board (the hardest exposure). If you bite off too much, you can always back down to something less disturbing.

As you go through the process of ERP, keep the following guidelines in mind:

>> Be on the lookout for subtle compulsions that you find yourself tempted to do in order to decrease your distress. You want to avoid coming up with a new compulsion, such as wanting to count in your head or repeatedly say a poem or prayer.

TABLE 10-2

Gil's "Checking Your ERP Progress" Form

Exposure Step	Ugh Factor Ratings
Picking up the mail	45, 50, 55, 55, 45, 45, 50, 45, 40, 30, 25, 20
Driving by a homeless person	20, 20, 10
Walking on lawns	60, 65, 65, 70, 55, 65, 70, 75, 70, 60, 50, 40
Walking on lawns	65, 60, 60, 65, 55, 45, 40, 45, 50, 40, 40, 30

>> Don't try to suppress your obsessions. Go ahead and let yourself worry about possible danger, contamination, or whatever. Notice the thoughts, but don't try to suppress them. In fact, it's a good idea to actively imagine the most feared and dire outcomes you can think of actually occurring — such as being stricken with a horrible disease and dying a slow, torturous death.

>> Sometimes you may be able to complete multiple exposures during a session. Other times, one step will feel like plenty. You may even need to stay with one trigger for several sessions. Use drops in your Ugh Factor Ratings as your guide — slow and steady works just fine.

>> Conduct at least two or three exposure sessions each week — the more the better.

Gil's OCD exposure practice began with three items that had Ugh Factor Ratings of 25, 30, and 30. He recorded each of these triggers in his "Checking Your ERP Progress" form. His first exposure session required about 2 hours, but he only needed to work on his next trigger for about 30 minutes for his Ugh Factor Ratings to drop a great deal. His third exposure trigger took him two separate sessions that each lasted close to two hours. You can see Gil's progress in Table 10-2.

Gil's "Checking Your ERP Progress" form demonstrates several important issues:

>> Sometimes your initial Ugh rating is inaccurate, and you discover that your distress is considerably higher (or lower) than you thought it would be. That's no problem. If any trigger is utterly too intense for you, try to come up with another, easier one. If it's way too easy (such as Gil's trigger involving driving by a homeless person), move on to another trigger quickly.

>> Your Ugh Factor Ratings will likely go up and down during your exposure session, though they will generally diminish over time.

>> Notice that Gil's third exposure session (involving walking on lawns) did not result in a significant reduction in his Ugh Factor Rating. Therefore, he repeated the session on another day.

>> Gil found that tracking his progress in this manner gave him incentive for continuing his exposure sessions.

Managing the ERP Process

Successfully carrying out ERP involves paying attention to a variety of important issues. It's easy to find yourself tempted to cheat, so you need to know what's cheating and what's not. You'll probably want to enlist support from a helper so you need to keep a few things in mind when you do (see Chapter 22 for more information about bringing family and friends into the picture). When things go wrong, I'll give you some tips for dealing with the problems. And don't forget to pat yourself on the back when you pull all this off, ERP is hard work, and you deserve some credit.

Knowing what's cheating and what's not

Your OCD mind will want to come up with clever ideas for helping you deal with the distress that ERP involves. Consuming alcohol, smoking pot, or taking other drugs to numb you before engaging in ERP are definitely forms of cheating. So are relying on lucky charms, security blankets (or their equivalent), or religious symbols. But you also need to be on the lookout for other interesting, but misguided, strategies. Ultimately, caving in and using any of these tactics will sabotage your efforts at ERP.

Staying above the fray with dissociation

You may attempt to neutralize or diffuse your distress by *dissociating* or finding ways to remove yourself psychologically from what's going on. Some people try to numb their feelings. Others imagine that they're removed from their bodies and are viewing the ERP process from a distance. Both techniques may make you briefly feel a little better, but they block ERP's benefits.

Getting propped up with reassurance

You may want to seek reassurance from other people that everything will be okay. This strategy seems reasonable and helpful, but it's actually just like the other forms of cheating. Obtaining reassurance makes you feel better, but only briefly, and it utterly ruins the effects of ERP. So, if you're using a friend or helper with your ERP (see Chapter 22 for much more information about how helpers can do and say the right things), ask them specifically *not* to reassure you by saying things like, "It will be alright," "You're perfectly safe," and so on.

Dabbling in distraction

I generally recommend that clients not use distraction to keep themselves from engaging in mental compulsions. So, you typically want to avoid watching television, talking on the phone with a friend, or surfing the net during exposure tasks. Distraction that almost completely takes you away from feeling any discomfort is not a good idea. You don't learn to break the associations between your OCD triggers and the discomfort if you aren't really "there."

However, if all else fails, distraction is better than using the compulsion. So, if you have an uncontrollable mental obsession (such as constant images of germs invading your body), studies say that using simple distraction by focusing on everyday tasks is better than using your usual mental or behavioral compulsions, such as washing or repeating certain phrases. The key is that if you do use distraction, try to maintain at least some attention on the exposure task and your feelings of distress.

Finding fair relief

So, is there anything you *can* do to reduce your distress during ERP if it feels really awful? In a limited way, yes. If you're already on prescribed medication for OCD, keep taking it. Also, you may consider using a brief relaxation strategy, such as the following:

1. **Inhale slowly and deeply.**

   Do so by pushing out your abdominal muscles in order to fill the bottom part of your lungs first.

2. **Hold your breath for a few seconds.**

3. **Slowly exhale as you pull your abdominal muscles in.**

   Exhale to a slow count of eight while making a very slight noise with the air in between your lips.

4. **Repeat up to ten times or so.**

This brief breathing/relaxation strategy should be considered a temporary stopgap. You can use it for your initial contacts with any given step on your OCD trigger list. However, you want to stop using the breathing for subsequent contact. You should not use this breathing to eliminate your distress, but rather to merely help you cope with it for a little while.

WARNING

Brief breathing/relaxation can be an effective strategy for dealing with many feelings of stress. Thus, you may want to use it while stuck in traffic and feeling frustrated. However, you want to be sure not to allow this strategy to turn into a compulsive response associated with your obsessions and/or your OCD triggers.

Troubleshooting ERP

I wish I could tell you that ERP works, that it works every single time, and that it works extremely well each time. Ah, but this is the real world, isn't it? It's true that ERP usually works and, for the most part, improvement is quite dramatic when it does. But, just like your car and everything else in life, sometimes things misfire. This section is about knowing what to do when problems arise in carrying out ERP.

Struggling with getting out of the starting blocks

It's not uncommon for people with OCD to hear about ERP and respond, "Thanks, but no thanks." That's because it can sound pretty scary. I might say, "Trust me; it's not that bad, and you'll be able to do it," but I have a feeling you may not believe me.

So instead of just trusting me on this one, try something else first. If you find yourself unable to get out of the starting blocks with ERP, read or reread Chapters 8 and 9. These approaches may work for you by themselves, or they may simply help you feel more ready to tackle ERP. If that doesn't work, seriously consider medication for your OCD (which is, of course, always an option and an especially good one for severe cases).

In addition, if you find ERP particularly scary, see whether someone (such as a therapist or good friend assisting you) would be willing to model or demonstrate the ERP steps for you before you try them. If they do this, it's very important that you continue the work without their modeling at some point. However, a demo or two can provide a boost to get you started. The reason the demonstrations need to cease at some point is that you could easily start to rely on them for excessive reassurance (see the previous section, "Knowing what's cheating and what's not").

Finally, work on accepting the idea that nothing, not ERP, medication, or anything else will ever totally remove all uncertainty for you. The OCD mind desperately wants to eliminate uncertainty, and ERP looks pretty dubious and uncertain to many people. Remind yourself often (but not obsessively) that one must accept a certain amount of uncertainty.

TECHNICAL STUFF

If you are a therapist working with a client diagnosed with OCD, you may have to spend multiple sessions getting your client "ready" for ERP. That will likely involve cognitive therapy techniques, psychoeducation about the model, and demonstrations of the process. Be patient.

Constructing huge hierarchies

Many people with OCD construct excessively long exposure trigger lists. They want to be certain that they don't miss *anything* that could be relevant. I've seen lists that run many pages in length. However, ERP hierarchies work best when the number of items runs in the range of about 10 to 20.

So, what do you do if the length of your hierarchy has gotten out of hand? Try condensing your list. Select items that have high priority. *You do not need to include everything in order to make excellent progress.* When people make progress on one item, like doorknobs, they usually find that similar things, like shaking hands or touching plates, get a little easier, too. Finally, make sure that the items in your hierarchy all relate to a single OCD theme, such as contamination. If another theme appears to be involved, make a separate hierarchy for that theme.

Avoiding avoidance

Always be on the lookout for whether you're engaging in subtle forms of avoidance and/or reassurance seeking. Maybe you give your friend or therapist a "certain look" to solicit reassurance that things will be safe and okay. Or you may try to avoid ERP by putting it off and procrastinating for reasons that may seem good but are really designed for avoidance.

When progress bogs down

If your progress stalls along the way (or even if your progress is slow from the get-go), there are a few things you can do. First, make sure your ERP sessions are long enough and frequent enough. Sessions lasting 90 to 120 minutes usually work pretty well. I've found on occasion that prolonging the exposure even more can help — anywhere from half a day to several days straight in a few cases. With prolonged exposure sessions, you obviously won't remain in constant contact with your triggers, but you will hit many triggers repeatedly without engaging in your compulsions.

Another possibility for improving progress is to take a short step backward. In other words, go back to earlier steps and redo them until your Ugh Factor Ratings diminish even further. Then proceed ahead once more. If you find that one of the triggers involves much more distress than you anticipated, you can always design a new step to fit in between.

Sometimes progress slows because compulsions crop up despite your best efforts to refrain from them. Probably the most difficult compulsions to keep from enacting are the mental ones such as counting inside your head, repeating comforting phrases, or mentally trying to either burn or blow-up a disturbing obsessive image. In this case, your best strategy is to actively refocus on the disturbing obsessive image or thought.

REMEMBER

Mental compulsions are not the same as obsessions, which are unwanted, feel out of your control, and are highly disturbing. *Mental compulsions,* on the other hand, are the things you do inside your mind to reduce your distress and discomfort. The goal is to prevent mental compulsions, while remaining in contact with your mental obsessions.

If you get stuck and can't get going again, that's the time to get some help. Most people with OCD can use help — sometimes from family and friends and quite often from professionals. See Chapter 7 for more info on getting help.

Wavering motivation

If you find that your motivation for engaging in ERP wavers, jot out a cost/benefit analysis for doing ERP. Make a list of all the advantages and disadvantages of continuing with ERP. Your lack of motivation qualifies as a problematic belief. You may also want to read or reread Chapter 6 on overcoming obstacles to change.

Coping when bad stuff really happens

People do get robbed; illness happens; houses catch on fire; cars do run over people; people die, that's life, and such events cannot be avoided with or without OCD. However, if bad luck strikes during your exposure treatment, it can set you back. You may conclude that your OCD thinking was right on target after all. In such cases, a therapist can help you cope.

Rewarding yourself

Fighting OCD with ERP can be hard work. Appreciate yourself and your efforts. When you have completed a particularly difficult exposure or successfully resisted engaging in a compelling compulsion, do more than give yourself a pat on the back. Reward yourself with a treat.

Deliberately decide on a reward. Set a goal to complete two (or more) sessions of ERP, and then pay yourself. Think of some activities that are special, such as getting a massage, going out to dinner, watching a performance, or taking some time to relax, whatever gives you pleasure. Congratulations on your hard work, you deserve it!

Limiting ERP

The idea of ERP is to push yourself pretty hard and do some things you find quite difficult to do. You're expected to keep at it until you feel substantial improvement in your OCD, and then do a little more. However, don't include items on your trigger list that most people would find extremely difficult or dangerous. For example, it's not a good idea for you to lick public toilet seats or share needles with someone who has HIV. If you're unsure whether a given exposure item is "over the top," ask your therapist or a health-care provider.

Chapter **11**

Considering Medications or Brain Stimulation for OCD

Some of those suffering with OCD are good candidates for medication, and others are not. For those who are, certain antidepressant medications have been found to be effective in treating OCD. Fortunately, for those who either do not benefit from medication or cannot take it, alternative treatments are out there (see Chapters 8, 9, and 10). This chapter guides you through the information you need to make an informed decision about taking medication. In addition, I describe information about a recently approved treatment involving brain stimulation.

Many people are helped by psychotherapies that are useful in the treatment of OCD — such as exposure and response prevention (ERP), cognitive therapy, meta-cognitive therapy, and mindfulness, as well as various combinations of these strategies. Rest assured that the purpose of this chapter is not to pit medication against these treatment options. The use of medication doesn't preclude other treatments; on the contrary, many people combine the use of medication with psychological treatment.

TIP

In my experience treating people with OCD, I have found that medication sometimes helps those who are reluctant to try exposure and response prevention because of high levels of fear and anxiety. After becoming slightly more stable on medication, they return to therapy more able to benefit from ERP. Often, they then wean off of medications while continuing ERP or some other therapy for a while.

Deciding whether Medication Is Right for Your OCD

The decision to take medication for your OCD needs to be a cooperative effort between you and your health-care provider. So that you can play an active role in the decision-making process, you should be well-informed of the pros and cons involved. Your doctor needs access to your health history and will conduct a complete physical exam to assess your current health status.

Getting a thorough check-up

To help you determine whether taking medication is right for you, a thorough physical exam is the first step. Your primary health-care provider should coordinate a comprehensive evaluation of your current health and health history. Appropriate laboratory and diagnostic tests should be conducted to rule out physical causes or contributors to your OCD symptoms. You also can turn to your primary care doctor for advice and recommendations for specialists (psychiatrist, prescribing psychologist, or psychiatric nurse practitioner) in treating OCD.

TIP

Some primary care providers do not feel comfortable prescribing medications for OCD because they have limited experience in dealing with the problem. Be sure to ask your primary care provider whether it would be a good idea to refer you to a specialist who has knowledge about OCD medications.

Coming clean with your doctor about your health and medications

Medications that affect your mind and your mood are powerful agents. If you and your health-care provider decide to use them as a tool to help alleviate symptoms of OCD, you must work in close collaboration. If you are honest and open, you can expect your doctor to be respectful and nonjudgmental.

Before you begin taking any new medication, talk with your doctor about the following:

>> Inform your doctor of any other health problems you have, including allergies, a history of heart problems, head injuries, seizures, problems with blood pressure, diabetes, glaucoma, or substance addiction.

>> Be open about other problems you may be having such as insomnia, poor appetite, or fatigue. Be sure to let your provider know if you have ever been diagnosed with a mood or anxiety disorder. Be sure to let your provider know if you have a history of suicidal thoughts or attempts.

>> Discuss worries you have about taking medication.

>> Provide a list of all other medications, either prescribed or over-the-counter, that you take. Include any herbs or supplements you are taking.

>> Tell your doctor if you are pregnant, considering getting pregnant, or breastfeeding.

>> Be honest about habits such as drinking, smoking cigarettes, marijuana use, or the use of other drugs.

If you decide to try medication, keep the following tips in mind:

>> Take your medication as prescribed. If you decide to discontinue your medication, talk to your health-care provider before you actually stop taking it. You may experience significant side effects from abrupt discontinuation.

>> Discuss any side effects you may be feeling. Let your doctor know if you are feeling more depressed, suicidal, agitated, or uneasy, or if you're experiencing any sexual side effects.

>> Be patient. Positive treatment effects may not be noticeable for a while — up to twelve weeks in some cases. Furthermore, your dosage may need to be adjusted, or you may need to try different medications before you find what works best for you.

TIP

When you start taking any medication that affects your mood or emotions, it is critical that you frequently communicate with your health-care provider. Medications are usually monitored closely until the effects are stable.

Looking at reasons for medicating your OCD

OCD experts agree that psychological treatment is the preferred choice for most cases of OCD, especially for OCD in children. However, in some cases, psychological treatment may not have the desired effect, or it may not be enough in and of itself. Medication may be a good choice when

>> **Your OCD is severe.** If your symptoms are ruining your life and you cannot work, function at home, or be independent, medication may decrease your symptoms enough so that you can start psychological treatment. You're still likely to benefit from ERP treatment (see Chapter 10).

>> **Your OCD is combined with depression.** Most people with OCD have at least some symptoms of depression, and about 2/3 of sufferers have had a major depressive disorder at some point in their lives. Depression alone can be treated by psychological treatment and/or medication. However, when you add OCD to the mix, both forms of treatment may prove to be necessary.

WARNING

>> **Your OCD is accompanied by suicidal thoughts.** If you feel hopeless and have thoughts of suicide, you must get help immediately. If you're unable to reach a mental-health professional, go to the emergency room of a hospital or call 911. Don't wait. Help is available.

>> **You have bipolar disorder.** Most people with bipolar disorder need medication management. Your best bet is to consult with a health-care provider who has expertise in both OCD and bipolar disorder.

>> **You see or hear things that others do not see or hear.** These symptoms are quite serious and almost certainly require medication. You likely need a psychiatrist, psychiatric nurse practitioner, or prescribing psychologist to evaluate your condition and prescribe treatment.

>> **Your thinking is very confused.** If you can't seem to concentrate or think rationally, medication may be appropriate. I still recommend a mental-health therapist to support you with psychotherapy.

>> **You refuse to try ERP.** A significant number of people with OCD can't stand the thought of ERP. For those people, medication may help take the edge off so that later they can try exposure. Or, in a few cases, they may discover that medication works so well that they feel little need for ERP.

>> **You've tried therapy, and it hasn't worked.** Some people don't benefit from the various OCD-specific psychotherapies (see Chapters 6, 8, 9, and 10). Medication can sometimes decrease symptoms sufficiently so that therapy can work.

>> **You can't find a therapist nearby or one whom you can afford.** Unfortunately, some areas do not have sufficient numbers of trained therapists who can do ERP or cognitive therapy. Some insurance plans do not pay for mental-health services.

TIP

If money is a factor in your treatment, you may be able to find a university, community mental-health clinic, or a few private practitioners who provide services on a sliding fee scale — you just have to ask.

>> **You can't find the time in your schedule for psychotherapy.** I hope this isn't the case. But, unfortunately, some people don't have the time. Frankly, if you can't find a couple of hours a week for therapy, that may be part of the problem. Stress can certainly make OCD worse. Furthermore, OCD steals considerable amounts of time from your day. Think of how much more time you will have without obsessions and compulsions. That said, medication, if it works, usually takes less time.

The story of Max illustrates a positive use of medication. Max's thinking was too confused for him to benefit from psychological treatment. For Max, taking medication was necessary to get him on the path to recovery.

Max believes that food purchased at restaurants and grocery stores is contaminated by fecal matter in the groundwater. Max used to think shopping at an organic grocery store was safe, until a couple of years ago, when he read about organic spinach being contaminated by fecal matter. Max's OCD has caused him to lose his job and his friends and to isolate himself from his family.

One day, his brother shows up at his apartment and is appalled to see Max, emaciated, with several pots of boiling water on his stove. Max has restricted his food intake to boiled potatoes and boiled ground beef. He boils each for 45 minutes. Max seems to be out of touch with reality, so his brother takes him to the emergency room.

There, Max is given a prescription for an antidepressant and an appointment with a psychiatrist. Family members make sure that he keeps his appointments. After two months, Max no longer believes that the food supply is contaminated. However, he still has many OCD symptoms. The psychiatrist keeps him on the medication and refers him to a psychologist for ERP.

Understanding the side effects and risks of medications

If popping a pill once or twice a day can help rid you of OCD, why not? There are downsides to taking medications, which can vary from person to person. Here are some issues for you to ponder before starting medication:

>> **Side effects:** Antidepressants can have very distressing side effects. Dry mouth, weight gain, constipation, tremors, diarrhea, insomnia, nausea, headaches, and dizziness are all commonly reported. For most people, these

effects decrease over time. And your doctor can sometimes recommend other medications to decrease your discomfort. Unfortunately, the side effects cause many people to stop taking medication before it has a chance to work.

» **Sexual problems:** This side effect can be pretty bothersome. Some people report loss of sex drive, and others have trouble achieving an orgasm. These symptoms usually go away or can be treated with other medications.

» **Discontinuation syndrome:** People on antidepressants sometimes have a difficult time stopping their medication. Some report feeling out of sorts or anxious; others feel like they have the flu. These symptoms can usually be avoided by slowly tapering the dosage of the medication under the guidance of your health-care provider.

» **Pregnancy and breastfeeding:** No long-term, well-controlled studies have been done on the effects of many medications during pregnancy or breastfeeding. I urge caution. Psychotherapeutic alternatives should be considered first.

» **Concern about relapse:** When medications work for treating OCD, they generally work very well, though rarely do they accomplish a complete remission of OCD symptoms. And if a person decides to stop medication, the symptoms usually return. Psychological treatments, on the other hand, provide greater protection against relapse.

» **Suicide risk:** The FDA warns that there is some increase in the risk of suicidal thoughts in children, adolescents, and young adults who start antidepressant medication. Because of this risk, people who start on antidepressant medication should be seen regularly and encouraged to call their health-care provider if they experience any of the following:

» Thoughts about dying

» Thoughts about suicide

» Worsening depression

» Agitation

» Hopelessness

» Irritability

» Aggression

» Unusual behaviors

» Inability to sleep

YIKES! I FEEL A YAWN COMING ON

Decreased libido and inability to have an orgasm are quite common side effects of many medications for OCD. However, extremely rare, unexpected, spontaneous orgasms have also been linked to certain antidepressant medications. Some researchers suspect that many of these cases aren't being reported to the prescribing doctor. No kidding.

Case studies reported in the *Canadian Journal of Psychiatry* and the *Journal of Biological Psychiatry* have documented these unusual side effects. One woman reported a three-hour orgasm while shopping! Wow. She found the experience pleasurable, but a tad socially awkward. Incredibly, there have been numerous reports of yawning spells with simultaneous orgasm while taking antidepressants. Yawning can occur at any time, and the orgasm appears to be uncontrollable. This can be particularly uncomfortable for men when accompanied by ejaculation. On the other hand, obviously this reaction can also be quite pleasant. So, if you are being treated with antidepressants, and you want to feel good, try watching reruns of *Green Acres*. Yawn.

Examining Your OCD Medication Options

Medications that are used to treat OCD are all antidepressants that increase the availability of serotonin and, sometimes, other chemical messengers, or *neurotransmitters*, in the brain. Serotonin supports communication between neurons in the brain. It affects your mood, your level of anxiety, your perception of pain, your memory, and your ability to control impulses. See Chapter 4 for more information about the brain's role in OCD.

People with OCD usually require higher doses of these drugs than the amounts typically prescribed for treating depression. Prescriptions are often started at a low dose and gradually increased. Furthermore, medications for OCD frequently require six to twelve weeks to significantly improve OCD symptoms, whereas these same medications sometimes work a little faster when used for depression.

Generally, medication treatment continues for about a year, after which a gradual discontinuance is sometimes attempted. However, many people find that they need to go back on medication, frequently for a lifetime, for successful OCD treatment. The odds of long-term success with medication withdrawal are improved greatly if ERP has been provided at some point.

SSRIs

The first choice of medication for most people with OCD is one of the selective serotonin reuptake inhibitors (SSRIs). SSRIs appear to work by increasing the level of serotonin that's available to the nerve cells. Exactly how that increased availability impacts OCD specifically is an unresolved issue. These drugs have been extensively studied and found to be effective in decreasing symptoms of OCD

New drugs are constantly being developed for emotional disorders. The effectiveness of these medications compared to each other has not been thoroughly studied. However, some of the more commonly prescribed SSRIs for OCD include the following:

>> Prozac (fluoxetine)

>> Luvox (fluvoxamine)

>> Zoloft (sertraline)

>> Paxil (paroxetine)

>> Celexa (citalopram)

>> Lexapro (escitalopram)

Tricyclics

An older antidepressant, Anafranil (Clomipramine), was the first antidepressant medication found to be effective for OCD. Clomipramine is still used, especially when other SSRIs have not worked. The primary reason that Clomipramine is sometimes avoided is that an overdose can be fatal. It is at least as effective as the SSRIs, but it has more unpleasant side effects. Clomipramine also carries some risk of inducing seizures, increased heart rate, and problems with withdrawal.

Clomipramine belongs to the class of antidepressants known as tricyclics. *Tricyclic* refers to the chemical structure of the drugs in this class rather than the effects they have on neurotransmitters, as is the case with SSRIs. Clomipramine appears to affect various neurotransmitters, including serotonin and norepinephrine.

WARNING

Other than Clomipramine, tricyclic antidepressants (such as Imipramine or Amitriptyline) do not appear to be helpful in the treatment of OCD, nor does the class of antidepressants known as MAO inhibitors.

Other medications

Prescribing medicine is part science and part art. At this point, the understanding of exactly how antidepressants work and which one is best for a particular person is surprisingly primitive given that they have been available for many decades. Patients frequently have to try multiple antidepressant medications to find the one or the combination that works for them. For unknown reasons, one SSRI may do nothing for a particular individual, yet another one will prove to be quite helpful.

Sometimes, other medications are added to augment the effects of the first medication. Furthermore, many people with OCD have other problems such as depression, attention problems, or an anxiety disorder (see Chapter 3). In those cases, other drugs may be used to treat the co-occurring disorder. Be willing to work with your doctor to find the best regimen for you.

Directly Altering the OCD Brain

A few people with OCD are not able to benefit from standard treatments. These people are often severely impaired and virtually unable to function because of their disorder. In these cases, health-care professionals have tried multiple trials of antidepressant medications and other types of medications. For some of these people, ERP and cognitive techniques have been tried without success. This type of OCD is called *treatment refractory,* meaning it is resistant to ordinary means of treatment.

When *all else* fails, brain surgery is a highly controversial but possible option. These surgeries are rare and involve destroying a small amount of brain tissue. This destruction interrupts the circuit of the brain that has been implicated in OCD (see Chapter 4).

TECHNICAL STUFF

Newer techniques of brain surgery allow procedures to be performed without opening the skull. A gamma knife surgery sends gamma rays to destroy targeted tissues in the brain. This surgery allows quick recovery and does not damage surrounding tissues.

For obvious reasons, there are no "controlled" studies in which people with OCD are randomly assigned to brain surgery or other treatment. Therefore, the success of these surgeries is based on case reports. Treatment of this type has been found to improve symptoms for many. Unfortunately, at least half of those treated with brain surgery continue to have OCD.

Another option for treatment of refractory OCD is deep brain stimulation. In this procedure, holes are drilled in your skull so that electrodes can be implanted in areas of the brain that are believed to be implicated in OCD. A battery and pulse generator is surgically implanted in your chest wall and sends signals to the electrodes in the brain. Side effects and complications from this surgery can be significant, and recovery can take weeks.

This technique has been used for people with advanced Parkinson's disease to treat tremors for many decades. Again, although people have improved after deep brain stimulation, the research is sparse and based on case reports.

Understanding how deep brain magnetic stimulation works

A much less extreme option to brain surgery also involves deep brain stimulation. The Food and Drug Administration (FDA) cleared deep transcranial magnetic stimulation for the treatment of OCD in August 2018. Deep transcranial magnetic stimulation (dTMS) consists of sending a short electric current to the brain. This noninvasive technique has been found to change the neuronal activity of targeted areas of the brain. For some people who have not experienced relief with traditional treatment (therapy or medication), dTMS decreases OCD symptoms.

Patients attend sessions in an outpatient clinic with a dTMS-trained health professional. Sessions generally last 20 to 30 minutes and are given frequently over the course of weeks or months.

People with the following are not good candidates for dTMS:

>> Those with devices or plates in their heads containing metal

>> People with bullet fragments or shrapnel near or in their heads

>> People who have had seizures or are at risk of having a seizure

>> Those who have another brain disorder such as traumatic head injury, epilepsy, brain tumors, or dementia

>> Those who have implanted electronic devices such as pacemakers, defibrillators, or nerve stimulators

>> Children or pregnant or nursing mothers

TIP

Now that dTMS has been approved by the FDA, some insurance companies will pay for treatment. Make sure that you check your coverage prior to starting dTMS. Many insurance companies require that you have attempted other therapies for OCD, such as exposure and response prevention or medication before they will approve payment.

Looking at the evidence

Both research and real-world clinics have found that dTMS patients benefit from treatment. A study published in the *American Journal of Psychiatry* found that symptoms of OCD were reduced by 30 percent in a significant number of study participants. Some studies suggest longer treatment is more effective. Unfortunately, not enough studies have followed up on these improvements for more than a few weeks or months. So, there is very little evidence on the staying power of dTMS.

In addition, side effects can be uncomfortable. Following treatment, some complain of headaches, facial twitching, temporary hearing loss, and occasional painful scalp sensations. A more dangerous but rare side effect is an increased risk of having a seizure.

TIP

The bottom line, I suggest you try the least invasive treatment first (psychotherapy). If that works, great. If not, consider medication. After much perseverance, I recommend that you use messing with your brain as your last strategy.

Chapter 12

Responding to and Recovering from Relapse

R elapse is a normal part of the treatment process for OCD. Most sufferers experience a recurrence of obsessions or compulsions at some point during or after their treatment. But take heart: Relapses should be expected, and with patience and persistence, you can continue on your road to recovery.

By the conclusion of treatment, many people have successfully reduced their OCD symptoms by 50 to 75 percent. Occasionally, people succeed in completely eliminating their symptoms. Even moderate reductions in symptoms usually result in more time for pleasurable pursuits, enhanced relationships, and a substantially higher overall quality of life. With appropriate treatment, these benefits are obtainable for most folks with OCD, even for many whose symptoms are severe.

Regardless of where you are in treatment, the information in this chapter can be useful. Maybe you want to know about relapse risks before you even begin treatment for your OCD. Or perhaps you know someone who is recovering from the disorder. After all, forewarned is forearmed!

In this chapter, I provide you with a realistic picture of relapse and OCD, such as which treatments have a higher rate of relapse, what to do if relapse comes knocking at your door, and how you can reduce the risk, duration, or intensity of relapse.

Understanding the Steps of Recovery and the Risks of Relapse

Relapse occurs with varying frequency after successful treatment of most emotional disorders, and OCD is no exception. Relapse from OCD treatment can be very high, but the risk greatly depends on the type of treatment you receive as well as how you handle your relapse. The sections that follow give you an idea of what you may encounter regarding OCD relapse rates and challenges. The following concepts are useful to consider first:

>> **Treatment response:** A response is an improvement, exacerbation, or reduction in symptoms following treatment. With OCD treatment, that response can vary from one person to another.

>> **Remission:** Following treatment, a person no longer can be thought of as having OCD. They may continue to have symptoms, but those symptoms are mild and do not interfere with daily life.

>> **Recovery:** At this point symptoms are generally not present, and treatment can be discontinued.

>> **Relapse:** Symptoms return to close to the level of severity that occurred before treatment. The person again meets the diagnostic criteria of OCD.

TECHNICAL
STUFF

People depend on research studies to make decisions about what treatment to seek, medications to take, potential risks and benefits, and relapse rates. One problem with research is that it is often conducted over relatively short time periods. Drug companies want to know if a medication is safe and effective so that they can offer their products for sale. Researchers of therapy techniques need to publish their results in a timely fashion. Although a few well-funded longitudinal studies last for decades, these are the exception. Therefore, it is difficult to specify how long remission or recovery lasts because of the lack of data specific to OCD and evidence-based treatment strategies.

Medication relapse rates

As discussed in Chapter 11, various medications have a good track record for demonstrating the ability to greatly reduce OCD symptoms. But for a host of reasons, many people with OCD choose to discontinue their medications. Sometimes they want to become pregnant and worry about possible effects on the developing fetus. Other times, they experience distressing side effects, such as weight gain, dizziness, nausea, loss of sexual desire, and/or inability to experience orgasms.

And for some, discontinuing medication simply reflects a personal philosophical preference.

If you have experienced success with medications and decide to discontinue them, you should do so only under a doctor's supervision. That's because abruptly stopping certain medications can cause discontinuation syndrome, which involves various distressing physiological reactions, depending on the type of medication prescribed and the individual person.

Be prepared to experience an increase in your OCD symptoms, especially if medications were the only thing you used to treat your OCD. Relapse rates following medication discontinuation are disturbingly high. Estimates of relapse vary widely but can run from 75 to 90 percent or so if you *have had* no other type of treatment for your OCD.

If you choose to go off your medication, you can reduce the risk of relapse by heeding the following advice:

>> Continue medication for at least a year or two before considering discontinuance. Taper off your medication slowly and under your doctor's supervision. If symptoms return, consider going back on medication, perhaps even for a lifetime.

>> Seriously consider exposure and response prevention (ERP) therapy, either while you're on medication or when you start to taper off of it. Studies suggest that if you combine medication with ERP, your risk of relapse plummets.

ERP relapse rates

There is some pretty good news about ERP and the risk of relapse. If you successfully treat your OCD with ERP therapy, your odds of relapse are fairly low. A number of large studies have shown that if you respond well to ERP, you have a very good chance (perhaps as much as 70 to 80 percent) of maintaining your gains after treatment is completed, possibly for several years. Your improvement may even last much longer. The true relapse rate is not known because there are simply no studies that follow participants over years after treatment.

If you took medication in combination with ERP, no problem. Most studies suggest that medication does not increase your risk of relapse following successful combined treatment. It's possible that your odds of maintaining gains may improve somewhat if you remain on medication for a lifetime.

CBT, metacognitive therapy, and mindfulness relapse rates

Cognitive behavioral therapy (CBT), metacognitive therapy, and mindfulness techniques (see Chapters 8 and 9) are three approaches that have many similar strategies and goals. Unfortunately, the data on relapse risk with these approaches is rather thin. More long-term studies are needed before it will be possible to make definitive statements about the relapse risks associated with these forms of OCD treatment. Given that early studies have shown that CBT, metacognitive therapy, and mindfulness appear to work pretty well for OCD, at least in the short term, future research is likely to show that they help reduce relapse risks as well.

This is particularly true if the track records of these treatments' success in treating depression are any indication. When used to treat depression, CBT has been shown to substantially reduce the risk of relapse as compared to medication. Similar evidence suggests that mindfulness may also reduce the risk of depression relapse.

Responding Well to Relapse

Only a few people who are treated for OCD are truly, 100 percent cured. Just because a degree of relapse happens doesn't mean your treatment was not successful. The vast majority of people continue to have some mild symptoms that are occasionally irritating or annoying. Others have a few lapses here and there, especially when under stress. Another group of people (long-term studies don't exist to say exactly how many) suffer a full-blown return of their OCD. (See the later section, "Knowing the difference between a lapse and a relapse," for a more detailed explanation.) So, what should you do if your OCD symptoms return? Here are three approaches for dealing with relapse:

>> **Do what worked for you before.** If you used ERP, do that again. You can try ERP on your own or go back to a therapist. Treatment is usually more efficient the second time around because you already know what to expect. If you took antidepressant medication, try going back on it.

>> **Try something new.** If you go back and find that what worked before is no longer effective, other treatment alternatives are available. From what research suggests, ERP is probably the best bet for long-term management of OCD. So, certainly, if you were only taking medication and you experience a relapse, I strongly suggest trying ERP (see Chapter 10). If you've previously done ERP, consider reviewing Chapters 8 and 9 for additional ideas. If you've tried ERP and/or CBT but not medication, by all means, review Chapter 11 for medication options.

>> **Accept a little OCD in your life.** Is OCD always bad? Not necessarily. Millions of talented people — artists, writers, scientists, and other good people all over the world — have OCD. If OCD is not making you miserable, try accepting it without becoming overwhelmed. You have made progress in the past. A little OCD can encourage creativity, hard work, and carefulness.

TIP

OCD can be an enemy of well-being. But a little OCD once in a while can be okay. The more you can embrace OCD as a friend, maybe as a pesky friend, but nevertheless a friend, the less OCD will overtake you.

Strategies for Reducing Relapse

The best defense against relapse is getting the right treatment (or combination of treatments) for your OCD to begin with. Although medication alone works well (see Chapter 11), you can reduce your relapse risk substantially by either remaining on your medication for a very long time (perhaps for life) or by combining medication with ERP. Also, combining ERP with CBT, metacognitive therapy, and/ or mindfulness can help.

Nevertheless, relapse happens no matter what the problem is or what therapy is being used. The following sections discuss steps you can take, or at least be aware of, to help you guard against OCD relapse.

Knowing the difference between a lapse and a relapse

Chapter 8 tells you that the way you interpret events makes a huge difference in the way you end up feeling. That principle holds for an occasional return of obsessions and compulsions. A lapse can be defined as a bit of a slip involving a mild increase in symptoms. By contrast, a relapse is considered to be a major regression toward pre-treatment functioning. I provide examples of each of these in the following sections.

Looking at a lapse

A lapse is usually mild and transient. In the following example, Jeremy gets treatment for his OCD and then experiences an occasional obsession, which indicates a lapse.

Jeremy suffers from OCD that centers on the theme of contamination. He avoids public restrooms and restaurants. He is first referred for help when his primary care provider notices that his hands are raw and bleeding. Jeremy confesses that he often spends an hour showering and washes his hands literally hundreds of times during the day.

After 12 sessions of ERP, Jeremy's symptoms come under control. Jeremy continues to have moments when obsessive thoughts return. He reminds himself that the obsessions are normal and to be expected. He purposely waits until the thoughts pass and does not engage in compulsive washing. Most days Jeremy feels that he is leaving OCD behind him.

Jeremy had been told by his therapist that thoughts that seem like obsessions occur in everyone from time to time (see Chapter 2 for information about how people without OCD frequently have thoughts that look much like obsessions — but they just don't take them all that seriously). And Jeremy had been informed that such thoughts would no doubt pop back into his mind from time to time. Armed with that information, Jeremy understands that his obsessions are normal, expected, and something that he can handle. He knows if they happen to worsen, he now has skills and tools for dealing with them. Such brief visits from his old obsessional thoughts are merely mild, temporary lapses, not a full-blown return of his OCD.

Revealing a relapse

A relapse can begin with a lapse and then spiral downward from there, resulting in a full-blown return of obsessions and compulsions.

In the following example, Todd initially makes a good decision to seek help for his compulsive handwashing. However, when he encounters a normal uncomfortable situation — the flu — his obsessions return.

Todd has OCD focused on contamination concerns. He is a compulsive washer and avoids public places as much as he can. His washing takes up hours of his day. Todd talks about this with his primary care doctor, who tells Todd about different kinds of treatment. Todd and his doctor choose to try an antidepressant to see whether that will help. Todd's doctor reminds him that the medication can take a while to have an effect. Todd is relieved to know that he may get better. After about eight weeks, his symptoms seem to lessen. He doesn't always think about contamination, and his compulsions to wash have lessened.

An early flu season hits, and Todd comes down with the flu. He finds himself obsessing about what may have made him sick. The more he thinks about it, the more he begins to avoid public places and engage in compulsive washing. Todd calls his doctor to complain that the medication is no longer working. The doctor encourages Todd to stay on the medication and consider seeing a psychotherapist for ERP therapy. Todd throws the pills away and hangs up the phone. Within a few weeks, Todd is back where he started with OCD controlling his life.

Todd's story illustrates how a lapse can turn into a relapse. The lapse began when Todd started to obsess a little about how he got the flu. The relapse came when he became discouraged and threw away his pills, resulting in a return of his symptoms with a vengeance. Todd would probably have benefited from psychological treatment in the form of CBT, metacognitive therapy, mindfulness, or ERP in order to help him understand and deal with his setback.

REMEMBER

An OCD lapse need not turn into a full-blown relapse. It all depends on what you do with it.

Prolonging treatment

Realtors have a saying that success all comes down to three words — location, location, location. When it comes to OCD treatment, I like to say success boils down to persistence, persistence, persistence — no matter where you are in your treatment process. As I explain in the section "Medication relapse rates," if you choose medication to treat your OCD, you should be willing to continue taking it for at least a year or two, and perhaps a lifetime.

If you treat your OCD with ERP, CBT, metacognitive therapy, mindfulness, and/or medication, with persistence and considerable effort, you will likely see a great deal of improvement within a few months. Many people obtain significant, sustained improvement within four or five months. On the other hand, sometimes severe cases and/or OCD that's combined with other problems can require prolonged treatment. Some people benefit from working on their problem over several years. In almost all of those cases, a multi-pronged treatment plan involving most of the strategies can be the best way to recover.

Phasing out your sessions gradually

The relationship between you and a therapist is unique. Therapy is a time when you can be open about your weaknesses, fears, and secrets. Within this relationship there is trust, confidentiality, and safety. You have the undivided attention of someone who wants to help. That can feel pretty good.

However, usually a point is reached when therapy can and should be terminated. Most of the time, this happens when the client and therapist agree that the goals of treatment have been met. Nevertheless, when you realize that progress has been made, you may worry that you won't be able to maintain it on your own. When that time is approaching, the following suggestions can ease the process.

>> **Taper off the frequency of your sessions slowly.** When you're close to reaching your goals, try seeing your therapist every other week and then monthly.

>> **Have your therapist help you develop a relapse plan.** How will you handle upsetting times or increased symptoms?

>> **Be sure to talk about how you can be your own therapist.** You can engage in ERP on your own. You can also return to using other CBT strategies, such as cognitive therapy and mindfulness described in Chapters 8 and 9.

>> **See whether your therapist can offer you limited contact.** Some therapists will agree to an occasional e-mail contact, text, or a brief follow-up phone call. These can cut off trouble before it gets out of hand.

TIP

You should also know that you usually can return to therapy for a tune-up. The nice thing about a brief return to your previous therapist is that you don't have to start from square one.

Staging a fire drill

If you work in a school or hospital, you probably run through fire drills from time to time. That way, if a real fire ever breaks out, everyone knows what to do. You can do the same preparation for your OCD.

Fire drills for OCD start with making a list of high-risk situations, those are any situations that may trigger a return visit from your OCD obsessions and compulsions. Depending upon the focus or theme of your OCD concerns, the following may trigger your OCD:

>> A burglary occurs in your neighborhood, causing obsessions about checking your locks.

>> A fire breaks out somewhere and triggers obsessions about your home's fire-safe worthiness.

>> You are having a particularly stressful time in your life and feel exhausted.

>> You have a thought about harming someone and fear you may act on it.

>> You run over an unexpected bump in the road that you didn't see and fear that you may have run someone over.

>> You experience a sudden loss such as from death, divorce, or economic loss.

>> You shake hands with someone you later learn has cancer and fear you may have caught it (even though cancer isn't transmitted this way, those with OCD sometimes have this fear).

>> You step in a pile of dog poop and worry about becoming contaminated.

As you can see, I could list dozens, hundreds, maybe thousands of such items. The point of making such a list is to be prepared. Expect to encounter such situations. When you expect the inevitable, you won't be shocked or surprised when it happens, and you can have a plan ready. Perhaps you'll want to try some metacognitive techniques, mindfulness, or a brief regimen of ERP (which are covered in Chapters 9 and 10).

Finally, it's not a bad idea to read about all the various types of OCD themes discussed in Chapters 13 through 19. You're not very likely to develop a new type of OCD, but it can happen. If it does, you'll already have some ideas about how to handle it.

Remaining vigilant

Very few people will eliminate their OCD virtually 100 percent and not experience an occasional setback. You can nip these setbacks in the bud if you catch them early. Therefore, I suggest that following successful treatment: You actually create a log and track your obsessions and compulsions. Please don't get obsessive about tracking! You don't have to keep this log all the time; you can start by tracking once a month for a few days at a time.

If your symptoms remain low, that's great. You may then reduce your monitoring to a day or two every few months. If your obsessions and compulsions even start to creep up, take them seriously. Check out the earlier section "Responding Well to Relapse" for ideas.

Zeroing in on especially problematic beliefs

Two specific beliefs frequently creep into the mind following successful OCD treatment, and these beliefs can pave the way for relapse. So, it's good to be on the lookout for them. (See Chapter 8 for more info on beliefs that provide fuel for OCD.)

Feeling as if something is true when you know it isn't

After your symptoms have been substantially reduced, you very well may find yourself thinking things like:

>> "I don't believe that using a public restroom is a threat to my health, but it still *feels* like it could be."

>> "I understand that walking into an Alzheimer's memory care facility isn't going to make me demented, but it *feels* like it might."

>> "Well, sure I now know that I can't really get toxic contaminants into my body by touching drywall, but I *feel* like I can."

REMEMBER

Obsessions and compulsions love to try sneaking in the back door. And it's easy to have thoughts like, "Big deal, so what if I cave into a few of my obsessions?" On the one hand, it isn't a huge problem if you slip a little. On the other hand, if you start having strong feelings that run counter to what your observant, rational mind tells you (see Chapter 9), this contradiction can serve as an important warning sign that your OCD mind is attempting a comeback. Conduct a cost/benefit analysis of buying into the OCD part of your mind rather than the observant, rational mind. See Chapter 9 for information about how to conduct such an analysis.

REMEMBER

You may also find it useful to ask yourself whether these feelings are based on clear evidence that most people would agree is valid. Generally speaking, such evidence should be based on things that you can clearly see, touch, hear, smell, or taste.

Feeling as if you must avoid all negative feelings

Please realize that negative feelings absolutely cannot be avoided in life. If you try to avoid all such feelings, relapse is likely waiting around the next corner, ready to pounce. Think of physical training. Working out provides an excellent analogy for helping you think about this issue.

Most people find that intense physical exercise causes a few discomforts — shortness of breath for a while, soreness, stiffness, sweating, and so on. However, the more you exercise, the more you feel the benefits — including fewer negative feelings. These benefits include:

>> Enhanced sense of well-being

>> Increased endurance

» Increased flexibility

» Increased mobility

» Increased strength

» Reduced pain

Tolerating the discomfort associated with obsessions works exactly the same way. In the short run, you feel distress, anxiety, and frustration. Sometimes those feelings can be quite intense. But the more you resist caving into the discomfort with your usual compulsions, the more your tolerance increases and the less discomfort you feel.

Recognizing events that trigger relapse

There are no guarantees in life. Roadblocks, setbacks, detours, and crashes inevitably occur. When these events happen, OCD symptoms may return. Increased stress decreases your ability to stay mentally healthy. Watch out for times of high stress that could trigger relapse, such as:

» Getting sick or injured

» Losing a friend

» Losing a job or failing to get an expected promotion

» Sleeping poorly

» Suffering a loss

» Watching the stock market tank and your 401K evaporate

» Working too hard

What some people don't realize is that even positive life events and changes can also trigger relapse. Whenever the status quo changes — even for the better — don't be shocked if some of your symptoms return. Most people with OCD struggle with the unpredictability and uncertainty that come with almost any type of change. The following events can trigger stress, and therefore, OCD:

» Getting married

» Graduating

» Having a baby

» Getting a new job

» Retiring

If a major life transition occurs shortly before a return of your OCD symptoms, you may find that it's very important to deal with the implications of that event prior to working on your OCD again.

Just because a negative or positive event occurs doesn't mean you are compelled to respond compulsively.

4

Targeting Specific Symptoms of OCD

Chapter **13**

Sanitizing Risk: Contamination OCD

More than one-half of all people with OCD worry about becoming contaminated. These worries often include feelings of disgust. Disgust is an emotional response that occurs universally across cultures. It has the survival function of warning people that something might be unsafe. Frankly, it's actually helpful to be disgusted by spoiled food, putrid water, or nauseating smells. But in those with OCD, the disgust system is stuck on overdrive.

This chapter delves into some of the most common contamination fears. The list is incomplete, however, because people can imagine an infinite variety of unusual, theoretically possible, contaminates. Following the descriptions of these obsessional fears, the chapter takes a look at the compulsive actions people use to protect or decontaminate themselves. Finally, strategies are offered on how to address contamination fears and the compulsions that follow.

Considering Contamination Obsessions

When people first think about OCD, they automatically think of the classic germaphobe. Although a good number of people with OCD are, in fact, concerned about getting sick, the variations of contamination OCD are revoltingly numerous. Frequently, people have more than one contamination obsession.

Obsessions are the unwanted intrusive thoughts or images that repeatedly invade your mind throughout the day. Obsessions create strong urges to do something (a compulsion) to get rid of the discomfort they produce.

People with contamination obsessions are driven by two faulty beliefs. The first belief is that brief or superficial contact can transmit contamination. For example, a brief contact of an insect on a plate makes the plate seem dirty even after washing it off. The second belief is that if something looks slightly similar to something disgusting or grossly disturbing, it really seems gross and unacceptable. For example, if a piece of candy is made to look like a bug, it becomes disgusting and inedible.

The term *sympathetic magic* describes the process by which unlikely beliefs about how pathogens are transferred and how neutral but similar-looking items can both pose a threat increases fear and disgust reactions in those with OCD.

Germs

People who obsess about germs may fear either catching something or spreading their own germs to innocent people. They become preoccupied with imagined risks from everyday life events such as the following:

>> Using public toilets

>> Being in crowded places

>> Believing that certain people are contaminated for no logical reason

>> Getting sick from potentially unsanitary food

>> Seeking routine health or dental care

>> Sleeping in hotel beds

>> Eating in a restaurant

>> Shaking hands

>> Touching items that were handled by others

>> Giving or receiving a hug

>> Touching money

>> Using a towel in a guest bathroom

>> Kissing a relative on the cheek

>> Touching a doorknob or elevator button

People with these specific obsessions believe that they may contact highly dangerous and infectious diseases through ordinary contact. They may believe that a small spot of grease or dirt on the counter is filled with killer microbes. Their lives can become extremely restricted, and they engage in a variety of compulsions to mitigate their fears (see the section "Staying Clean: Contamination Compulsions").

The disgustingly gross

As noted previously in this chapter, disgust often accompanies contamination OCD. Although all humans have the emotional response of disgust, those with OCD are more disgusted more of the time. Research has found that people with contamination OCD have a stronger sense of revulsion to disgusting situations than those without. In addition, they are more likely to find a wider range of things disgusting.

Disgust reactions are again related to everyday life. People with OCD and elevated disgust may go to great lengths to avoid touching or even looking at potential "threats" such as

>> Vomit

>> Feces

>> Garbage

>> Diapers

>> Spoiled food

>> Dirty bathrooms

>> Roadkill

>> Semen

>> Hair in the drain

>> Sticky or slimy foods

>> Sweat

>> Saliva

>> Fingerprint smudges on silverware

>> Lipstick residue on a glass

>> Pus

>> Dandruff

>> Hair in food

Yuck. The list is disgustingly endless. Disgust is also thought to be involved in some other types of OCD, such as feeling ashamed or disgusted by one's own thoughts. And the feeling of disgust usually shows up on the face of the person experiencing it. The typical facial expression of disgust consists of wrinkling of the nose and brows and raising of the upper lip. This facial expression may derive from an evolutionary way to protect the nose and eyes from real contaminates.

Unusual contamination fears

Contamination fears can range from the ordinary to the bizarre. Emotional contamination occurs when someone believes that personality traits, sexual orientation, or something dreadful is magically passed on from one person to another. This form of contamination obsession can occur by coming into contact with a person thought to be contaminated, by being close to another person, by talking to the person on the phone, or even through texts or emails.

Some with emotional contamination fears believe that watching certain shows can cause contamination. A frequent fear is one of being contaminated by something related to death such as seeing or walking by a cemetery. Another common contamination fear is that walking near a hospital makes it possible to catch cancer or another deadly disease.

Other unusual contamination obsessions may come from merely seeing a neutral object that has some vague similarity to a feared contaminant. For example, someone with a fear of being dirty may be triggered by a stain on someone else's shirt. The site of the shirt alone can cause overwhelming feelings of disgust and danger.

Still others with contamination OCD fear that they are somehow contaminated themselves, and they are very likely to spread it to others. So, they may avoid getting close to people around them for fear of harming them. This can also lead to ritualistic cleaning or decontaminating compulsions to protect others.

Pandemic contamination

Imagine planning a trip to get groceries. Your stomach feels a bit off, a sense of doom fills your mind. You put rubber gloves in one pocket and a spray bottle of hand sanitizer in the other. You put on two handmade masks, hoping they will keep germs away. Your fear rises as you double lock your apartment door. You use your elbow to push the elevator button. When the elevator arrives, you check to see who your companions will be for the 12-story descent. You're grateful the elevator holds only two others and hope that not many more passengers will invade your car. You push the ground floor button, again using your elbow, and begin the silent ride. Perhaps you hold your breath and try to breathe shallowly.

As you leave your building, you try to maintain as much distance as possible from others. You enter the store and carefully scrutinize people around you, constantly worried about getting contaminated. You might be watching to make sure they have masks on and whether their masks cover their noses. You stealthily put on your rubber gloves, quickly grabbing a few items and get ready to check out. You see a line of three people ahead of you, and your anxiety increases. What if they are carrying the virus? Will you get sick? You hear sirens in the distance and picture the dead and dying being sent to overflowing hospitals and morgues. You're overwhelmed with dread.

This hypothetical story could be a truthful accounting of the thoughts and feelings of quite a few New York City residents in the spring of 2020, when vaccines, adequate masks, or treatment were not yet available. It also reflects everyday experiences of people with OCD. However, imagine if you already had OCD and then had to live through a worldwide pandemic. How did those people fare?

Not well, according to the surveys of people who previously had OCD before the pandemic. Most people with any type of OCD reported worsening of symptoms. However, those who typically were afraid of contamination and had compulsions to wash or clean fared the worst.

Imagine watching the news and discovering that what you feared most — that danger lurked on every surface and even in the air — was, in fact, true. Many people watched the news about COVID with horror. Some became overly obsessed with the statistics and compulsively reviewed multiple sources of infection rates, hospitalizations, and deaths.

Staying Clean: Contamination Compulsions

When there is fear of contamination fear, worry, and anxiety increase. Compulsions follow to reduce the fear. People may go thought very extreme and elaborate routines in order to rid themselves of these possible dangers.

Note, many of the compulsive acts overlap, and people with OCD have a wide variety of routines. However, the following sections describe some of the more common compulsions related to contamination.

Washing

Excessive handwashing is a common compulsion. The hands of washers are usually rough, dry, red, and sometimes have open sores from their repeated abuse. Many variations of washers exist. Some simply wash their hands hundreds of times a day. Others use special soaps that are thought to clean better. Some have washing routines that must be followed such as first using cold then warm water or washing using a brush to get the cleanest possible result.

Taking long showers or baths is also common. Forty-gallon water heaters run out of water during one shower. Cleaning supplies damage skin from overuse or harsh chemical ingredients.

Cleaning

Not all compulsive hand washers engage in additional cleaning routines, but some do. These routines may include sterilizing, disinfecting, and scrubbing. Many with cleaning compulsions have strict routines for sorting and washing clothes or packing the dishwasher, or they must perform certain movements while cleaning to satisfy their need to clean just right. Cleaning supplies often become a large part of the budget for those with cleaning compulsions. Compulsive cleaning frequently takes hours a day. Items must be cleaned over and over to maintain the right amount of cleanliness.

The actions of health-care professionals can serve as an example. For instance, when arriving home from a shift at the hospital, it's common for people to shed their clothes directly into the washer and then immediately take a shower. That's perfectly normal for people whose jobs regularly expose them to disease. However, when a compulsive washer returns from the mailbox, a health-care appointment, or the grocery store and strips off clothes, throws them into the wash, and immediately showers, that likely indicates a cleaning and washing compulsion.

Avoiding

Avoidance is a common way of handling any difficult feelings. People with OCD go to extreme measures to avoid. Some become homebound because of fears that the outside world is full of contamination potential. Others wear protective clothing in situations that don't really qualify as potentially dangerous.

The OCD mind sometimes determines that there are inherently clean and dirty areas in their lives. They become contaminated in the so-called dirty areas and must carry out certain rituals when they arrive in clean areas. What constitutes clean or dirty is rather idiosyncratic to each person.

Rituals

Many cleaning compulsions have a rigidly ritualistic flavor to them. Hand washers may have a certain order to follow. Showers may have to be completed according to strict routines. Surfaces might have to be scrubbed in circles or for a certain length of time. There may be counting, or chanting involved. When rules are not followed, then the compulsion must be repeated until the actions meets the high standards of the ritual.

Discarding

Certain items become so "contaminated" that they must be destroyed. For some, simply throwing away suffices. Therefore, an article of clothing that could have come into contact with germs needs to immediately be tossed in the trash. For other people with OCD, contaminated items have to be buried or burned.

Reassurance seeking

With contamination obsessions, most compulsions involve cleaning or rituals to decontaminate. However, some people with these obsessions ask others to participate and help reassure them that things are okay. Unfortunately, loving family members often get pulled into elaborate rituals themselves in order to reassure those with OCD.

Parents are especially vulnerable to the reassurance trap. They often cooperate with whatever tactics it takes to make their OCD child feel better. This complicity actually makes things worse. For example, I have seen families with children who have OCD engage in extreme cleaning rituals to please their children. These rituals disrupt normal family life and lead to resentment and stress for the entire family.

REMEMBER

When you give people with OCD reassurance, they usually experience a brief positive feeling. That feeling makes them more likely to increase the desire for reassurance in the future. This can lead to repeated feelings of insecurity and a vicious cycle of reassurance seeking.

Confronting Contamination OCD

Exposure and response prevention (ERP) is the most effective treatment for contamination OCD. ERP involves gradually exposing a person to their fears and helping them to delay or eliminate compulsive behaviors. As the person practices this approach, they slowly learn that nothing much happens. In addition, the therapy empowers and educates OCD sufferers that their feelings of disgust and worry are not dangerous and actually decrease in intensity over time.

Medication is sometimes used in tandem with ERP. Medication should be prescribed by a provider experienced in working with people who have OCD. See Chapter 11 for more information about medication.

Making a list

The first step in treating contamination-related OCD is to sort out the facets of your own OCD. This process usually should be done in concert with a mental health professional. However, it can be useful to begin the task on your own. Ask yourself the following questions:

>> **What triggers my OCD cycle?** Is it a specific situation or place that I think is contaminated? Do I have intrusive, obsessive thoughts? Or do I just have the feeling that something is contaminated?

>> **What do I think might happen if I get contaminated?** Will I get sick? Will I die? Will I get others sick? Am I really afraid of feeling dirty or disgusting? I am just not sure but know it will be awful?

>> **What do I do to prevent myself from getting contaminated?** Do I wash or clean objects that might be dirty? Do I avoid certain situations that seem unsafe? Do I have rituals or routines that I must follow? How long every day do I spend on either cleaning up from or avoiding being contaminated?

It helps to write (or type) out your answers to these questions. Spend some time thinking about each one. You might ask a trusted friend or family member their thoughts and insights concerning the preceding list of questions if you feel comfortable.

Make a list of at least 10 triggers for your OCD. Then rate them for their difficulty (I call that an Ugh factor) from 0 for little distress to 100 for extreme distress. For more information see Chapter 10.

Here's an example of **Atticus,** a young man with OCD. He answered the preceding questions in the following way:

> When I get near any strangers, I start to worry about what sort of diseases they may have. I never get close to anyone I don't know really well because I am afraid that if they touch me, even just briefly, I could get sick. I used to be able to go to one neighborhood store that I got used to, but now I get all of my groceries delivered. It's getting easier to avoid strangers. I work from home, do my banking online, and if I need takeout, it's delivered. But deliveries scare me, too. I'm even starting to worry about getting messages from strangers. I know this sounds weird, but I'm starting to get freaked out by email and texts.

> If I get contaminated, I will certainly get sick. I might get something really serious and die. I have a sense of dread in the pit of my stomach, and I worry it might be the start of a fatal illness.

> I do many things to keep me safe. If I think I've been contaminated, I take repeated showers. The first shower is to get the dirtiest germs off. I have special soap that is kind of hard on my skin, but that's the price I pay to get clean. After I towel off, I return and rinse off. The next shower might be after I get dressed and do a bit of work, but then I start to feel dirty again. I also have daily routines of cleaning all of my devices. I use both air and alcohol on my keyboards and phone, especially after I get a message from someone I don't know. I'd guess my cleaning only takes a few hours out of most days. But if I have to leave the house, they take much longer. I spend a bunch of my money on getting things delivered.

> Atticus developed a list of triggers and their relative level of difficulty. A few examples are depicted in Table 13-1.

TABLE 13-1

Atticus's OCD Trigger List and Ugh Factor Ratings

OCD Trigger	Ugh Factor Rating (On a Scale of 0–100)
Getting close to strangers	80
Going into a store	70
Picking up take out	50
Touching my phone or computer after I get an email or text	60
Eating at a public restaurant	95

Setting a goal

The broad goal is to feel better and not be a prisoner of OCD. However, that goal needs to be broken down into doable steps. Most people prefer to start with a relatively easy task and build from that point; however, what you start on is entirely up to you. Hopefully, you will be consulting with a therapist.

To illustrate the possible process, consider the preceding example of Atticus, who is worried about being contaminated by any stranger. After reviewing his answers he decides that he needs to start saving some money by going to the grocery store and to restaurants when he wants takeout. He realizes that he is spending hundreds of dollars a month in delivery fees.

Exposure and response prevention (ERP)

Over the course of my work with OCD clients, I have had many yucky experiences with ERP and contamination fears. That's because the therapist often becomes the model of bravery to show the client that their fear is pretty harmless. I confess, I have a pretty low threshold for disgust, and these exposures probably helped me reduce my own tendency to avoid disgusting situations. I've flushed and cleaned hundreds of toilets, rubbed the inside of garbage cans, eaten off of the floor, held onto countless doorknobs, crumpled dirty tissues, touched dried bird poop, gotten dirty oil on my hands, and even rubbed sap from trees onto my hands.

After being able to observe the model, clients are usually more willing to try it themselves. The next step also involves self-control. After doing all of these disgusting things, the client must refrain from the compulsive behavior that usually follows. During many exposures, I would use a timer to gradually increase the time following the exposure until the client is given the go ahead to clean up.

However, part of the exposure also involves eliminating, shortening, or modifying the amount of compulsion. For some of the messier exposures, it's perfectly okay to wash hands, but only for 20 or 30 seconds.

REMEMBER

Exposure involves getting into the dirt, and response prevention means to stop engaging in compulsions to clean up the mess.

Using the example of Atticus, recall that he wanted to get out more to stores and restaurants — partly to save money. He decided to start exposure and response prevention with a psychologist who offered telehealth. Although he was extremely nervous about talking to someone, after a few sessions, he agreed to a plan. Here are a few of the exposure and response prevention activities they came up with:

- ►► Atticus would walk to the closest restaurant in the morning and look at the menu posted on the window. He would return home and not take a shower for at least 4 hours. He would repeat this exercise daily until his anxiety decreased.

- ►► Atticus would order online and pick up his food at that restaurant. He would return home and resist wiping the counter with disinfectant after eating. Also, he would still not shower for at least 4 hours. He would do this activity weekly until his anxiety decreased.

- ►► Meanwhile he would continue to walk by the restaurant on the days he did not order take out and extend his walk so that he walked by his neighborhood grocery store. He would return without showering for at least 5 hours.

- ►► After several weeks of exposure, he was feeling pretty confident. So, he was able to go into the store and buy a few groceries. He felt pretty anxious, but also proud. He started showering no more than once a day.

Atticus and his therapist continued to work on increasing the difficulty of his exposures. Atticus was doing very well in therapy until the spring of 2020. Then, he had a setback.

COVID complications

When COVID hit, people with OCD were especially impacted. Contamination fears were the most challenging to treat with exposure and response prevention. Especially in the early months of COVID, someone who feared touching doorknobs was not advised to go around touching doorknobs. If someone had a fear of getting sick by being in large, crowded places, it would have been malpractice to assign a client to attend an event when COVID rates were significant. Instead, therapists had to use common sense and help their OCD clients navigate through an unusually trying time.

Basically, therapeutic recommendations included finding reliable sources of information such as the Center for Disease Control (CDC), World Health Organization, and prestigious medical centers such as Johns Hopkins. When sources were identified, clients were encouraged to follow established guidelines. That was also hard because people with OCD crave certainty, and there was little certainty in the scientific community. Guidelines changed over time. However, that was also an opportunity to help people learn about the scientific method and changing guidelines were based on new information.

In dangerous times, it is important to look to both mental and physical health professionals for guidance.

WARNING

Alternatives to ERP

Alternative treatment for OCD contamination fears generally includes using techniques from cognitive therapy to rethink risk, accept a degree of uncertainty, and see what seems catastrophic more realistically (see Chapter 8). In addition, looking at the distinction between feelings, thoughts, and actions may help you to take a broader look at your thinking style. Finally, learning to accept and embrace the present moment without judgment, gives you the grace to live through difficult times (see Chapter 9).

Cognitive therapy, metacognitive therapy, and mindfulness can help you get to a place to do ERP if you find ERP too difficult at first.

Chapter **14**

Dealing with Doubting and Checking OCD

Worry wears you out. People with the doubting and checking type of OCD feel uneasy and worried much of the time. Many of their concerns have a remote chance of happening, but a few are extremely bizarre and wildly unrealistic. More than a few people focus on worries about illness and disease. Normal body fluctuations, such as muscle soreness after exercise, turn into an esoteric, degenerative neurological disease in their minds. Others imagine their homes being burned down because they left on an appliance. For those with this type of OCD, these fears and behaviors commonly occur hundreds of times each day.

Doubting comes in the form of an *obsession:* an unwanted image, urge, or thought. The doubt is intense, seems realistic, and vivid. These obsessions center on things such as damage being done to their house or harming someone, all through some imagined negligence on their part.

Checking is the compulsive part. There is a compelling need to see whether the lights are on, the door is open, the stove is turned off, or someone got hurt. See Chapter 2 for more information about the differences between obsessions and compulsions.

This chapter provides more details about doubting and checking types of OCD. I offer specific strategies for dealing with doubt and resisting checking.

Defining Categories of Doubting

Doubt means uncertainty. Doubt leads to questions, hesitation, and, in the case of OCD, checking. Doubt is associated with many of the other types of OCD, but in the doubting and checking type, doubt towers over reason and logic. The individual, specific doubts of doubting and checking OCD vary endlessly but tend to cluster together into several areas of concern:

>> Obsessions about the home

>> Worry about harming others

>> Obsessions having to do with unintentionally running someone over

>> Personal health concerns

The next sections give examples of each area of concern.

Harming your home through negligence

One area of doubting involves concerns with harm occurring where you live. People with this concern worry about something terrible happening to their homes because of their own carelessness. The feelings of doubt are so intense that they lead to nearly endless loops of compulsive checking.

Those who are obsessed with such matters worry about fires breaking out, roofs falling in, and termites consuming their walls until they collapse. They worry about explosions from gas leaks and asphyxiation from carbon monoxide. They obsess about faucets that may have been left turned on, resulting in flood damage. This type of OCD is difficult to overcome because you can never absolutely rule out the possibility of damage or harm occurring to your home, no matter how many times you check.

The following example illustrates the vicious cycle of doubting and checking OCD as it relates to household safety.

> **Carl** turns the oven knob to the off position. Actually, he turns it on, then off, then on, and then off. He looks to make sure it is still off. He leaves the house. But he fears the knob may have slipped back on. He goes back inside and checks. It's off.

He leaves the house and gets in the car. But as he pulls out of the driveway, he wonders whether there's a chance that the oven could still be on. Maybe, just maybe, he thinks, it is. He pulls back in, gets out of the car, and goes back in the house. Checks the knob. It's off. Whew! He opens the oven door to see whether the oven is warm. He thinks it is. He checks the knob. He closes the door. He checks the knob. He leaves the house. Gets into the car. Starts the car. Looks back. Was that smoke? Is the oven on? He stops the car. Goes back to the house. And checks everything all over again.

Just reading about Carl's doubting is exhausting! The pattern is difficult to stop. Doubt, check, doubt, check . . .

Harming others through negligence

Another concern of people with doubting and checking OCD is fear that their behavior or negligence will somehow harm someone else. The specific content of the fear ranges infinitely. But the belief is one of hyper-responsibility for other people's welfare and safety. The afflicted person must constantly be on guard to make sure that something really bad doesn't happen.

This type of OCD worry escalates, with sufferers taking more and more drastic steps to keep others safe. Their attempts to protect others consume more of their time as the concerns go on. The following example illustrates how someone with this type of OCD concern attempts to protect people but actually accomplishes little or nothing for her efforts.

Naomi believes that she is responsible for warning her friends and family about bad weather. This problem gets worse after she hears about a child dying in a tornado that briefly touched down in her town. Her obsession causes her to constantly monitor the weather station. When there are reports of storms in the area, she sends text messages to each person on her list of 14 family members and friends. At first, she only texts when the storms are serious and imminent, but after a while she texts when there are mere threats of rain.

Friends and family no longer answer their texts when they see her number on their phones. However, she leaves phone messages when they fail to answer her texts but worries that the voice mail won't get picked up in time. And if it isn't, and someone might possibly get hurt, she feels she will be personally responsible. She literally begins driving to the house of multiple people on her list who don't answer. Upon arriving, if no one answers the door, she leaves a note warning of the impending doom.

Naomi's story shows how the sense of responsibility inflates to incredible proportions. There is virtually no end to the efforts people with this type of OCD will make in order to protect the safety and well-being of those they love. Sometimes they expend this energy on protecting perfect strangers. But these efforts require huge amounts of time and fail to add significant safety to the lives of those they worry about.

Parents with OCD might have thoughts about potentially harming their children. This can happen during a child's infancy (see Chapter 2 on perinatal OCD) or throughout their lifetimes. Over-the-top parental worries often results in over-protection of children. These kids can become overly anxious themselves or eventually rebel with recklessness behavior. Needless to say, treating the OCD of the parent is crucial for the healthy development of their kids.

>> A mother frequently fears she may poison her children by undercooking their meat, so she routinely burns their dinner.

>> A parent does not allow his teen to wait at the bus stop, even though they live in a safe environment, therefore he drives the boy to school every day.

>> A father worries about his kids' health so much that he home-schools them to avoid exposure to contagions.

Harming others with your car through negligence

The hit-and-run focus is actually a variant of the "harming others through negligence" concern discussed previously. However, hit-and-run is such a common form of doubting and checking that it deserves special attention. Those who dwell on hit-and-run issues greatly fear hitting someone with their car. Therefore, they interpret every bump in the road, unexpected honk, or random movement detected in their peripheral vision as evidence that they have run someone over.

After they make that interpretation, they feel driven to go back and check on the victims or, more hopefully, find evidence that they did not actually cause a horrible accident. Sometimes they go back to the scene dozens of times often causing them to be late to their destinations and sometimes engaging in dangerous driving. Additional ways these folks check on possible hit-and-run accidents include

>> Asking for reassurance from passengers in their car

>> Calling hospital emergency rooms to inquire about recent arrivals

>> Carefully rubbing the surface of their cars for signs of dents from an impact

>> Listening to police scanners for calls on accidents

>> Reading obituaries in the newspaper

>> Scrutinizing the exterior of their cars for any signs of blood

No one really knows why this concern appears so often. Some have speculated that it stems from the importance of cars in modern society as well as the fact that automobiles cause many thousands of deaths and injuries each year.

Another contributor to the cause of hit-and-run OCD may be the fact that every so often a news story about someone backing out of the driveway and running over a child pops up in the newspaper or on TV. Almost always the person driving was unaware of the child's presence, and the act was a tragic accident.

The following exercise asks you to put yourself in the shoes of someone who has actually experienced such a tragedy. Doing so gives you an idea of what this type of OCD feels like to those who have it.

> Imagine you are backing out of your driveway, maybe thinking about a grocery list or a dinner date. You feel a slight bump of the wheels. Then you hear the screams of neighbors. People are running toward your car, pointing. The realization that something is horribly wrong floods your mind. You desperately wish that you could go back in time, but you can't. You stop the car, open the door, and there, on the driveway, lies a lifeless child.

People with hit-and-run OCD repeatedly have such images, with feelings to match, most days of their lives. The horror *seems* real and the urge to check irresistible. Paradoxically, a few people with hit-and-run OCD have been hurt or caused real accidents because of their compulsive need to stop and turn around in traffic to check.

Harming your health through negligence

People with doubting and checking OCD frequently have excessive concerns about their own health or sometimes the health of loved ones. The health fear usually is specific to one condition or disease and often makes little sense to others. The following example shows you how someone with this OCD concern thinks.

> **Jack** believes that fibers from synthetic clothing contain carcinogenic material. He avoids wearing anything except natural cotton or wool. He calls stores and clothing manufacturers around the country asking about what types of thread they use for sewing on buttons. He asks about the machines used to cut and sew the material to see whether they are also used on the dreaded synthetic fabrics. If he is not fully assured that the machines are used only to manufacture natural materials into clothes, he won't buy the brand in question.

In addition to the fabric, Jack obsesses about the plastic holders used to attach price tags to clothes. He cuts each off and checks to make sure that no plastic piece remains hidden in the garment. He also washes new clothes several times before he wears them.

He checks all fabric tags repeatedly before he puts on his clothes. He gets very upset when someone walks by too closely, fearing that synthetic fibers from clothes can jump from person to person. He monitors his body constantly for what he believes are possible signs of cancer, such as bloating, blemishes, swollen sinuses, and headaches.

Jack's story may seem pretty wacky to you. But that's how OCD works sometimes. OCD stories don't always make a whole lot of logical sense. Other examples of people with OCD health concerns include the following:

>> A teenage boy obsesses about being killed by natural disasters. He convinces his parents to buy enough supplies to last for two months in case of an emergency. That's not such a bad idea, but his OCD is revealed by the fact that the boy does an inventory of the supplies each day. He also pressures his parents to move to Nevada because it has a lower incidence of natural disasters than California, which is where they live.

>> A woman fears getting attacked by killer bees. She constantly looks up news about killer bees around the world checking to see if any are possibly on their way. She rarely goes outside in the summer and wears long sleeves shirts and pants even on the hottest days of summer.

Getting stuck on unanswerable questions

Sometimes called existential OCD, this category of checking refers to the frequent obsessive questioning of unresolvable issues. Questions that many people ask at different times in their lives ruminate throughout the day. For example:

>> Do I exist?

>> What is the purpose of life?

>> Why am I here?

>> Is there a god?

>> Are people good or evil?

These questions cause worry, and the compulsive activities that follow are constant asking for reassurance, attempting to find answers by researching these questions, discussing these issues with others, or other idiosyncratic methods.

For example, an adolescent with OCD may be particularly concerned about the environment. Climate change is a perfectly reasonable worry. However, the teen is constantly searching for whether or not the Earth will still be inhabitable during his lifetime. He worries excessively about that possibility, and that unanswerable question dominates his conversation with anyone who will listen. He does not participate in any proactive activities to preserve the environment but is stuck in a loop of questions and worries. Eventually the people around him grow tired of his obsession and avoid him when possible.

During the COVID pandemic, there were many unanswerable questions. One common and understandable set of questions for many was

>> Will I get COVID?

>> How bad will it be?

>> If I get it, will I die?

For those with normal worries, the initial response was to watch the statistics, likely quite a bit in the beginning, but with somewhat less frequency over time. However, for some of those with OCD, COVID checking became a compulsive response to obsessive, unanswerable questions. Many spent hours watching the news and checking sources of statistical information about COVID, hoping to add certainty to an uncertain world.

Categorizing Approaches to Checking

The compulsion to check momentarily decreases doubt, and that feels like a relief. But the doubt quickly returns. That's the nature of OCD. Checking is a very temporary solution because absolute certainty *never* replaces doubt. To the OCD mind, there is always a chance that something bad might happen. Over the long haul, continued checking produces increased uneasiness, frustration, and doubt.

Checking usually happens when the person with OCD is alone and further increases when the person feels stressed or unhappy. Checking falls into one of three forms: obvious or overt, mental, or assisted. The following sections describe each form in more detail.

Obvious or overt checking

These compulsions are active and can be seen, like clicking the car key fob again and again to make sure the car doors are locked or checking over and over to see that the dryer is turned off. Obvious checking is also apparent when a driver turns around and goes back to the area where a bump in the road seemed suspicious. Another example of this type of checking is when a person scans the news for accident victims or repeatedly calls friends to make sure that they are okay.

Mental checking

Mental checking refers to thinking about or reviewing something over and over. Someone may think about all the details of driving to work repeatedly to check for the possibility of harming someone. Or one may mentally review each step taken to make sure that the windows at home are closed. People obsessed with health concerns may scan the internet or social media for information about their obsessions. Still others may repeatedly review each conversation from the day in order to be sure that they said nothing offensive to anyone.

Getting others to check

One way to get others to help check is simply to ask. A person might call their roommate and ask them to check and see that the stove is off. Another person might ask a passenger in the car if they felt that bump. Another way of getting others involved is through *reassurance seeking* (covered in Chapter 5). Someone might ask their spouse if they think they look sick. A child might repeatedly ask their parents whether they think the house will be safe from intruders.

Taking Steps to Defeat Doubting and Control Checking

Treating doubting and checking OCD is relatively straightforward. However, it takes effort, a willingness to do a few uncomfortable things, and perseverance. In addition, you need to be very self-observant in order to pick up on all the important nuances that your OCD may involve. The following five sections take you through a typical treatment game plan, step by step.

If you don't feel ready to tackle your doubting and checking OCD, seriously consider first reading Chapter 6 on overcoming resistance. If the material in that chapter doesn't make you feel fully prepared, consult a mental-health professional for assistance. You should also make an appointment with a professional if your own efforts stall at any point.

Note: You need to open a file or find something to write on as you work through the following steps.

Step 1. Searching for signals, triggers, and avoidance

The first step in treating doubting and checking OCD involves a little detective work. You must monitor your environment, actions, and behaviors carefully in order to determine what *triggers* (problematic situations and events) set off your doubting and checking cycle. Assessing and listing anything and everything that you find yourself avoiding is a good way to discover these triggers. But try not to be too obsessional in your search.

For example, if you have trouble leaving your home due to fear of burglaries, the need or desire to go out into the world may trigger a cascade of obsessions about the security of your doors and windows. Similarly, if you avoid watching television out of fear that you'll fail to hear someone breaking in, then turning on the television and perhaps other noisy appliances may trigger your OCD. Additional common triggers for doubting and checking OCD include driving, traffic, being in crowds, sneezing, feeling nauseous, and listening to news stories. Actually, the list of possible triggers goes on and on and on, but for now, choose ten or so items from your list so you won't feel overwhelmed. Write these items in your notebook or file.

Occasionally, your problematic triggers may seem to strike from out of the blue. However, usually when you look hard enough, you find something that likely triggered your OCD cycle. Typically, the trigger is a fairly clear-cut event or happening. Other times, it may be something a little vague such as increased stress at work or having had a poor night's sleep.

Step 2. Identifying obsessional doubts

The second step in treating your doubting and checking OCD is to figure out what you fear will happen if you stop avoiding your OCD triggers. These fears constitute your obsessions or doubts. Usually, whatever consequence you fear is rather horrible. That's why it's so hard to give up on checking.

For example, if you went ahead and drove in congested areas and over speed bumps, what do you think the consequence would be? If you have hit-and-run worries, the consequence is likely to be pretty clear, you fear that you will cause someone's death or serious injury. Write down the obsessions or feared consequences of encountering your triggers in your notebook.

Step 3. Compiling compulsions

A critical component of your doubting and checking OCD treatment is making a list of your compulsions. These compulsions include checking and safety behaviors. Checking compulsions involve all the things you do to see whether your worst fears have actually occurred or not, such as:

>> Checking your locks

>> Returning to the scene of a feared accident

>> Going to the doctor to check out your latest physical symptom

>> Checking to make sure the stove is turned off

>> Reviewing the newspaper for stories about car accidents you may have caused

Ritualistic safety behaviors are another type of compulsion and encompass things you do to prevent your fears from occurring. These include rituals such as checking your stove exactly 14 times while counting out loud from 1 to 14. Other safety compulsions include repeating certain words or phrases to prevent bad things from happening and carrying lucky charms to accomplish the same goal. Safety behaviors often have a superstitious or magical flavor to them (see Chapter 17 for OCD that focuses on superstitions and other magical thinking). Write down your list of compulsions and safety behaviors in your notebook.

Robyn's story illustrates how someone with severe doubting and checking OCD goes about finding the triggers, obsessions (feared consequences), and checking compulsions for her OCD cycle.

Robyn has doubting and checking OCD that focuses on worries about harming others with her car (see the section "Harming others with your car through negligence"). Her OCD has progressively worsened over the past few years. Today, she can rarely manage to drive anywhere at all. Robyn identifies the actual events, situations, and triggers for her hit-and-run concerns. She comes up with this list of triggers:

- Driving in congested areas
- Driving near bike lanes
- Driving near crosswalks
- Driving near sidewalks
- Driving on bumpy roads
- Driving with passengers in the car due to the distraction
- Going over speed bumps

Robyn ponders the obsessional fears that she believes will occur if she stops avoiding her OCD triggers. The answer is pretty obvious: She assumes that the likelihood of her harming or killing someone with her car will skyrocket.

She reflects on the following obsessions or feared consequences of encountering her OCD triggers:

1. She runs someone over.

2. The police pull her over and arrest her.

3. She is driven to jail in handcuffs.

4. She appears in court.

5. She is found guilty of negligent manslaughter and is sentenced to ten years in jail.

These obsessions cause Robyn to engage in an array of compulsive checking. She does this by

» Returning to the place of the perceived accident over and over again until she feels she can go on

» Examining the exterior of her car for an hour twice each week

» Having her car washed twice a week to facilitate her examination of her car

Her compulsions also include safety behaviors:

» She drives only on certain uncongested roadways.

» She repeats the words "break a leg" as she drives.

» She drives five miles an hour below the speed limit.

With these lists of triggers, obsessions, and compulsions in hand, Robyn is prepared to take on the next step in her OCD treatment — disputing doubts.

Step 4. Disputing obsessional doubts

If you suffer from the doubting and checking type of OCD, it is distressing for you. This type of OCD centers on obsessional worries about caring for others, keeping the home safe, and staying healthy. Checking feels like a logical response because the imagined consequences of harming others, watching a home burn down, or becoming seriously ill are harsh. The fact that you and others with this type of OCD may resist direct challenges to these worries is understandable.

Resistance is a common response to exposure and response prevention (ERP) therapy (see the next section).

However, if you start by learning to rethink the way you view doubt, you may feel better prepared to undergo ERP (which is the next step). OCD doubts are not based on evidence. In contrast, realistic doubts stem from logical information. To help you figure out whether your doubts are realistic or based on your OCD, ask yourself the following questions (see Chapter 8 for more on this and other strategies for rethinking doubts):

>> **Are your doubts based on direct information from your senses (sight, sound, smell, taste, or touch)?** Most OCD doubts are not based on one's senses.

>> **Does your doubt seem to have a life of its own and keep coming back, even without new evidence to support it?** OCD doubts typically do continually return over and over without fresh evidence.

>> **Is there anything about your doubt that other people would see as illogical?** If your doubt is OCD, people likely see it as very illogical.

>> **Is there anything that would convince you that your doubt is likely false?** If you have OCD, you likely can't be convinced that your doubt is false, no matter what the evidence says.

REMEMBER

Obsessional doubts come from your OCD mind. Doubts are not grounded by rational thinking. If your doubts persist in spite of contradictory evidence, then OCD is at work.

For example, in the preceding section I discussed Robyn, whose obsessional doubts center on the fear of running someone over with her car, being arrested, and going to jail. Following are her answers to these questions:

>> **Are your doubts based on direct information from your senses (sight, sound, smell, taste, or touch)?**

I've never experienced hitting someone with my car, so I guess I don't have any direct information about these doubts.

>> **Does your doubt seem to have a life of its own and keep coming back, even without new evidence to support it?**

Yes, my worry continues even when I avoid lots of dangerous intersections and congested traffic. I've had no accidents and nothing has happened that logically would suggest that I might be at special risk for running someone over.

>> **Is there anything about your doubt that other people would see as illogical?**

I don't talk about this with most people. But my close friends think it's pretty crazy. I guess I don't talk about it with more people because I know they would think it's crazy.

>> **Is there anything that would convince you that your doubt is likely false?**

I've never thought about this question before. I guess I can't think of anything that would make me stop believing in my worries.

Robyn reviews her answers and concludes that it's pretty obvious that her doubts are coming from her OCD mind. She still feels wary but is now more willing to consider that these doubts are groundless. And she feels more prepared to engage in ERP, as discussed in the next section.

Step 5. Applying ERP to doubting and checking

REMEMBER

Chapter 10 discusses ERP in depth. Please read that chapter prior to attempting to use ERP for your doubting and checking OCD. It contains step-by-step ERP instructions and guides for troubleshooting problems.

Here are three sample trigger lists relevant to doubting and checking OCD. See Chapter 10 for more about constructing trigger lists and assigning Ugh Factor Ratings to obsessions for virtually any OCD concerns.

Hit-and-run OCD trigger list

As discussed earlier in this chapter, the fear of hitting someone with your car is a relatively common form of doubting and checking OCD. Robyn's example in the preceding two sections is typical of this concern.

She and her psychologist work out a trigger list together, as shown in Table 14-1. Notice that they include a couple of imaginary steps. Obviously, someone with this OCD concern cannot use exposure steps of actually running over a pedestrian! After she completes her list, she carries out ERP as discussed in Chapter 10.

Burning down the house

Fears about home safety dominate the thoughts of some people with doubting and checking OCD. If this reflects your concerns, see Table 14-2 for an example of a few triggers and their Ugh factors. Please realize that your own OCD trigger list could contain a very different list of specific items with different Ugh Factor Ratings.

TABLE 14-1

Robin's OCD Trigger List and Ugh Factor Ratings

OCD Trigger	Ugh Factor Rating (On a Scale of 0–100)
Driving to the grocery store near a congested intersection	70
Driving while other people are in my car (because of distractions)	60
Driving near school crossings	90
Driving near narrow bike lanes	95
Imagining hitting someone with my car	99 plus

TABLE 14-2

OCD Trigger List and Ugh Factor Ratings for Home Safety

OCD Trigger	Ugh Factor Rating (On a Scale of 0–100)
Imagine leaving the coffee pot on	60
Only checking the door locks once before leaving	90
Not checking that all of the windows are closed at night	50
Not rechecking that the stove is turned off before bed	80
Not checking to see that the faucets are turned off	65

Healthy or not

Fears about the state of one's health plague the minds of some of those with doubting and checking OCD. Table 14-3 gives you some sample triggers for this concern. Your particular list could contain very different items and ratings.

Check once with your health-care provider on what symptoms suggest the need for an appointment. Many health insurance companies have helplines with nurses available to answer basic questions about when to see a primary care or urgent care provider. But don't become a frequent checker on the helpline, that could easily become a compulsion.

TABLE 14-3   ## OCD Trigger List and Ugh Factor Ratings for Health Concerns

OCD Trigger	Ugh Factor Rating (On a Scale of 0–100)
Imagine dying from cancer	95
Volunteering at a hospice	90
Not checking your blood pressure daily	50
Seeing a red spot on your face and waiting to make an appointment for a week	70
Going for a week without asking anyone for reassurance about your health	65

Chapter **15**

Subduing OCD-Driven Shame

G enerally speaking, those with OCD are unusually caring, moral, kind, and decent folks. Unfortunately, those with a type of OCD called shaming OCD *believe* quite the opposite of themselves. Their minds fill up with obsessional images involving blatantly immoral, shameful, inappropriate, and humiliating actions. They believe that because those images enter their minds, they will actually put those thoughts into actions.

People with shaming OCD feel so ashamed of their thoughts that they often keep them secret. Therefore, many people with this problem suffer for years and fail to seek help. That's a shame because treatment works.

This chapter describes the major themes of shaming OCD and tells you how to go about treating this problem. I include a discussion about ways to think differently about your worries. Then I show you how to behave in ways that help tackle your shaming OCD.

REMEMBER

This chapter includes examples involving gruesome and horrific scenes. This is not meant to be sensational or to shock you. The reason this material is included is because people with OCD often have these terrible thoughts and worry that this means they may be dangerous or crazy. If you are plagued by gruesome obsessions, realize that you are not insane or a terrible person, you probably have shaming OCD.

Surveying Shaming OCD

Shaming OCD draws on a deep well of self-distrust. People afflicted with this problem vary greatly in terms of the specific themes upon which they base their concerns. However, they all share a profound fear that they may act in ways that will bring them great shame. Thus, one person may believe that they are likely to kill all their loved ones, another may think they will sexually abuse children, and someone else may imagine that they are an immoral sinner who offends God.

The sections that follow reviews the three most common areas of concern for those who suffer from shaming OCD. Those concerns are

» Fearing loss of control

» Questioning sexual identity

» Adhering to extreme religious rules (scrupulosity)

SHAME VERSUS GUILT

Feelings of shame and guilt are reminders that some action or behavior is not acceptable — either morally, legally, or ethically. Although both emotions are negative, they help people know when they have done something wrong. Most people use the words shame and guilt pretty much interchangeably. However, social scientists usually make a distinction between the unpleasant emotions of shame and guilt.

Shame is a personal feeling about oneself and is usually all-encompassing: "I am ashamed of myself," thus means, "I am a bad person." People who are ashamed tend to avoid others, get angry, or become depressed. They appear less likely to do something positive to make up for their deeds. On the other hand, guilt is more specific and adaptive: "I feel guilty that I ran that red light. Next time I'll try to pay more attention," or "I feel guilty about getting angry with my brother." Those who feel guilty are more likely to try to fix the problem or do something to make amends.

The bottom line is that a little guilt isn't all that bad as long as it motivates you to do better in the future. If you feel guilty here and there, you probably have a good, well-functioning conscience. By contrast, shame is rarely helpful because it doesn't point the way to improved behavior.

Being afraid of losing control

Many of those with shaming OCD fear that their thoughts will ultimately turn into actions. They envision themselves acting out uncontrollably. Three areas stand out as concerns for those with the losing-control issue — aggression, sexually acting out, and losing control of bodily functions in public.

When horrible thoughts come into their minds, people with this type of OCD become very judgmental and self-critical. They often say to themselves, "If I have these bad thoughts, then I must be a bad person."

Struggling with thoughts of aggression

Thinking you may be a mass murderer is a whole lot better than actually *being* a mass murderer. But even the contemplation that you may lose control and harm someone else can be quite disturbing.

People with this concern worry that they will snap and do something terrible to someone else. The target of the aggressive impulse could be a stranger or a loved one. Some common worries include

>> What if I am swimming, and I hold my child's head under water?

>> What if I kill my pet?

>> What if I push down someone who is handicapped?

>> What if I slap my boss?

>> What if I walk near a knife, pick it up, and stab someone?

Wrestling thoughts of acting out sexually

One common concern of those with shaming OCD is the fear that they may act out sexually deviant behavior at some point. I'm not just talking about acceptable, though perhaps unusual, sexual practices between consenting adults. When OCD is involved, the feared sexual acts are typically considered highly immoral by the sufferer and even dangerously illegal. Some of the top worries of those with shaming OCD involving sexual concerns include

>> **Thoughts about pedophilia:** This issue involves worrying that one may sexually abuse a child. Mind you, these people do not *want* to abuse a child and actually find the idea utterly abhorrent. However, they have obsessional thoughts about the possibility and constantly check on themselves to

determine whether this could really happen. They interpret minor, meaningless bodily sensations in the genital region as proof positive that they actually are aroused by children. These concerns often cause them to avoid being around playgrounds, schools, and other places where children congregate.

>> **Thoughts about rape:** Those with this concern fear that they may lose control and rape someone. Although occasional rape fantasies are not uncommon, most people don't worry that they'll actually act them out. Those with shaming OCD who have this problem have a different perspective. They believe that even a brief image of a rape scene floating through their minds means they are at real risk of acting it out. Therefore, these folks often avoid being around anyone they can imagine raping.

>> **Thoughts about bestiality:** People who worry about this issue believe that they actually may engage in sex with an animal. They respond to any thought or image about sex with animals as though it means they are actually sexually attracted to animals. Like those with concerns about rape and pedophilia, these people find their thoughts about sex with animals disgusting. They typically avoid being around animals in order to control their imagined urges.

Worrying over losing control of bodily functions

Another interesting theme among those with shaming OCD is the fear of losing control of bodily functions. Those with this affliction fear doing one of the following two distressing things:

>> **Losing bladder or bowel control in public.** People suffering with this OCD issue constantly fret that they may wet or mess themselves in a public place. This feeling of uncertainty plagues people with elimination obsessions. The thoughts and accompanying feelings become so pressing that going out is avoided as much as possible. They monitor their bodies for slight changes and believe that they won't be able to control themselves.

When forced to leave the house, their first step is to find the nearest bathroom. They end up going to the bathroom at every opportunity — even when it's completely unnecessary — just to avoid having a humiliating accident.

>> **Vomiting spontaneously in public.** Others with shaming OCD obsess about the possibility of vomiting in public. Images come into their minds of uncontrollable projectile vomiting in crowded restaurants, at work, or in class.

To avoid such horrific happenings, those plagued with this concern often stop eating out. They also avoid other possible triggers for their concerns, such as opening their mouths to speak in public. These avoidance behaviors can make them seem strange. Finally, they commonly resort to safety behaviors such as taking antacids and anti-nausea drugs prior to going out.

REMEMBER

Some people have medical conditions that could realistically cause loss of control over body functions. They, too, have fears about losing control in public, however this is not considered OCD.

Questioning established sexual identity

The sexual identity theme in shaming OCD calls the very essence of a person's sexuality into question. Unlike the fear of sexually acting out, this worry does not involve aggressive or illegal acts. However, those with this torment feel considerable shame and distress, because the obsessional fears raise questions about their established sexual identity. These fears and thoughts are irrational and come out of the blue.

The example that follows describes someone with this issue.

> **Estabelle,** a happily married woman, begins to wonder whether she's gay. The woman enjoys a healthy sexual relationship with her husband but worries that she is attracted to other women. She starts to study herself for signs that she is aroused by women. She begins looking at lesbian pornography to see whether she finds it arousing and interprets almost any thought or bodily change as evidence of her newfound orientation. She constantly asks her husband for reassurance that he finds her attractive. She is so self-conscious about her sexuality that she finds herself distracted during sex. For the first time, she is unable to have an orgasm. This problem gives her OCD more fuel to question her sexual orientation.

Estabelle's example portrays someone who feels ashamed and extremely confused by the possibility that she may be gay. She is not aroused by thoughts of sexual encounters with women. These thoughts seem to have come out of the blue. Her obsessions are unwanted, frequent, and uncontrolled. And she's not gay.

Being heterosexual, homosexual, bisexual, transgender, or queer are not signs of an emotional problem. However, having obsessional worries about being sexually different — when you're not — is considered a form of OCD. People with this problem usually have some strategies to deal with their obsessions. Some repeatedly ask for reassurance from others about their potential sexual differences. Others challenge themselves by looking at pornography or going to certain types of bars or night clubs. Many avoid situations in which they think they may be tempted to act on their thoughts. These coping strategies can be considered compulsive.

Taking religious or moral beliefs to the extreme

The category of shaming OCD that deals with religion involves adhering to an overly demanding religious or moral code. Those with this form of "religious" shaming OCD, which is also known as *scrupulosity*, obsess over perceived sins, fear losing control of their behavior in religiously inappropriate ways, or endlessly fret over failing to please God. They attempt to relieve the obsessions through compulsive acts such as praying, chanting, asking for reassurance, or confessing. Scrupulosity takes many forms; the following are a few examples:

>> A woman repeats Bible verses over and over because she doubts that she says them correctly.

>> A man at church sees a statue of the Virgin Mary and imagines having sex with her. Now he finds that every time he goes to church, he has similar thoughts and images. He believes that merely having these thoughts is blasphemous. He frequently goes to confession for reassurance, which helps for only a short time.

>> During Yom Kippur, a woman discovers that she has mindlessly chewed on the end of her pencil. Because her religion calls for fasting during this time, she believes that she has sinned. She views many such "transgressions" similarly.

>> During daily prayers, a Muslim man sometimes has sexual thoughts. He views himself as evil.

>> A teenager sits through church service believing that he will suddenly shout out obscenities against God. He resists going to church because of this fear, but then feels he has committed a horrible sin by not going to church.

Scrupulosity can also involve slavish adherence to moral codes that are not based on religion. These codes of conduct go far beyond what most people consider necessary. Thus, those with this concern may review all their actions for the slightest hint of a possible indiscretion or wrongdoing. Some rebuke themselves for giving a compliment that is not 100 percent true. Others think they've committed an *unforgiveable* act if they fail to count their change from a cashier and later realize that they walked away with a nickel too much change.

Treating Shaming OCD

Shaming OCD involves thoughts, feelings, and behavior. The thoughts are usually distorted and highly judgmental. The feelings include self-disgust, shame, humiliation, anxiety, and guilt. Rarely, if ever, does anyone actually act out the behaviors they fear they will. Instead, they avoid situations they think could lead them into trouble. They engage in various safety behaviors and compulsive attempts to neutralize their obsessive thoughts.

Treatment targets both thoughts and behaviors, with the result being an improvement in the way the person feels. The following two sections discuss specific strategies designed to treat shaming OCD thinking and behaving, respectively.

Changing OCD thinking by challenging the evidence

The primary approach to changing your shaming OCD thoughts is what's known as "checking the evidence." This strategy has also been successfully applied to other emotional problems, such as depression and anxiety. It is particularly useful for shaming OCD because the thinking component of this type of OCD is prominent.

Checking the evidence involves carefully reviewing and responding to a variety of questions that help you to challenge your OCD-related thoughts. These questions include the following:

>> Do people I like and respect sometimes have shameful thoughts, too? (*Hint:* If you don't know, consider asking a few very trusted friends.)

>> Have any of my obsessions gone up and down in frequency and intensity over time? If so, what happened in terms of my actual behavior, and why do I think my obsessions vary over time?

>> How many times have my thoughts actually caused me to engage in unacceptable behavior?

>> What would happen if I used the same standards for myself that I have for other people?

>> What would I tell a good friend of mine who told me about having thoughts just like mine?

>> When I am excessively critical of myself, do I end up feeling better or worse?

Take some time to consider these questions and write out your answers. Keep a copy of your answers handy. When you have an obsessive thought, take a look at your responses. Read them out loud. Don't expect an immediate change; continue to work by completing the behavioral exercises in the section that follows on ERP. Here's an example that represents how someone with shaming OCD may respond to the questions:

Tamara, the mother of a 10-month-old boy, was treated for contamination OCD as a teenager and had recovered. She began having strange thoughts shortly after the birth of her baby. She changes a diaper and notices a rash. The thought that the rash is caused by her sexually abusing him flashes in her mind. After that first thought, she feels disgusted and repulsed. But why would that thought come to her mind? Maybe she wants to abuse him, or maybe she is sexually aroused by him. She starts to avoid looking at his genitals when she changes him, but this leads to her not getting him clean, and his rash gets worse. He gets more and more fussy. Tamara can barely make herself hold him because she fears that she will act on her obsessions. Tamara's mind floods with horrible images and thoughts.

Her family members notice how disturbed she is becoming and suggest she check in with her former therapist. Her therapist explains that she has had a relapse of her OCD. He tells her that because she responded to treatment before, she will likely get better quickly. Together, they collect evidence regarding her new obsession. Here are her answers:

>> **Do people I like and respect sometimes have bad thoughts, too?**

I know a lot of people have OCD. And I read somewhere that most people sometimes have thoughts that are just like the thoughts that those of us with OCD have. So probably most of my friends have similar thoughts here and there. They just don't take them as seriously as my OCD mind does.

>> **Have any of my obsessions gone up and down in frequency and intensity over time? If so, what happened in terms of my actual behavior, and why do I think my obsessions vary over time?**

Oh, yes. At one time I was afraid of contamination from all kinds of things — dirt, oil, food, you name it. I think stress had something to do with it. In any case, I guess I can see it's "all just OCD."

>> **How many times have my thoughts actually caused me to engage in unacceptable behavior?**

Well, in truth, it's never actually happened. I can't absolutely know that it won't, but it hasn't yet.

>> **What would happen if I used the same standards for myself that I have for other people?**

I never thought of that. I suppose it would make me less self-critical. Maybe my OCD would drop a little too.

>> **What would I tell a good friend of mine who told me about having thoughts just like mine?**

I would tell a friend that she was just having OCD. My OCD from the past tells me that much. I'd tell her to repeat "There goes my OCD again" each time she had those thoughts.

>> **When I am excessively critical of myself, do I end up feeling better or worse?**

Definitely worse. My OCD jumps up and I just spiral down. I guess trying to be more self-forgiving might help.

After completing the "checking the evidence" questions, Tamara feels significant relief. She still has work to do in therapy but feels more emboldened to take on her OCD. She and her therapist work on some of the techniques described in the next sections.

Using ERP to change shaming OCD

Changing your OCD related behavior is probably the most powerful way to combat your shaming OCD. The primary tool in your OCD toolkit discussed throughout this book is exposure and response prevention (ERP).

ERP is covered in considerable detail in Chapter 10. Please read that chapter thoroughly before you proceed further. There you will see exactly how to carry out ERP and what to do if and when you encounter trouble.

The purpose of this section is to present you with several ERP trigger lists for use with ERP. ERP trigger lists rate the intensity of discomfort (Ugh factor) for those situations that start your OCD thinking.

You won't know what to do with these lists unless you read about ERP in Chapter 10 first. If you were to attempt something without that information, you could easily make things worse for yourself. And please see a professional trained in ERP if you encounter any snags or difficulty. Finally, consult a professional if you have scrupulosity OCD or any shaming OCD issues that concern illegal or highly immoral acts. You need a proper diagnosis as well as careful guidance — but you can be helped! For religious issues, your therapist may want to collaborate with a spiritual advisor.

Losing bladder or bowel control in public

If worries about urinating and/or defecating in public pervade your mind, here's an ERP trigger list involving this theme. Please realize that your personal concerns will vary somewhat (or even greatly) from these items. However, reviewing this sample should help you devise your own set of triggers.

Some people struggle with various medical conditions that may cause actual embarrassing moments. If that's the case for you, various medical treatment options may be available. Unfortunately, for some, the only solution is the use of adult diapers. These do manage to control the embarrassment but check into medical treatments first.

Some people with this form of OCD wear adult diapers not because of any medical condition, but to protect themselves from their worries about accidents, which they typically have never experienced. That's why going without adult diapers is on this list; this is *not* advice for someone with a true medical condition to follow. See table 15-1 for some possible ideas.

TABLE 15-1

Losing Control OCD Trigger List and Ugh Factor Ratings

OCD Trigger	Ugh Factor Rating (On a Scale of 0–100)
Imagine peeing in my pants and everyone stares	95
Traveling on the subway without adult diapers	50
Drinking more than one glass of water at a restaurant	65
Not checking for the location of bathrooms in an unfamiliar mall	75
Taking a long airplane trip without diapers	99 plus

WARNING

Don't get so compulsive with your ERP that you actually cause yourself severe pain and distress from avoiding voiding.

Notice that a trigger list can contain items that occur only in the mind as well as some that you actually carry out. That's because carrying some of these situations out with real actions would indeed be pretty darned embarrassing! Fortunately, you don't have to venture out into the world and truly pee in your pants.

Vomiting in public

Now it's time to review a nauseating trigger list. Just for the record, I'm pretty sure that most people don't especially enjoy vomiting. However, those with this kind of shaming OCD worry about vomiting every day. They avoid eating out and anything else that could possibly make them feel nauseous and vomit.

WARNING

It is *possible* that carrying out some of these triggers in Table 15-2 could result in you becoming somewhat nauseous and even vomiting. If a given item starts to make you quite nauseous, you may want to back away and try an easier one. However, it's okay if you get nauseous or vomit. People do vomit, and the consequences of doing so are not nearly as horrific as your OCD mind tells you. If you find the asks too scary, enlist the help of a professional.

TABLE 15-2

Vomiting OCD Trigger List and Ugh Factor Ratings

OCD Trigger	Ugh Factor Rating (On a Scale of 0–100)
Putting vomit soup in your mouth (see sidebar for recipe) and spitting it out	99
Pull your abdomen muscles in and out rapidly	55
Imagine being on an airplane with severe turbulence and having to vomit in a bag	45
Walking in an alley late at night and smelling urine and vomit	80
Watch videos of vomiting repeatedly	75

EEEW, GROSS: VOMIT SOUP

If you can carry out this instruction, you're very likely to make great strides with your vomiting-in-public worries. Note that this item will likely be extremely difficult if vomiting in public is your primary OCD worry. Some therapists with considerable expertise in treating this issue concoct a brew that has much the same look and feel of vomit. Here's our own recipe.

The base of any good vomit recipe is soup. You can choose your own brand. I recommend a vegetable soup such as green pea, minestrone, or plain old vegetable. Make sure the soup has some color and good chunks in it. Next, you need a little more

(continued)

(continued)

texture. Soft curd cottage cheese is always good. Exact portions are not important, but a little more than a quarter cup is enough. Add a little carbonated beverage of your choice to give the mix a few bubbles (I don't recommend champagne for this one unless you're also trying to give that up).

Mix up some of this lovely potion. Then fill your mouth with it while in a bathroom. Roll it around, make a good gagging sound and spit it out into a toilet. If you spill a bit on the toilet seat, that's great. This is true exposure. Repeat as needed until your anxiety drops significantly or until you can't stop laughing. Yum.

Complementary Treatments for Shaming OCD

The preceding strategies are your primary tools for use against shaming OCD. However, a few techniques can be useful add-ons. You can think of these techniques as experiments. Try them out and see what data comes in.

Revealing to others

Those with shaming OCD usually hide their OCD thoughts from others. They work hard to conceal what they label as their hidden shame. That's because they're convinced that others would be repulsed and/or would reject them outright.

However, hiding your shaming OCD prevents you from hearing a more reasonable perspective. Therefore, I suggest that you start by marshaling your courage and finding a therapist. Therapists are highly trained in being nonjudgmental.

After you reveal your hidden thoughts to a therapist, the two of you can work out a plan to open up with a few highly trusted people in your life as well. Doing so enables you to see whether they interpret your OCD thoughts in a more benign, less judgmental way. If you open up with three or four close, trusted friends, the odds are you'll see that they attach less significance to your thoughts than you do. Hopefully, this information will help you see that your thoughts are not as meaningful as actions and that they stem from the OCD part of your mind.

REMEMBER

Of course, it's always possible that you may pick a judgmental, rejecting person to reveal your thoughts to. But accepting a degree of uncertainty is part of treating OCD. If you do encounter a bad reaction, a therapist can help you work through the incident. And one final word of advice: Don't *continually* seek the counsel of others because doing so can morph into reassurance seeking, something I frequently warn against.

Experimenting with being "off duty"

Most people with shaming OCD vigilantly monitor their thoughts and behaviors in order to prevent themselves from actually carrying out their feared, shameful actions. They mistakenly believe that it is only this monitoring that stands in the way of them engaging in one of these acts, such as shouting out obscenities in church, acting out sexually, or vomiting in public.

Try experimenting with periods of "off duty" for this type of OCD. "Off duty" is a time span during which you consciously cease vigilant monitoring of yourself for the possibility that you might engage in some shameful act. You can start with an hour in which you decide not to monitor yourself at all. Then try extending that time period to three hours, a full day, and so on.

After each "off duty" period, jot down whether anything catastrophic occurred or whether you actually lost control. Then try experimenting with times of "ultra-vigilance." During those times, try to control and actively monitor every single thought and action. After the "ultra-vigilance" period, jot down whether you felt safer and whether you felt more in control or out of control.

Most of the time, this experiment leads people to conclude that their excessive vigilance does nothing to protect them. It doesn't make them feel safer or better. In fact, most people feel much worse during their periods of "ultra-vigilance." The paradoxical lesson from this exercise is that *you will feel more in control as you let go of your need to be in control.*

Experimenting with self-critical versus self-accepting views

Those afflicted with shaming OCD almost always believe that they suffer from severe deficiencies in control and morality. They seem to believe they are inherently defective as human beings. They manage to "prove" their inherent defectiveness by examining everything they do from a highly critical, judgmental perspective.

But what would happen if you experimented with turning this cycle on its head? That's what I ask you to do here. First, designate a full day to engaging in harsh, critical scrutiny of each and every thing you do. For example, right now, I could beat up on myself for not typing fast enough or failing to word each sentence in the best possible way. Similarly, you could berate yourself for failing to read quickly enough or understand the full meaning of each word and sentence.

Jot down notes here and there during your "critical" day. Notice how you feel and whether your shaming OCD concerns increase or decrease. I'm betting that your concerns will rise.

Then choose a full day in which you decide to view yourself in a neutral, benign way. When you have OCD thoughts, merely say to yourself, "There goes my OCD mind again, how interesting." If a disturbing image floats through your mind, do the same. If you make a mistake, say, "I guess that makes me human." View all your OCD thoughts as though they are as meaningless as particles of dust.

Again, jot down notes on how you feel during your neutral, self-accepting day. See if you feel better or worse when you drop your self-critical stance. If you feel better, and I think you will, consider extending these periods to a week, then a month, and, ultimately, for the rest of your life.

Chapter **16**

Messing with "Just So" OCD

Symmetry refers to pleasing balance and proportionality. Symmetry is found in classical art and architecture. Faces, leaves, and butterfly wings are generally balanced and symmetrical. People normally feel comfortable when surrounded by order and symmetry. Having a place for everything and seeing everything in its place can be reasonably satisfying. But life has a way with messing with neatly ordered garages, kitchens, and office desks. Most people are okay with this.

Some people with OCD crave order and symmetry in everything all the time. They are not satisfied or comfortable until certain things are done or ordered correctly, precisely, or "just so." Their concerns vary; some arrange books or cupboards; others rewrite letters or numbers. However, they share the same feeling of discomfort when things don't feel right, just so, or complete.

This chapter describes the common concerns of those with what I call *just so OCD*. I tell you how to change your thinking surrounding this type of OCD. Changing your thinking helps you prepare for changing your behaviors. After you've changed your thoughts and behaviors, you're likely to start feeling better, even when things are out of place.

Being Driven to Make Things Just So All the Time

Just so OCD frequently begins in childhood. You can see elements of this issue in many normal childhood activities. Lots of children arrange their toys in special ways, enjoy reading the same book over and over again, and have bedtime rituals. Usually, these patterns, which help provide a needed sense of security and comfort, slowly fade over the years. As children grow and mature, they recognize that the comfort and security they experienced was not created by the patterns, but rather by parents and caregivers. But in some children, either because of biology or learning (see Chapters 4 and 5), OCD takes over.

For children with the just so type of OCD, the urge to find symmetry, order, and feelings of just so increases over time instead of fading. Their lives begin to fill with distress and rituals designed to make them feel better. This pattern can continue for a lifetime.

Just so OCD often exists along with other forms of OCD. For example, someone may believe that arranging the closet just so is necessary to please God. This driven, excessive need to please God stems from shaming OCD that focuses on religious issues (see Chapter 15). Another person may arrange the closet just so in the belief that it's necessary in order to keep the family safe. In this case, the person has the doubting and checking type of OCD along with the just so type. Finally, people with *just* the just so OCD may arrange their closets because they feel driven to have their clothes just so.

Unfortunately, research is currently lacking for the treatment of just so OCD. In part, this neglect in literature appears to be due to the fact that many of those with this type of OCD don't seem as interested in changing as those afflicted with other OCD types. They view their need for symmetry and order as the right way to be. This belief may be held in spite of family and friends complaining, teasing, or even getting angry with the just so behaviors.

Yet, some folks with this problem do want to do something about their OCD. They may want to change because they realize how much time their need for order and symmetry takes or because they are responding to others' complaints. If the desire to change describes you or someone you care about, read on. On the other hand, if you have this type of OCD and don't want to do anything about it, maybe you'll find what comes next in this chapter interesting.

SHIFTING GEARS AND SYMMETRY

The symptoms of OCD are quite varied. Some people with OCD have obsessions and compulsions about harming others; others collect useless junk; others have obsessions and compulsions requiring order and symmetry. These forms of OCD may involve different areas of the brain.

A study reported in the journal *Neuropsychology* looked at the way people with and without OCD were able to shift their attention from one thing to another. They also looked at how types of OCD differently affected the performance of tasks that required this ability. Shifting attention or set shifting involves responding to information from the environment by changing your focus. Set shifting is involved when you learn from your mistakes or solve problems through trial and error.

What they found was that people with the need for order and symmetry, what can be called just so OCD, had more trouble than others shifting attention. So how might this play out in real life? People with trouble shifting attention may have difficulty changing from one activity to another, multi-tasking, using feedback, or solving problems. And perhaps some of them have trouble shifting away from the need for order, symmetry, and having things around them just so.

TECHNICAL STUFF

Most obsessions and compulsions are not welcome by the person who has them. The technical term for this offensiveness is *ego-dystonic.* On the other hand, *ego-syntonic* refers to the feeling that one's obsessions and compulsions are appropriate and merely reflect one's values. Symmetry, or just so OCD, is often ego-syntonic.

The rest of this section looks at the two primary expressions of just so OCD:

>> **Arranging:** Seeking order

>> **Repeating:** Seeking perfection

Enforcing order and symmetry on life

If you suffer with the *arranging expression* of just so OCD, you are focused on arranging the environment in certain ways. You want particular things around you to be perfectly symmetrical, smooth, clean, or orderly. This need for order can take on any number of areas. Here are a few examples:

>> **Books:** Some people spend hours each day arranging their books by size and shape. Others consume time by precisely measuring the distance between the edge of the shelf and each book. Some order books alphabetically by author or, oddly enough, the first word that appears in the book. Still others dust each book every day or arrange them by color. There's no end to the permutations of these arrangements, but everyone with this concern feels driven to arrange books in some special, personally meaningful way.

>> **Carpet fibers and fringe:** This concern is surprisingly common. More than a few folks straighten the fringe on their rugs many times each day. You can imagine how easily a few pieces of fringe can be disturbed by a cat, the wind, or people walking around. Others repeatedly vacuum and pick at any stray fibers. They want each and every strand of carpet to stand up straight and in the same way. Yikes.

>> **Food:** People with this focus arrange food in their refrigerators, cupboards, and pantries in various and sundry ways. The arrangement may be alphabetical or by size, shape, color, nutritional content, or weight. Another food-related compulsion is the need to arrange food on the plate or table in very specific ways. I'm not talking about a "nice presentation" here, but a precise, rigid pattern based on unusual rules. And after sitting down to eat, some people feel driven to eat in a fixed pattern — again, based on arbitrary ideas about what constitutes the right order.

>> **Money:** Of course, many people like to arrange their wallets with the ones, fives, tens, and twenties in consecutive order. However, people with this OCD concern repeatedly arrange, smooth, and check their bills. Sometimes they even iron them each day. Others keep their change on their dressers in peculiar, precise, patterns.

>> **Other stuff:** As noted earlier, the particular items that must be arranged, straightened, ordered, or made just so varies greatly. Pictures on the wall must be perfectly level and aligned. The hangers in the closet must be evenly spaced. Clothes, whether on hangers or in drawers, may have to be arranged in special orders by color, function, or texture. Decorations throughout the home have their specific spaces, which cannot be altered. Pillows on the couch must be arranged in certain ways. Items on a desk may need to be arranged in idiosyncratic ways. Shoes must shine without the slightest scuff.

REMEMBER

In order for concerns about symmetry and keeping things just so to be considered OCD, they must consume a significant amount of time and interfere with your life significantly. Many people have a dollop of fussiness without having OCD.

Trying to get it right by repeating and redoing

If you suffer with the *repeating expression* of just so OCD, you focus on the need to repeat and redo actions until they feel just right. There are no objective criteria for what constitutes just so because it's based on a purely subjective feeling. If you ask people with this type of OCD how they know when something is just so, they're likely to answer, "I just know; I can feel it." Sometimes the repeating and redoing goes on for hours. Examples of the repeating and redoing expression include:

>> **Dressing:** This routine involves dressing and arranging one's clothes over and over again, until it all feels and looks just right. Picking just the right clothes can be part of this pattern, but the person may not know what's going to feel just right until everything is on. Then, if it doesn't feel just right, they may start their dressing routine all over again.

>> **Evening up:** This issue has to do with a need for achieving a feeling of evenness. Someone with this concern may feel a need to open doors with the left hand as often as the right hand. Some people feel driven to chew their food as much on the right side of their mouth as the left side. Still others work hard to make sure that their socks come up to exactly the same height on each ankle. A few folks try to keep conversations evened up by tracking how long each person speaks and trying to match them in duration. All of these actions require lots of repeating and redoing before that perfect feeling of evenness is achieved. And, of course, the feeling doesn't last.

>> **Reading and writing:** Reading redoing entails the need to read, reread, and reread until the person feels that the material has been completely and fully absorbed and understood. Mind you, the person probably understands the material well enough on the first read; it's just based on a "feeling." Worry about the slightest ambiguity or imperfection in one's written work can cause someone to redo his or her writing many times over. It's a darn good thing I don't suffer from this problem!

>> **Cleaning routines:** OCD categories tend to overlap. Some people have ritualistic cleaning compulsions to alleviate their need to have perfectly cleaned homes (just so). This differs from the emotionally driven cleaning of someone who suffers contamination fears. People who engage in this type of cleaning need specific order and cleanliness because of craving perfection.

>> **Showering or washing routines:** You may think that long cleaning rituals sound like contamination OCD (see Chapter 2 and 13). But in this case, the worry isn't so much about contamination as it is in getting things to feel right. Therefore, the person scrubs and washes different body parts in certain sequences and ways until the feeling of just right occurs. This process can take hours.

The list for repeating and redoing potentially goes on and on and on. I could include more items, but this list feels just right.

Taking Steps to Change Just So OCD

Earlier in this chapter, I note that many people with the just so type of OCD waffle on whether or not they want to do something about the problem, or whether they view it as a problem at all. If that description fits you, I recommend that you read Chapter 6 first on the topic of overcoming OCD obstacles. That's where you find ways of exploring and possibly enhancing your motivations for change if you indeed want to consider changing. If loved ones or others around you are indicating that you may have an issue, then working with a therapist to determine your need for change may be helpful.

Assuming you do find the motivation for change, you should know that there are two primary approaches to treating just so OCD:

>> By addressing ways to change your OCD thinking

>> By tackling your OCD behavior

I generally recommend employing both strategies for this and other types of OCD. Medication is also an option (see Chapter 11), though medications may not be quite as effective for this specific type of OCD.

Rearranging your thinking

Chapter 8 reviews many of the ways that the thinking of those with OCD becomes distorted. That distorted thinking usually worsens OCD symptoms. Interestingly, many of these thought distortions do not seem to play a large role in those plagued with the just so type of OCD. Thus, those with just so OCD do not tend to exaggerate risk, struggle with uncertainty, feel excessive responsibilities, or confuse their thoughts with what's real.

However, those with just so OCD do have some beliefs that get them in trouble and keep them bogged down. These beliefs are about

>> Self-image

>> Handling difficult emotions

Each one is discussed in the sections that follow.

Rethinking self-image

At some level, most of those with just so OCD feel that the directives from their OCD minds are the correct way that they should approach their lives. You may feel like you wouldn't be you without your order and symmetry or just so OCD. Papers *should* be orderly, books in their place, and everything smooth, perfect, and even. And within limits, a little order does feel good.

However, if you think that just maybe your just so issues have gone too far, try answering the following questions:

» Does the time I spend making everything just so take away important time for other, more meaningful activities such as my friends, family, work responsibilities, spiritual practice, hobbies, or other interests?

» Would I tell someone I care about that this (ensuring that everything is just so) is a good way to spend lots of time? Would I tell them that the OCD is about who they are as a person?

Heather's example shows how pondering these questions helps motivate her to work on this problem because she begins to see her OCD as OCD and not as herself.

Heather keeps a clean house. Each day, she cleans every room from top to bottom. Each dish, food item, decoration, picture, and book has its own place. All the closets in her house are organized by type of clothing, and hangers are 1/2-inch apart. Heather spends hours keeping her house clean; she rarely goes out. Her teenage children are never home because they prefer to spend time at homes where the parents are less uptight.

Heather is shocked to learn that her oldest son has been arrested for shoplifting. She is required by her son's probation officer to attend family counseling. Here are the answers she comes up with concerning her belief that she just wouldn't be herself without her just so OCD.

» **Does the time I spend on making everything just so take away important time for other, more meaningful activities?**

I'd estimate that my just so OCD takes me at least three or more hours each day. If I spent just a few of those hours each week on quality time with my family, everyone would be happier. The feelings are powerful, but so is the value in trying to overcome this problem.

I realize that I spend many hours yelling at my family to clean up that I could have spent doing something more meaningful. I feel pretty bad that my kids don't want to be home because I am so obsessed with housecleaning.

» **Would I tell people I care about that this (ensuring that everything is just so) is a good way to spend lots of time? Would I tell them that the OCD is about who they are as a person?**

No way. I'd tell my friends, my husband, or my kids to do anything and everything they could to stop spending time this way. I know doing the things I do is pointless and silly. I'd tell them that spending time this way will detract from their lives, as I can see it has from mine. This OCD stuff isn't about who they are or who I am as a person; it just feels that way to me sometimes.

These questions help Heather step back a little from the directives coming out of her OCD mind. She can now see that the time she spends on her OCD costs her a lot and that she would never recommend that anyone else do what she does. She can also see that the OCD is not about who she is as a person; it's just her OCD mind talking when she thinks otherwise. She starts making progress with her just so behavior.

Rethinking emotional responses

You may believe that you just can't tolerate having things unfinished, incomplete, or out of order. It no doubt does *feel* like you can't stand the feelings you have when things seem this way. If you have this problem, you likely feel unbalanced, tense, anxious, and out of it, along with a sense of urgency to bring your feelings back to "normal." When things are back in order, you feel significant relief for a while, but the out-of-sorts feelings soon return. Try answering these questions about not being able to stand these feelings.

» Have you ever had prolonged pain from an injury, dental work, or illness? If so, were you able to stand it, and was it as difficult as your OCD obsessions?

» Do you think the urges would continue at the same intense level forever if you kept yourself from caving into them?

» Were there ever things in the past that you detested doing, yet found ways to tolerate? Is it possible that your just so OCD urges could become tolerable over time?

Jackson's story involves a slightly different form of just so OCD, and he uses these questions to help him see that he probably can stand having some uncomfortable feelings for a while.

Jackson has just so OCD and focuses on a variety of ordering issues as well as redoing concerns. He has very specific ways that everything on his nightstand must be lined up, or he believes he cannot go to sleep. He also reads notes about his job assignment for the next day each night. However, he feels he must read and reread until he has completely understood each and every part of the assignment. He knows this reading should require about five or ten minutes, but he usually can't stop until he's read the material slowly at least ten times, a process that takes him an hour and a half most nights. He believes that stopping his driven OCD behaviors would drive him crazy and that he simply couldn't stand going through each day any other way.

» Have you ever had prolonged pain from an injury, dental work, or illness? If so, were you able to stand it, and was it as difficult as your OCD obsessions?

I remember playing on my college football team. I got injured often, but once I broke my ankle in two places. It hurt for weeks while I hobbled around. I'd have to say that the pain from that injury actually felt worse than the feelings of incompleteness I have when I resist my OCD for a while.

» Do you think the urges would continue at the same intense level forever if you kept yourself from caving into them?

It does sort of feel like they would continue forever. But now that I think about it, I can recall a few times when I resisted the urges for a few hours and the feelings actually started to come down a little. Maybe if I continued that work, the feelings would come down even more.

» Were there ever things in the past that you detested doing, yet found ways to tolerate? Is it possible that your just so OCD urges could become tolerable over time?

I remember that for years I absolutely hated paying bills and balancing my checkbook. I almost couldn't get myself to do it at all. It's funny, but now I don't mind those tasks. Sometimes I even look at balancing the checkbook as a challenge when it seems a little off at first. I get the point; maybe if I work really hard at it, my just so OCD could be a little like my hating to pay bills and balance my checkbook. Over time, it just might get better.

Jackson's work on these questions helps him to see that feelings can change over time. And he now realizes that he can stand all sorts of uncomfortable feelings for a while. He feels more confident that if he tolerates the discomfort, his urges will slowly but surely fade. He happens to be right.

Redoing your responses to repeating

Exposure and response prevention (ERP), described in Chapter 10, is widely considered the most effective treatment for OCD. Refer to that chapter for detailed instructions on carrying out ERP. Here are some sample trigger lists for just so OCD.

The example ERP trigger lists are just that — examples. The actual content for your particular list will vary considerably. However, these examples give ideas for how to construct your own.

Many people with just so OCD may need some extra support in their attempts at ERP. I suggest getting help from a mental-health professional trained in ERP.

In the sections that follow there are examples of ways to use ERP to address the two primary expressions of just so OCD: arranging and repeating.

Applying ERP to ordering and symmetry

Sometimes, being organized and having a place for everything is pretty nice. But when this type of OCD gets out of hand, life can become pretty miserable for the person with this arranging expression and any family members who are involved. Table 16-1 presents an example of an ERP trigger list for someone with order and symmetry concerns. In simple terms, you start with one item on your list and do it (or do it for increasing periods of time) until you feel that you can handle a bit of disorder in your life.

Applying ERP to repeating and redoing

Repeating and redoing can become time consuming and interfere greatly with functioning. This can be especially problematic if you are required to read or produce written products at school or work. Having to do things over and over again slows you down. See Table 16-2 for a sample exposure trigger list for this type of concern.

TABLE 16-1

Symmetry and Order Trigger List and Ugh Factor Ratings

OCD Trigger	Ugh Factor Rating (On a Scale of 0–100)
Leaving junk mail on the counter instead of immediately throwing it away	40
Waiting until morning to put dinner dishes into the dishwasher	90
Not making the bed perfectly in the morning	75
Leaving the blinds on the windows uneven	80
Messing up the fringe on the rug	65
Putting a few books out of order on the shelves	30
Not keeping the desk in the right order	50
Putting some clothes in the wrong spot	80
Not arranging the dishes in the dishwasher in the correct way	90

TABLE 16-2

Repeating and Redoing OCD Trigger List and Ugh Factor Ratings

OCD Trigger	Ugh Factor Rating (On a Scale of 0–100)
Writing an email and ignoring spellchecker	70
Writing a text and not rereading it twice before sending it	80
Getting ready for work in under one hour	90
Not brushing hair a certain number of times	80
Not reading the news in a particular order in the morning	45
Not brushing teeth in a certain way	50
Not repeatedly rereading work product (maximum of two times)	80
Showering without doing ritual washing from top to bottom	50
Picking out a greeting card to a friend in under 10 minutes	55
Washing clothes and mixing light colors with dark colors	55

Chapter 17

Shrinking Superstitious OCD

G od bless you! Gesundheit (which is German for "health")! These phrases are examples of the custom of giving a blessing to others after they sneeze. Most people say something when in the company of a sneezer, even if they aren't sure why. Such responses to sneezing, like many superstitions, probably have some origins that make a little sense.

The expression "God bless you" may have begun during the bubonic plague in Europe. Sneezing could be the first sign of an illness that often led to death. The blessing was an attempt to stop the disease or provide some spiritual comfort if, in fact, the sneezer was infected. Other beliefs about sneezing include that when someone sneezes, the soul tries to escape, the heart stops, or the devil tries to inhabit the body. What is really known about sneezing is that it causes zillions of germs to spew out of your nose at about 100 miles an hour!

This chapter discusses superstitious OCD. Lots of people have superstitions. I tell you the difference between "normal" beliefs, superstitions, and OCD superstitions. Next, I present the most common superstitions associated with superstitious OCD and give you techniques for challenging superstitious OCD thinking and behavior.

Seeing When Superstitions Constitute OCD

A popular old song asks the question, "Do you believe in magic?" You probably base most of your beliefs on what you observe, what you can prove, and what you have been taught. So, you observe that the sky is blue, you can prove that apples fall to the ground, and you have been taught that Abraham Lincoln was the president of the United States during the Civil War.

You've probably heard that some people consider the number 13 to be associated with bad luck. Do you believe that? If you do, then what do you base your belief on? If you think about it, you can't observe, prove, or base a belief that the number 13 is connected to bad luck on any real or factual evidence. When a belief is disconnected from any proof or facts, it is very likely a superstition.

Maybe the number 13 makes you a bit uncomfortable, but you really don't live most of your life thinking about the number 13. In fact, you probably rarely give the number much thought at all. If that's the case, your superstition about the number doesn't interfere with your life. Thus, you have a superstition, but it's not superstitious OCD.

If you have superstitious OCD and view 13 as something to be avoided, you may refuse to go outside on the 13th day of each month. You may feel compelled to avoid looking at the number 13 or refuse to exit the elevator onto the 13th floor. You may find yourself avoiding groups of 13 people at meetings or restaurants. You strongly believe that the number 13 must be avoided, or it will in some way hurt you or people you care about. You may struggle to get through this paragraph because of all the number 13s that appear in it. I thought about making this Chapter 13 but decided not to take the risk!

The difference between general superstition and superstitious OCD is that OCD consumes your mind and steals significant time from enjoying your life. Think of a continuum of belief. At one end is not taking something too seriously (like bad luck associated with the number 13); at the other end is believing in something wholeheartedly despite a lack of evidence or experience — and then taking time-consuming actions to avoid the superstition.

REMEMBER

Those with superstitious OCD have unwanted *obsessions,* which are thoughts, images, or urges about their superstition. They also have *compulsions,* which are mental rituals or patterns of actions, that they perform in order to neutralize or decrease the discomfort of the obsession.

REMEMBER

Various types of OCD overlap with each other. Seeing elements of superstitious OCD associated with other types of OCD is particularly common. However, I present superstitious OCD separately because some people suffer primarily from this type of OCD and show few or no signs of other types of OCD.

Revealing Common OCD Superstitions and Rituals

Like most expressions of OCD, those involving superstitions are infinite and mostly unique. Obsessions and compulsions often start with common superstitions, such as thinking that 13 is unlucky, but become odder and increasingly complex. A few superstition themes are particularly common. Here are some examples, along with a few of the ways that people try to neutralize them through various compulsive rituals:

>> **Cats:** Cats are a common worry among those with superstitious OCD. Black cats, of course, stand out and are seen as inflicting bad luck or harm when they cross one's path. Some also believe that cats can suck the breath out of babies if left unattended for even a moment around an infant. Those with superstitious OCD sometimes feel inclined to "undo" the effects of cat encounters by carrying lucky symbols, turning in circles seven times, or saying "tac" seven times in their minds in order to cancel out the cat because tac is cat spelled backwards.

>> **Cemeteries and death:** Cemeteries, words related to death, and symbols of death often create consternation for many of those with superstitious OCD. These folks typically avoid driving by funeral homes and cemeteries. They try to avoid passing by a hearse or even letting their eyes pass over the obituary section in a newspaper. When they do have the misfortune of confronting one or more of these death-related objects or symbols, they feel driven to neutralize the event. Some may need to chant the word "life" over and over again. Others may need to plant nine new flowers in their gardens. You can imagine how full those gardens become.

>> **Colors:** For many, black means death and evil. Red represents blood and injury or ill health. If these colors are thought about or encountered, the person may feel a need to neutralize them by performing any number of rituals, such as tapping a foot, praying, imagining another color, or spelling the color backwards.

>> **Numbers:** Those with superstitious OCD commonly believe in lucky numbers and unlucky numbers. Numbers can have any kind of significance. For example, a man may read license plate numbers and have to stop his car whenever he encounters a plate with the number three in it. A woman may fear the number four and worry that thinking about the number or encountering it in her daily life will cause harm to herself or her family unless she finds a way to neutralize the number. When she sees or thinks about four, she must walk in counterclockwise circles eight times to neutralize the number's effects.

>> **Symbols:** Some carry around grave concerns about the meaning of various symbols that, like certain words, can convey either positive or negative powers. Symbols frequently associated with positive energy and good luck include four-leaf clovers, rabbits' feet, ankhs, horseshoes, rosary beads, shamrocks, and swallows. Symbols viewed as bad or evil include the inverted pentagram, the zodiac, a goat's head, an upside-down cross, and a hand held in a horned position. When people encounter negative or evil symbols, they often feel compelled to neutralize their effects either by bringing out a positive symbol or by engaging in one or more rituals, such as chanting "God please protect me and those I love" 14 times.

>> **Words:** Some people believe that certain words transmit good energy and other words have bad, or even evil, power. Words often thought to be infused with inherent good energy include: "good," "God," "beneficent," "love," "sharing," "kindness," "soothe," and "relax." Sometimes bad words actually have no inherently negative meaning at all for most people. They become seen as bad because they are associated with an unpleasant event in the person's life. For example, a woman may associate the word "table" with hearing about a loved one's death because she was sitting at a table when she was told about the death. Thus, she may feel compelled to cross herself three times whenever she hears that word.

The preceding list is very incomplete. Superstitions come in a dizzying array of forms. Following are just a few miscellaneous superstitions to give you an idea:

>> Breaking a mirror brings seven years of bad luck.

>> Leaving your shoes upside down causes bad luck to visit.

>> Dropping a pair of scissors causes your spouse to be unfaithful.

>> Failing to compensate anyone who gives you a knife or anything sharp causes harm to come to you.

>> Walking under a ladder brings bad luck.

>> Failing to lift your feet up when driving over a railroad track causes bad luck.

Those with superstitious OCD take these superstitions seriously and feel compelled to do all kinds of strange things to undo them when the feared events occur. I give you only a few sample rituals so that you get the idea. Trying to think up a ritual that no one actually uses is a little like trying to find a username that no one else has ever used.

When people use neutralizing rituals, they typically believe that they must be performed with perfect precision. If anything goes wrong in the execution of a ritual, it must be repeated over and over until it feels perfect. This repeating until perfect is similar to "just so" OCD, which is discussed in Chapter 15.

EVIL IN WASHINGTON, D.C.?

The *Washington Post* reported on a superstition that some people believe about the capitol of the United States — Washington, D.C. Apparently, these folks believe that the city harbors profound satanic forces because one can draw a demonic pentagram by connecting the dots formed by these important landmarks: Dupont Circle, Logan Circle, Mount Vernon Square, the White House, and Washington Circle. Others add to this "evidence" by pointing to the fact that the Freemasons had an important hand in designing major structures throughout the city. They assume that the Freemasons collaborated with Satan. Like many Americans, I'm not always that pleased by some of what goes on in Washington, but I sort of doubt it has a lot to do with landmark configurations and Freemasonry. However, I won't presume to speak for Satan!

Changing Thinking About OCD Superstitions

People with superstitious OCD are pretty darned convinced that giving up their ways will result in harm to others or themselves. Because they believe that not adhering to their superstitious beliefs and behaviors will allow something bad to happen, they don't often volunteer for treatment. Why step on that crack when you never know if the one time you do . . . oops, there goes your mother's back. The point is that because people tend to avoid checking out, challenging, or testing the validity of their superstitions, they never find out whether or not they're true.

A problem with superstitious OCD is that the feared consequence is usually vague, can't be disproven, or lies in the distant future. Maybe you worry that opening an umbrella inside, seeing an open umbrella, or hearing the word "umbrella" in your home will cause bad luck. As a result, you basically never go out of the house when it rains and avoid watching the weather on the news.

On Tuesday, you hear the word "umbrella" on the lead-in to the local news; you immediately engage in elaborate exorcisms, turning on all the lights in the house, arranging the hangers in your closet in a particular way, and chanting a prayer 32 times. But, after all that, you go outside and see that the car has a flat tire. Your OCD mind convinces you that the flat tire was caused by hearing the word "umbrella." Wow. That brain is pretty clever. Even if your tire isn't flat, you aren't off the hook. You go to work, and at the lunch table, a colleague mentions that her cousin has been diagnosed with cancer. Your OCD mind tells you the cancer is caused by the utterance of "umbrella."

You can challenge superstitions in a couple of ways:

>> One way is to make up competing superstitions and create playful scenes.

>> Another is to learn to handle moderate feelings of discomfort.

Read about these two change strategies in the next two sections.

WARNING

All OCD change strategies have a slight risk of making you feel worse for a little while. That's especially true for exposure and response prevention (ERP), which I discuss in detail in Chapter 10. If you experience any excessive uptick in your distress or harbor any concerns or worries about conducting any of these exercises, please consult with a mental-health professional for additional help.

Creating competing superstitions

One way to challenge your superstitious OCD thinking is to make up competing stories and practice them. I assume that you have a few troubling superstitions in your head. When you are exposed to these superstitions, you feel uncomfortable. You have some neutralizing rituals like chants, tapping, and counter words.

The idea here is to create what essentially are "fake" superstitions. You choose the object of this fake superstition, and you decide how it works. Because you are making up these competing superstitions, you know they really can't impact you or anyone else. However, by examining these fake superstitions and pretending how you would feel if they were real, hopefully you'll gain insight into how to overcome your active superstitions.

TIP

Make this fun. Be creative and silly.

Get out your notebook and try the following exercise:

1. Pick a neutral word, event, color, or happening that is not connected to your superstitions in any way.

2. Write a few sentences (purely fiction) that turn these words, events, or happenings into superstitions.

3. Choose a few bad outcomes for encountering this word, event, or happening.

4. Write out the actions or mental rituals that are necessary in order to protect you from the new superstition.

    Make sure these actions are not ones you use for your current, active superstitions.

5. **After you've completed Steps 1 through 4, reflect on how you feel.**

Can you think differently about your active superstitions? Are your real superstitions any more logical than the fake one you made up? Yet, does the fake one feel a little less worrisome? If so, what does that tell you? Write down your reflections.

6. **Consider designing three, four, or more of these new, fictional superstitions.**

Being silly with neutral, fake superstitions can loosen up your thinking. You're probably not ready to give up your active superstitions, but maybe you're closer. The next example shows you how one woman used this exercise. It also illustrates how superstitious OCD can become quite quirky.

> **Kate** is required by her OCD to drive at a certain speed that always involves her lucky number 6. The speed depends on what is on the radio when she starts her car. If there is music, she drives 6 miles faster than the posted speed limit. If there is news or talk, she drives 6 miles slower than the speed limit. If she does not follow this rule, she believes her children will be kidnapped. You can imagine how many times she is harassed while driving, which increases her discomfort, as well as her certainty that many bad drivers out there may be watching her in order to take her children.
>
> Kate consults a psychologist who suggests that she try designing new superstitions. This idea sounds a little strange to Kate at first, but she decides to give it a try. Here are two brand new superstitions she comes up with:
>
> **New superstition #1:** Yellow and white lines must be avoided. This is because white lines are suggestive of cocaine, an illegal and immoral drug, plus, yellow is the color of urine. Yellow lines, therefore, are a double whammy. They are both contaminated and evil. If you encounter a yellow line, you must cross yourself eight times while thinking, "blue square, blue square, blue square . . . ." Saying "blue square" neutralizes the yellow line by symbolically blocking its path and turning it green.
>
> **New superstition #2:** If you go through the left door to a store, you will lose all your money. The reason? "Left" sounds like "leave." You may leave your wallet or purse in the store. So, you must enter through the right door. If that door is locked, you need to go to another entrance. If that isn't possible, you must not go to that store. Even when you go through the right door, you may have bad luck because some of your energy may have gone in the left door. Thus, you need to touch eight things using your right hand to prevent bad things from happening.
>
> Kate concludes by thinking about what this exercise has taught her. She tells her psychologist, "I can see how these new superstitions are almost identical to the nature of my real superstitions. I was surprised how easy it was to come up with

them. Yet, these new ones don't really bother me all that much because I know I made them up. In fact, they seem pretty silly. I guess the point is that my OCD mind came up with my original superstitions, too. Maybe I can start challenging these things."

Kate's story shows you how easily the mind can spin into superstitious thinking. You can make up these things out of thin air. If you try your hand at this, you're likely to see how creative your OCD mind really is. Creative, but wrong.

Managing discomfort differently

At the beginning of this chapter, I explain the way most people automatically respond when they hear a sneeze. Most people do some sort of blessing that does not really have much to do with religious belief, superstition, or consideration of the other person. Saying "bless you" when someone nearby sneezes is a habit.

Nothing is inherently wrong with habits. Habits can be useful. You may brush your teeth every day without really thinking about what you're doing. That's a good habit. If you're like most people, not engaging in a habit is somewhat uncomfortable. For instance, if you're unable to brush your teeth before you go to bed, you probably don't feel right. And if you have the habit of saying "bless you" after a sneeze, then stopping yourself from saying "bless you" after someone sneezes is difficult, if not uncomfortable — try it and see.

Smoking cigarettes is a habit and one that is very hard to break. People struggle for years and suffer significant discomfort when attempting to quit smoking, partly because smoking is a habit and partly because nicotine is highly addictive, which compounds the problem.

Superstitious OCD can be thought of as a habit, too. This superstitious habit is not so helpful. If you don't comply with what your OCD mind tells you to do, you're likely to feel some discomfort, sometimes a lot of discomfort at first.

To manage the discomfort you encounter while working to overcome your superstitious OCD, remind yourself of the following points:

>> All discomfort lessens as you continue to cease your old habitual rituals.

>> Tolerating discomfort is like building muscles — you have to feel the burn and increase weights slowly over time — no pain, no gain.

>> No one has ever died as a result of confronting their superstitions.

Yes, bad habits and superstitions are hard to break. But persistence and willingness to tolerate discomfort will eventually break them down. Consider reading Chapter 9 on mindfulness for ideas about how to tolerate discomfort.

Deflating the Power of OCD Superstitions with ERP

Exposure and response prevention (ERP) is the cornerstone for the treatment of most types of OCD. And that's the case for superstitious OCD as well. ERP involves facing your OCD triggers head on, but don't worry; you won't crash. Odds of success are high when using ERP. However, most people will experience greater success if they work in collaboration with a mental health professional trained in this approach.

TIP

Chapter 10 covers ERP in considerable detail. Please review that chapter prior to attempting ERP for your superstitious OCD.

Facing off with scary superstitions

Table 17-1 is a trigger list with Ugh Factors that exemplifies the use of ERP in dealing with suspicions. These triggers are all associated with a superstitious fear of death. The exact nature of your trigger list will depend very much upon the nature of your individual superstitious OCD. However, this example gives you an idea of how to proceed.

Defeating the power of superstitious charms

Not all superstitions are scary. For example, wishing someone good luck is not necessarily a bad thing, and it conveys a positive sentiment. Charms don't make luck, but many people carry them just in case.

Most people with superstitious OCD believe in the power of good-luck symbols. However, they often turn to good-luck charms in compulsive ways, as a means of reducing distress associated with their obsessional, superstitious fears. Since overcoming OCD typically involves letting go of compulsions, here's a strategy for dealing with these superstitious symbols — even though they may appear positive at first glance. This exercise could appear silly to those who don't have superstitious OCD, but those who suffer from it will find it difficult.

TABLE 17-1 ## Superstitions Trigger List and Ugh Factor Ratings

OCD Trigger	Ugh Factor Rating (On a Scale of 0–100)
Looking at pictures of funeral homes and cemeteries on the internet for an hour	60
Sitting in a cemetery for an hour and touching the headstones	99
Walking around the parking lots of several funeral homes for at least an hour altogether	75
Looking at the yellow page ads for funeral homes for an hour	80
Reading a collection of obituaries in the newspaper over and over	65
Discussing all the details of my superstitions with my therapist for 50 minutes	40
Walking in a cemetery for an hour without touching any headstones	90
Imagining scenes of people dying for 45 minutes with my therapist	80
Writing the word "die" on paper over and over for an hour	75

Figure 17-1 illustrates some good-luck charms, which are quite likely to apply if you have almost any type of superstitious OCD.

Do something very different than what your OCD mind wants you to do with these illustrations. Spend some serious time on the following exercise:

1. **Carefully look at, review, and read each and every symbol, picture, or word.**

2. **Say the words out loud.**

3. **When you feel ready, cross off the words. You may even consider cutting up a photocopy of the page.**

   (Please don't deface the book if it doesn't belong to you — for example, if you've borrowed it from a library.)

4. **As you cross the words out (or cut up the page), notice your feelings.**

5. **Stay with this exercise until your feelings of distress are reduced.**

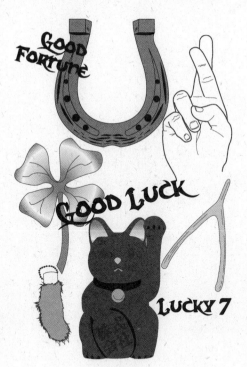

You can either make multiple copies of the page and slowly destroy each one, or you can continue to cross the words out, over and over. You can even repeat phrases such as "I don't want good luck!" again and again. Try to stay with the exercise until your stressful feelings come down by 50 percent or more.

6. **Consider making an alternative, bad-luck page with the help of a therapist.**

   You can make this page by surfing the internet for all kinds of bad-luck symbols and words that give you trouble with your superstitious OCD.

7. **After you've made your alternative page, expose yourself to each word and symbol the way you did with the good-luck symbols.**

   However, in this case, you don't destroy the page, but rather, you expose yourself to it. Read the words and observe the evil symbols. You may even consider rubbing the page over your arms and hands.

IN THIS CHAPTER

» **Counting compulsively**

» **Tapping and touching**

» **Dwelling on doodling**

» **Taking too long to get things done**

» **Getting a handle on hoarding**

Chapter **18**

Uncovering OCD Accomplices

C ounting, touching, doodling, and compulsive slowness often accompany the other specific types of OCD, which are covered in earlier chapters. For example, some people with hit-and-run issues who fear running someone over with their car may count compulsively while driving in order to shut out their obsessive images. Others with doubting and checking OCD may feel a need to repeatedly touch door handles in specific ways in order to check whether the door is locked. Or someone with contamination OCD may take slow, hour-long showers in order to feel clean enough.

In all such cases, the counting, doodling, touching, and slowness are not really distinctly separate types of OCD, although they occasionally present as the primary symptoms. These symptoms are quite common and often difficult to treat. Furthermore, counting, doodling, touching, and compulsive slowness tend to capture so much of people's attention and resources that they find themselves unable to carry out important tasks in their lives. So, I pay special attention to them in this chapter.

The next sections describe people who suffer from these particular OCD symptoms. Each of these four types of behaviors can be treated using a two-step approach that involves changing how the behaviors are done and then not doing them!

The last section in this chapter covers the special category of hoarding. Although no longer thought to be part of the OCD spectrum, hoarding merits a discussion because so many people who have OCD also have tendencies to hoard.

Concerning Counting

The staircase to my former private practice office has 19 stairs. How did I know this fascinating fact? Well, umm, as I was writing this chapter, I mused about how common counting compulsions are among those with and without full-blown OCD. In my mind, I realized that I count steps from time to time. And I recognized that I do so more often at times when I'm feeling a little worried about something, such as running late for an appointment or having work pile up on me.

Do I have OCD because I occasionally count? No. Many people count stairs, steps, and ceiling tiles. Frequently, counting does not result in a diagnosis of OCD because it doesn't take lots of time or cause major interference with a person's life. It may serve to reduce or distract people from worrisome, anxious thoughts, or it may just alleviate the boredom of sitting in a doctor's waiting room.

At other times, counting grows to the point that it greatly disrupts a person's life. Those who have this problem count all kinds of things, such as:

>> Books on a bookshelf

>> Cars passing

>> Change and money

>> Steps

>> Breaths

>> Letters in words, names, sentences, or paragraphs

>> Highway markings and signs

>> Lines in the sidewalk

>> Streetlights

Some people count consecutively; others like to count in sets of specific numbers, such as groups of four or seven. For example, a person may count four sets of seven steps. Or someone else may look out the window and feel compelled to count cars in sets of five until they have logged six sets.

Counting effectively blocks out other thoughts. That's not a problem as long as it's brief or occasional. When counting gets out of control, however, the person cannot focus on work or other important life tasks. Counting becomes a disturbing compulsion in those cases.

Preparation for combating compulsive counting involves self-monitoring. Jot down notes about what it is you actually find yourself counting and when you usually do it. You may need to spend a few days collecting data to catalog your counting.

After you've collected information about what and when you count, you're prepared to tackle your counting head-on. Here are a couple of strategies for you to try in the following two sections:

>> Misdirecting counting behavior through miscounting

>> Stopping counting by resisting counting

By the way, how many "c's" appeared in the past two paragraphs? Well, you probably shouldn't answer that question. I quickly counted 18 c's. But maybe I did that too quickly. Perhaps I should count them a few more times. Then again, maybe not.

Miscounting on purpose

One of the best ways to mess up your counting problem is to practice the art of miscounting. Miscounting involves intentionally screwing up. Thus, you could skip counting a few steps, count one step as three, or count totally out of order. The OCD mind doesn't like messing up in this manner. If you attempt this technique, be sure to

>> Miscount for increasingly longer blocks of time.

>> Expect some discomfort and rate that discomfort (see Ugh Factor Rating in Chapter 10) each time you miscount.

>> Pat yourself on the back for each successful attempt to miscount.

After you've experienced some success and a decrease in discomfort from miscounting, you're ready for the next step — resisting counting (see the next section).

If you do not experience success, consider seeking professional help.

Resisting the act of counting

Resisting counting is rather similar to exposure and response prevention (ERP — see Chapter 10 for details). However, unlike most other compulsions, counting crops up almost anywhere, anytime. This makes it harder to design a set of difficult steps for an ERP trigger list.

Instead, set aside blocks of time when you do not count. You can start with brief periods, perhaps as short as five minutes if you're currently counting almost all the time. Then aim for successively larger blocks of time in which you resist all counting.

Try to do this exercise as often as you can, at least several times a day. If you do find yourself starting to count, stop. Don't get upset with yourself; just gently remind your OCD mind that you are in charge and will not count for now. Remind yourself that the counting isn't "you," but merely a product of your OCD mind.

TECHNICAL STUFF

In Chapter 8 and elsewhere, I warn about not attempting to suppress obsessive thoughts because they will merely increase if you do. *Resisting* compulsive counting is not the same thing as thought *suppression*. That's because obsessions are unwanted, intrusive thoughts that really can't be effectively suppressed. However, counting is a mental compulsion that is designed to decrease anxiety and distress. This kind of compulsion can be effectively resisted or at least delayed.

Taking Charge of Touching

If you've ever watched the formerly popular television series *Monk,* you may have seen detective Monk touch various objects such as parking meters or posts while walking down the street. Many people without OCD ritualistically touch a series of items from time to time. Again, touching only becomes OCD when it takes lots of time or interferes with your life.

Troubling touching can consist of constant tapping of fingers in certain sequences, touching every third railing and needing to go back if one is missed, tapping wood ritualistically, rubbing smooth or rough surfaces over and over, or complicated combinations of foot tapping and hand movements.

TIP

Distinguishing between motor tics (see Chapters 3 and 19) and touching symptoms of OCD can be tricky. Motor tics involve quick, uncontrollable movements of various types, but are usually not accompanied by obsessive thoughts. You may want to consult a professional trained in OCD diagnosis and treatment for help with making this distinction.

The first step in taking charge of your touching is self-monitoring. Spend a day or two noticing all the ways in which you ritualistically touch, tap, or rub various items or surfaces. Take notes and record when, where, and how you touch. Then you can apply a two-step method for addressing OCD touching:

>> Mixing up your touching patterns

>> Stopping touching for increasingly longer lengths of time

Messing with your touching

Similar to miscounting noted earlier in this chapter, messing with your touching entails changing your touching patterns. Thus, you can:

>> Change the rhythm of your tapping.

>> Change the typical surfaces you rub.

>> Tap out of order.

>> Instead of tapping your right foot, try tapping your left foot.

>> Intentionally miss tapping a few items in a sequence (like lampposts).

>> Tap harder than usual.

>> Tap more slowly than you want to.

Notice how you feel when you change your touching patterns. Expect some discomfort at first and be aware that the discomfort is highly likely to decrease as you continue.

Discontinuing touching

After you've mastered messing with your touching, you're ready for the next step, discontinuing touching. When you feel like touching something, don't do it! Of course, it isn't quite that simple. You will probably find it useful to start by not engaging in your compulsive touching for an hour or so. Write down your success. Then up your goal to an hour and a half, then two hours, then three. You get the idea. Ultimately, your compulsion to touch will decrease after you've made it through an entire day or two. However, you will need to remain vigilant, because touching OCD loves to creep in through the back door when you're not looking.

Doing Away with Doodling

Everyone doodles now and then. Harmless, right? Well, yes, in most cases. But with OCD, things tend to run out of control. And it happens with doodling just like it does with other OCD symptoms. Compulsive doodlers sometimes have favorite themes for their doodling, such as circles, weapons, or mazes.

Those with a doodling problem often become so wrapped up in their doodling that the rest of the world is shut out. This symptom often shows up in students. They sit at their desks doodling and may not even hear the lecture they're attending. Even if they do, they certainly can't take notes. The same problem shows up at the office. Some office workers doodle their days away and run into trouble with their supervisors for a lack of productivity.

The techniques for doing away with doodling look much like the strategies outlined for counting and touching earlier in this chapter. Start by jotting down how often, where, and when you doodle. Get a feel for just how much trouble it causes you. Then try the following two techniques:

>> Doodle differently.

>> Don't doodle.

Doodling in different ways

Change your doodling patterns in every way you can think of. Most people who doodle compulsively have preferred pens, pencils, paper, designs, and patterns for their doodling. Regularly change all these things in some way or another. The goal is to make doodling as unsatisfying to your OCD mind as possible.

Denying the urge to doodle

Stopping doodling is best executed after you've been doodling differently for a time. The strategy of just saying no to doodling demands increasing amounts of time in which you consciously resist the urge to doodle. You slowly build up your tolerance while taking notes, working on your tasks, and so on. It helps if you monitor your successes as well as the amount of discomfort you feel when you don't doodle for each block of time (see Chapter 10 for details on the Ugh Factor Rating).

Speeding Up Slowness

OCD inevitably slows people down, if for no other reason than because it consumes so much of their time. However, sometimes slowness becomes the primary problem. Showering can take over an hour — or until the hot water runs out. Getting ready for work can require two or three hours, making you chronically late for work. Eating a meal can drag on and on, and not just because you're savoring the food. Some people with compulsive slowness speak . . . very . . . very . . . ever so very . . . slowly. You can imagine how slowness not only interferes with completing life's tasks, but also can be exquisitely annoying to others.

Those with this OCD symptom are not particularly slow thinkers *per se*. Typically, their slowness represents an attempt to reduce their doubts and uncertainty and/or obtain perfection. These people want to make sure they complete tasks in a correct or "just so" manner.

WARNING

A few neurological disorders include symptoms of motor slowness as a prominent feature. These include Parkinson's disease and Binswanger's disease, which is a form of vascular dementia. If you or someone you love demonstrates a change with problems involving compulsive slowness, check it out with your family doctor, who may refer you to a neurologist.

Compulsive slowness is a little tricky to treat with standard ERP. However, you can address the issues of doubting, uncertainty, and perfectionism (which frequently drive this problem) by working carefully through Chapter 8. Just don't take too long to work through your issue!

Two types of exposure strategies can be successfully applied to problems with slowness — mixing things up and speeding things up.

Mixing things up

Each person's slowness problem is unique. More variations on this theme exist than there are books in the library. However, most people who live in slow motion are looking for certainty and perfection. Therefore, it's often helpful to experiment with an ERP trigger list that pushes you to engage in the activities that you're slow at with increasing amounts of uncertainty and imperfection.

TIP

Before you begin, read Chapter 10 for important instructions on how to use exposure trigger lists within ERP. Austin's story illustrates how he uses an exposure hierarchy to speed up his life.

Austin is a freshman in college. He is gifted but graduated from high school with only mediocre grades because of his compulsive slowness. He's often late to class because he is so slow getting ready to leave — he combs each hair into place, straightens his clothes, and polishes his shoes to perfection. He takes notes slowly and retraces each word to make sure that it's clear. However, this note-taking strategy prevents him from getting much of the important material on paper.

He graduated from high school because he was bright enough to get away with this inefficiency. But now in college he finds that his notes don't give him the information he needs to pass his tests. His slowness also bogs him down because he reads and rereads all his textbook assignments out of fear of not understanding everything. He's behind in all his classes. He seeks counseling at the student mental-health center. His therapist persuades him to try exposure and response prevention. Table 18-1 shows what they come up with.

TABLE 18-1 **Mixing Things Up to Battle Slowness Trigger List and Ugh Factor Ratings**

OCD Trigger	Ugh Factor Rating (On a Scale of 0–100)
Polishing one shoe and not the other	60
Turning in a paper that I briefly edit only once	99
Intentionally mussing up my clothes	75
Taking notes quickly without tracing over letters	80
Reading a section in my textbook only twice	65
Not folding my underwear	40
Not combing my hair at all and going out in public	90
Taking really sloppy notes with misspelled words	80
Wearing one blue sock and one brown sock	75

Austin completes his trigger list over a few weeks, which helps him speed up because it gives him practice with making mistakes and engaging in imperfection — both of which fuel his slowness. Austin's treatment also involves talking about his experiences with the exposure exercises.

Speeding things up

Survey a few close friends or family members and ask them how long they spend doing basic tasks such as eating, showering, shaving, brushing teeth, getting dressed, grooming, or whatever it is that you're slow at. Then write down the average of their reports and make it your goal to meet or beat those lengths of time. Each time you succeed, be sure to reward yourself.

The key here is to try and not go um, er . . . too fast! What I mean is, try and speed up about 10 to 20 percent with each attempt until you've reached your goal. You don't have to accomplish the goals all at once, but neither do you need to take forever getting there.

Here are a few of our suggestions for goals on some basic life tasks. These are not set in granite and not based on scientific research — just common sense.

>> **Baths:** Under 20 minutes unless you're wanting an occasional relaxing treat

>> **Eating most meals:** 30 minutes

>> **Putting on make-up:** Under 15 minutes (except for a special occasion or if you're starring in a movie)

>> **Selecting clothes and getting dressed:** Under 15 minutes

>> **Showering:** Under 10 minutes

>> **Brushing your teeth:** 2 minutes (a typical electric toothbrush times out then)

Other tasks that involve slowness, like writing or reading, are more difficult to assign exact goals to. Review your own particular slowness issues and try to design some common-sense solutions. If you have trouble doing so, consider seeing a therapist for some help.

Handling Hoarding

Hoarding disorder is no longer considered a specific type of OCD; however, it is considered a related disorder. Those with hoarding disorder are usually quite content to be left alone with their collections. They believe that their collections have value, although in almost all cases, the collections are worthless. Hoarders hoard because they strongly believe that they must keep things such as junk mail, old newspapers, broken appliances, string, and bits of wire, because they are sure they might need them sometime in the future. Although they may have some insight into their problems, they experience little anxiety about their excessive acquisitions.

Collections that have true value such as coins, stamps, sports memorabilia, or other collectibles are not considered problematic. However, some people collect so many different things that their homes are stuffed with stuff. There is a continuum of normal to hoarding that cannot always be clearly defined.

In addition to those who have hoarding disorder, some people with OCD also hoard. They usually have highly distressing obsessions that require them to hoard. For example, a mother may believe that throwing away the school papers from her children will lead to bad outcomes. So, she saves all of the papers from preschool through high school, unable to throw out any for fear of harming her children.

Other OCD type hoarding can relate to certain superstitious numbers, for example buying multiples of 6 or 12. Contamination fears can also result in hoarding behavior. Some items become contaminated and, therefore, cannot be touched and must remain in one spot.

Some OCD hoarders fear that they may discard something that will be needed in the future. These collections are born out of obsessive anxiety and result in stuffed homes, basements, garages, and sometimes rented storage units. The main difference between hoarding disorder and OCD hoarding is the strong emotional distress that OCD hoarders experience.

Hoarding, whether accompanied by OCD or not, is a very difficult problem to treat. If you or a loved one has trouble with hoarding, seek an experienced mental health professional for help.

Researchers have found that people with OCD who hoard are more likely to have just so (symmetry) type obsessions and have repeating and counting compulsions. They also tend to be more severely impaired than those without hoarding compulsions.

Chapter **19**

Dealing with OCD-Related Impulsive Problems

Tics, Tourette's syndrome, trichotillomania, skin-picking, and nail-biting all fall under the category of *impulsive problems* — tics and habits that are driven by sudden impulses. Tics are repetitive, rapid vocalizations or movements that are difficult to suppress. Such noises include grunts, groans, barks, and swear words, whereas movements may involve rapid head jerks, eye blinks, facial grimaces, and so on. Impulsive habits are repetitive and difficult to suppress, including pulling out one's hair (trichotillomania), picking at one's skin, and biting one's nails. (See Chapter 3 for more detailed descriptions of each of these disorders.)

Many experts believe that these problems have some connection to OCD, but they are not officially considered to be part of OCD at this time. They do, however, frequently co-occur with OCD. Like OCD, people report that they have great difficulty stopping these behaviors. Unlike OCD, these behaviors are largely thought to occur as a way of self-soothing or obtaining a pleasurable feeling rather than reducing fear, anxiety, and distress. However, some people with these habits report engaging in them as a way of reducing distress, so the distinction may not hold for everyone.

This chapter reviews the primary strategies for undoing these problematic behaviors and habits. Most importantly, I describe a treatment that was developed in the 1970s by Drs. Nathan Azrin and Gregory Nunn called Habit Reversal Training (HRT). Today HRT remains one of the most widely employed treatment approaches to these issues. The chapter concludes with a discussion of important thinking habits to acquire in order to succeed and maintain your gains.

TECHNICAL STUFF

I review other cousins of OCD in Chapter 3 that I do not discuss in this chapter because treating them entails greater complexity. These problem areas include body dysmorphic disorder, hoarding disorder, olfactory reference disorder, eating disorders, pathological gambling, kleptomania, compulsive buying, somatic symptom disorder, pyromania, and various paraphilias. If one of these problems seems to apply to you, I recommend that you seek professional help for diagnosis and treatment.

Changing Behavior to Reduce Impulsive Problems

Addressing OCD-related impulsive problems can be difficult. That's because these impulsive habits tend to occur with little or no conscious thought or awareness. They are well-ingrained habits, and most people have them for years before they attempt to change them.

Habit Reversal Training (HRT) has been the most heavily researched strategy for these problems and usually works quite well. HRT, like exposure and response prevention (ERP) therapy (see Chapter 10), involves extended periods of time in which the person refrains from the problematic behavior. However, unlike ERP, it attempts to instill a new behavior that competes with the habit.

HRT consists of four major components:

>> **Increasing your awareness of when your problematic behaviors and habits are occurring.**

Many people report that they are almost completely unaware of when they have tics, pull their hair, or pick at their skin.

>> **Learning how to relax as a way of handling stressors that sometimes set off problematic behaviors and habits.**

>> **Learning new, alternative behaviors.**

   This strategy is particularly important.

>> **Seeing how to keep yourself motivated with self-rewards.**

**TECHNICAL
STUFF**

Some professionals used to believe that if you eliminated problematic behaviors such as tics and hair pulling, you would simply find another bad habit to replace it. However, studies have consistently failed to verify this concern. Thus, if you succeed in ridding yourself of a problem behavior, you are good to go.

Increasing awareness of your impulsive problems

Increasing awareness of your tics and habits prepares you for the rest of HRT. I recommend at least a week of careful monitoring. Although it's something of a pain, make note of the following during that time:

>> The time of day you feel an urge.

>> Where you are when an urge strikes.

>> How you feel when you have an urge (happy, sad, anxious, angry, and so on).

>> What you are doing when you feel an urge (watching television, scrolling through social media, and so forth).

>> How you feel after you engage in your tic or habit, or how you feel if you don't engage in the problematic behavior.

>> Describe your behavior in detail. If it's a tic, note which part of the body is moving or what sound is made. If it's hair-pulling, note where you're pulling the hair from and whether you use one hand or two.

TIP

Some people worry that increasing awareness of their tics, urges, and habits will make them all increase. If you have that concern, relax. Studies show that increasing awareness does nothing to increase symptoms and sometimes reduces them somewhat, at least for a while. However, you need to carry out the rest of HRT in order to reduce symptoms permanently.

Relaxing away impulsive problems

The second step in HRT is what's known as progressive muscle relaxation training. Dr. Edmund Jacobsen developed this strategy more than 50 years ago. Literally hundreds of studies have shown that this technique can improve anxiety and health in numerous ways, although among the four components of HRT, relaxation may be the least important. Here is a set of instructions for progressive muscle relaxation:

1. **Take a deep breath, hold, imagine, and let the tension go.**

Pulling the air in from your abdomen, breathe deeply. Hold your breath for three or four seconds and slowly let the air out. Imagine your whole body is a balloon losing air as you exhale and let tension go out with the air. Take three more such breaths and feel your entire body getting more limp with each one.

2. **Squeeze your hands tight and then relax.**

Squeeze your fingers into a fist. Feel the tension and hold it for six to ten seconds. Then, all at once, release your hands and let them go limp. Allow the tension in your hands to flow out. Let the relaxation deepen for 10 to 15 seconds.

3. **Tighten your arms and relax.**

Bring your lower arms up almost to your shoulders and tighten the muscles. Make sure you tense the muscles on the inside and outside of both the upper and lower arms. If you're not sure you're doing that, use one hand to do a tension check on the other arm. Hold the tension a little while and then drop your arms as though you cut a string holding them up. Let the tension flow out and the relaxation flow in.

4. **Raise your shoulders, tighten, and then relax.**

Raise your shoulders as though you were a turtle trying to get into its shell. Hold the tension and then let your shoulders drop. Feel the relaxation deepen for 10 to 15 seconds.

5. **Tighten and relax the muscles in your upper back.**

Pull your shoulders back and bring your shoulder blades closer together. Hold that tension a little while . . . and let it go.

6. **Scrunch up your entire face and then relax.**

Squeeze your forehead down, bring your jaws together, tighten your eyes and eyebrows, and contract your tongue and lips. Let the tension grow and hold it . . . then relax and let go.

7. **Tighten and relax your neck in the back of your head.**

Without causing any pain, gently pull your head back toward your back and feel the muscles tighten in the back of your neck. Notice that tension and hold it, let go, and relax. Feel relaxation deepening and repeat it if you want.

8. **Contract the front neck muscles and then loosen.**

Gently move your chin toward your chest. Tighten your neck muscles and let the tension increase and maintain it; then relax. Feel the tension melting away like candle wax.

9. **Tighten the muscles in your stomach and chest and maintain the tension. Then let it go.**

10. **Arch your back, hang on to the contraction, and then relax.**

Be gentle with your lower back and skip it entirely if you've ever had trouble with this part of your body. Tighten these muscles by arching your lower back, pressing it back against the chair, or tensing the muscles any way you want. Gently increase and maintain the tension, but not too much. Now, relax and allow the waves to roll in.

11. **Contract and relax your buttocks muscles.**

Tighten your buttocks so as to gently lift yourself up in your chair. Hold the tension. Then let tension melt and relaxation grow.

12. **Squeeze and relax your thigh muscles.**

Tighten and hold these muscles. Then relax and feel the tension draining out; let the calm deepen and spread.

13. **Contract and relax your calves.**

Tighten the muscles in your calves by pulling your toes toward your face. Take care; if you ever get muscle cramps, don't overdo. Hold the tension . . . let go. Let tension drain into the floor.

14. **Gently curl your toes, maintain the tension, and then relax.**

15. **Take a little time to tour your entire body.**

Notice whether you feel different than when you began. If you find any areas of tension, allow the relaxed areas around the tense areas to come in and replace them. If that doesn't work, repeat the tense-and-relax procedure for the tense area.

16. **Spend a few minutes enjoying the relaxed feelings.**

Let relaxation spread and penetrate every muscle fiber in your body. Notice any feelings you have. You may feel warmth, or you may feel a floating sensation. Perhaps you'll feel a sense of sinking down. Whatever it is, allow it to happen. When you want, you can open your eyes and go on with your day, perhaps feeling like you just returned from a brief vacation.

Recordings of progressive muscle relaxation techniques are available online. Some people like to record their own version; if you want to go that way, feel free to use or change the wording and make your own, personalized recording.

Practice relaxation every day for at least a couple of weeks. As you get more skilled, you may discover that you can relax more quickly by condensing several muscle groups into one. For example, you could tighten your hands, arms, and shoulders together and relax them at the same time. Then you could tighten your upper back, face, and neck muscles simultaneously and relax them. After a while, you may find that you can completely relax within a few minutes.

TIP

Recent research has found some positive results from using mindfulness-based strategies (see Chapter 9) with Habit Reversal Training. It makes sense that adding mindfulness might improve relaxation and emotional regulation. What's important is finding a strategy that really works for you. Feel free to experiment.

WARNING

If your impulsive problem involves any kind of intentional cutting on your body until bleeding occurs, you should seek professional help for the problem. HRT may ultimately play some role but consulting a trained mental-health professional will likely be essential. Furthermore, I also recommend professional consultations if you do not make good progress on your own for any of the problems described in this chapter.

Sidetracking impulsive problems with something different

Possibly the most crucial aspect of HRT is designing a new response to compete with the old habit or behavior. Ideally, this new response uses virtually the same muscles as the tic or habit. It also needs to be something you can do in public without appearing obvious. It's best to take each tic or habit one at a time; after you've succeeded with one, you can move on to another one.

You may wonder what these competing responses look like. Table 19-1 shows you an array of possibilities. You may want to use one or more of these, but your own particular tic or habit may not be included. In that case, you can probably design your own by using these as a guide.

After you've designed and planned your competing responses, you're ready to start using them. Whenever you feel an urge or strong desire to engage in a tic or habit, immediately begin your competing response. Maintain that response for several minutes; later you can shorten the time to a minute or less. Try not to stop until the urge has lessened.

TABLE 19-1

Examples of Impulsive Problems and Suggested Competing Responses

Compulsive Problem	Competing Responses
Hair-pulling (habit also called trichotillomania)	Make a fist; squeeze a soft ball; squeeze the arms of your chair
Facial grimace (tic)	Tighten your lips together; clench your teeth
Eye-blinking (tic)	Open your eyes as wide as possible
Nail-biting (habit)	Make a fist; squeeze a soft ball; squeeze the arms of your chair
Noises — grunts, groans, barks, and so on (tics)	Keeping your mouth closed, inhale slowly and deeply through the nose, then exhale slowly
Shoulder shrugs (tic)	Push shoulders back against chair; make a fist and push it into the palm of the other hand
Head jerks (tic)	Tilt head down toward the chest
Hand and arm jerks (tic)	Make a fist and push it into the palm of the other hand with some force
Skin-picking (habit)	Make a fist; squeeze a soft ball; squeeze the arms of your chair

REMEMBER

While you are doing your competing responses, don't forget to practice your previously learned relaxation technique.

Reinforcing positive gains in overcoming impulsive problems

Now for the good part. Reinforcing or rewarding your good efforts is important. Of course, you can always treat yourself in various ways such as indulging in a favorite food, going out to a movie, reading a great book, or buying yourself something special.

However, the best way of keeping your motivation high is to enlist the help of some trusted friends or family. Tell them what you're doing and ask them to encourage you and remind you to keep at it. See Chapter 22 for ideas about how to use coaches and support people — you certainly don't need them nagging you!

Changing Thinking to Reduce Impulsive Problems

Tackling tics and habits doesn't make any "Top Ten" lists of the "Easiest and Most Fun Things You Can Do." Rather, ridding yourself of these scoundrels takes hard work and determination. It helps if you tinker with your thinking as a way of obtaining and maintaining momentum. In the following sections, I recommend a little work on four particular areas of thinking. These areas are

>> Choosing to change

>> Confronting hopelessness

>> Setting unfairness aside

>> Being self-supporting

Finding reasons to change

Many people report that their tics or habits have hung around their necks since they were bordering on pubescence. And they decide to get help when they are middle-aged adults, meaning they have waited several decades or longer to finally deal with the issue. Such long delays in seeking treatment usually occur due to deep shame over the problem. Other people wait because they attempt to minimize the issue and pretend that it's no big deal.

In either case, you're likely to benefit from developing a list of reasons for dealing with your problematic habit or tic. Think of every imaginable motivation you have for finally loosening the chokehold your habits and tics have on your life. Here are a few such incentives that people have mentioned to me:

>> I hate it when someone notices my problem and asks me about it.

>> I live in constant fear of embarrassment and rejection.

>> I no longer want to feel the constant pressure to hide and cover up my problem.

>> I want to feel in charge of my life rather than feeling like my tics (or habits) have the upper hand.

>> These habits distract me from tasks that I need to accomplish.

You get the idea. You likely have many reasons for making these changes. Remind yourself what those reasons are as you proceed. If your motivation happens to wane at any point, consider reading or rereading Chapter 6 for ideas on how to overcome obstacles and resistance to change.

Pushing hopelessness aside

Many people report slipping into thoughts of hopelessness when they try to break stubborn habits. If you find yourself having thoughts such as, "I'll never overcome this," "I thought I was getting somewhere, but this slip obviously means I haven't learned a thing," or "I can't even imagine getting over this problem," you need to jump on such self-defeating thoughts. You can start by answering the following questions:

>> Have I ever tackled my tics or habits with professional assistance before?

>> Have I ever experienced an extended time when I successfully dealt with my habits? If so, is it possible I can build upon that experience?

>> Have I ever succeeded at anything that seemed impossible at the time?

>> Have I ever tried HRT or ERP for these problems?

Scott has a vocal tic in which he constantly clears his throat, and he bites his nails. He has had both of these problems since he was an adolescent and feels terribly embarrassed about them. He used the preceding questions to overcome his thoughts of hopelessness because he'd made a number of attempts to overcome these problems but had failed each time. Here are Scott's answers to these questions:

>> **Have I ever tackled my tics or habits with professional assistance before?**

My doctor put me on medication for smoking, but it didn't help. I have never seen a therapist for this stuff, but maybe that could help.

>> **Have I ever experienced an extended time when I successfully dealt with my habits? If so, is it possible I can build upon that experience?**

I did manage to quit smoking after about 20 tries. And I did stop my nail-biting for three months once. So maybe if I keep at it . . .

>> **Have I ever succeeded at anything that seemed impossible at the time?**

Yes, I recall getting through graduate school. I never thought I'd make it.

> **» Have I ever tried HRT or ERP for these problems?**
>
> *I'd never heard of HRT or ERP before. Maybe it can help.*

Answering these questions helped Scott realize that changing habits is not a hopeless undertaking. He now feels more optimistic about making difficult, but desired, changes.

Undoing unfairness worries

Sometimes people defeat themselves by dwelling on how terribly unfair and unjust it is that they have one or more of these problems and have to work so hard to change them. They typically feel angry about the fact that the world has dealt them such a lousy hand.

If any of this thinking sounds like something you hear rattling around in your head, try to reconsider. Almost every person I've ever known struggles with difficult issues. Traumas, death, financial setbacks, and emotional struggles present formidable foes for everyone at one time or another throughout a lifetime. Focusing on the unfairness and injustice of it all merely takes your eye off the ball. Remind yourself, "Of course it isn't 'fair' that I have this problem, but I need to dwell on doing something about it, not on how unfair it is."

Designing supportive self-statements

Sometimes preparing a few straightforward self-statements helps you stay focused. Self-statements are simply thoughts that you say to yourself as reminders and motivators. Here are a few that you may find useful. Feel free to use these examples, change the wording a little, or design your own:

> **»** I know I am entering a situation that sets my habit off; get ready!

> **»** Urges are tough, but each and every time I resist them, I build up more strength.

> **»** I want to take charge of my life again!

> **»** Control takes time; patience is the key.

> **»** When I "fail," I can still learn from the process if I simply don't beat up on myself.

Consider jotting down one or more of these statements on an index card or keep it handy somewhere on your phone. Carry the card or look at your phone to remind yourself. You can do this!

Applying ERP to Impulsive Problems

Although far less studied than HRT for tics, ERP has shown promising results for this problem. Essentially, people with tics are asked to undergo multiple two-hour sessions in which they are exposed to situations that represent a high risk of causing tics to occur.

During these exposure sessions, the individuals try to suppress the tics and are also asked to concentrate on the body areas involved with their tics. Therapists usually act as coaches at first, and then clients are asked to practice faithfully at home.

Treating Impulsive Problems with Medication

WARNING

If you are considering taking medication for an impulse control disorder, make sure you go to a physician who has training and experience in managing these problems. The doctor may have to try several different drugs or drug combinations before finding the best treatment for you.

Tourette's syndrome and tics are difficult to treat with medication. Antipsychotic drugs are sometimes helpful in controlling tics. However, the long-term use of these drugs can result in *tardive dyskinesia*, a serious disorder characterized by involuntary movements. These movements are repetitive and may include facial grimacing, sticking out the tongue, lip smacking, or purposeless movements of the arms, legs, or fingers. You can imagine that a person who already has tics is not going to want to suffer from these side effects.

Other newer drugs called *atypical antipsychotics* are also used. Side effects appear to be less severe, but concerns about the long-term use of these medications still exist. Clonidine, a drug designed to lower high blood pressure, sometimes works to control tics. The side effects can include fatigue, dry mouth, and dizziness.

Hair-pulling, skin-picking, and nail-biting have not been as well researched as tic disorders. Often, people with these habits have other problems going on as well, such as social anxiety, depression, or OCD. Selective serotonin reuptake inhibitors have been used with some success to treat the latter conditions, but not so much for hair-pulling, skin-picking, and nail-biting.

TIP

The best advice: Try working on your impulse control problem by using a behavioral treatment such as HRT. Work hard and get help from a therapist. If that doesn't work, then consider consulting with a psychiatrist, neurologist, or other physician who specializes in these problems.

5

Assisting Others with OCD

Chapter **20**

Wondering about Children and OCD

Millions of adults throughout the world suffer from OCD, and for most of them, the signs and symptoms began in childhood or adolescence. Unfortunately, OCD is under diagnosed in children, just as it is in adults. Because kids with OCD often go untreated, they frequently experience bullying and social rejection by peers. Other kids often label their behavior "weird" or "crazy." The time consumed by obsessions and compulsions and their highly distracting nature often cause kids with OCD to do poorly in school.

This chapter gives you information about what OCD looks like in children and points out some common childhood disorders that can be confused with OCD. If you think your child may have OCD, I give you suggestions on how to find help.

WARNING

It's not a good idea for parents to try to diagnose their own children. However, if you believe that your child has some of the symptoms listed in this chapter, you should definitely consider checking them out with a professional.

Understanding Childhood OCD

Kids don't go to their parents saying, "I've been having lots of trouble with terrible obsessions and compulsions." In fact, they typically try to hide their symptoms out of shame and embarrassment. Sometimes they even think they might be crazy.

REMEMBER

Obsessions are recurrent, unwanted thoughts, images, or urges. Compulsions are the actions (either mental or behavioral) that are practiced to decrease distress or neutralize obsessive thoughts.

Children may not be able to talk about obsessions because they don't have the vocabulary or insight necessary to do so. They describe obsessions only as powerful feelings of fear or of things just not being right. Compulsions are more likely than obsessions to be observed by parents.

Recognizing possible symptoms

If kids aren't likely to discuss their obsessive worries or compulsive actions, how can you, as a parent, know whether your child has OCD? Well, you can look for various signs. Don't become too obsessed with this list. All kids have a few of these sorts of problems from time to time. Nevertheless, the following signs and symptoms may be worth checking out:

>> Asking parents or family members to repeat a phrase over and over

>> Counting out loud repeatedly

>> Demanding symmetry in objects, dinnerware, and furniture

>> Being excessively concerned about their appearance and clothing

>> Having strict rituals about cleaning or organizing that must be followed

>> Spending an excessive amount of time getting ready for bed at night

>> Worrying excessively about religion or going to hell

>> Being overly superstitious

>> Displaying extreme irritability or anger when their usual routines are disrupted

>> Fearing unlucky numbers and showing considerable interest in lucky numbers

>> Needing frequent reassurance regarding their own health

>> Worrying frequently about the fire alarms or home safety

- » Making lots of erasures on schoolwork

- » Worry that they might do something to hurt a family member

- » Being overly concerned with getting dirty

- » Questioning parents about sanitation or cleanliness

- » Checking door locks or windows repeatedly

- » Asking questions repeatedly about parents' health and well-being

- » Going through doorways over and over

- » Touching items repeatedly in a ritualistic way

- » Asking for constant reassurance that they are loved

- » Tracing over words repeatedly on schoolwork

- » Repeating the same phrase over and over

- » Needing an increasing amount of time to get ready in the morning

- » Having trouble completing tests on time at school

- » Spending unusually long periods of time washing hands or showering

- » Adhering very strictly to routines

- » Worrying about contamination from radiation or other toxins

WARNING

This list is not exhaustive, nor does a single item allow for a diagnosis of OCD to be made. The difference between OCD and normality can be subtle. Plus, a fair amount of subjectivity is involved in discerning what is excessive or unusual as opposed to what's reasonable and normal. The key is to *determine whether these issues are starting to interfere with your child's or your family's life.* If you feel worried about the signs your child is demonstrating, you need to consult with a mental health professional.

Ruling out normal growth and health issues

Rituals that are transient (meaning they fade over time) are a normal part of childhood around the ages of three to seven. For example, most kids enjoy specific bedtime routines. They also like to line up toys in specific patterns and even "order" their parents to sit in certain seats. Other little kids like to repeatedly turn on and off lights and fans, to see what happens. Children typically outgrow these behaviors, and the behaviors don't significantly interfere with the family or the children's lives.

THESE PANDAS ARE NOT CUTE

Antibodies are designed to attack germs and aid in recovery. Sometimes these antibodies get out of control and attack normal, healthy parts of the body. The result of this phenomenon is called autoimmune disease. Strep throat, a common childhood illness, can produce antibodies that attack normal, healthy structures. This attack may result in PANDAS or pediatric autoimmune neuropsychiatric disorders associated with streptococcal infection. Although no specific lab tests for PANDAS are available, a positive strep throat culture is one of the diagnostic criteria.

The symptoms mimic OCD. They come on quickly after the infection, are usually severe, and often include tremors, twitches, clumsiness, sensitivity, eating problems, bedwetting, and extreme fear and anxiety. PANDAS can be successfully treated with medication and cognitive behavioral therapy (CBT). However, in several successful clinical trials, children have received treatment that removes the strep antibodies, resulting in a dramatic reduction of symptoms.

Childhood OCD most often starts before adolescence. In boys, it usually starts showing up by around the second or third grade. Girls typically show signs of OCD a little later. If symptoms start before the age of five, something else may be going on (see the sidebar "These PANDAS are not cute"), and you should check with your pediatrician.

Sorting through other childhood disorders

Diagnosing OCD can be complicated because the symptoms of OCD can look like symptoms of other childhood disorders, and children with OCD are likely to have other problems. That's why it is especially important to have your child assessed by a mental-health professional experienced in the diagnosis and treatment of OCD. OCD can either accompany or sometimes be confused with the following:

>> **Anxiety disorders:** Although OCD is no longer considered to be one of the anxiety disorders, other problems like separation anxiety (extreme fear of leaving a parent), social anxiety (extreme shyness and fear of rejection), or generalized anxiety (excessive worrying about many things) frequently accompany OCD.

>> **Attention Deficit Hyperactivity Disorder (ADHD):** When children are con-sumed by obsessive thoughts and compulsive rituals, they fail to pay attention. Children are commonly given a diagnosis of ADHD when OCD is the real culprit. ADHD can also accompany OCD. Common symptoms of ADHD include distract-ibility, impulsivity (talking and behaving without thinking), and inattentiveness.

>> **Behavior disorders (including oppositional defiant disorder and conduct disorders):** Kids with one of these problems demonstrate defiance, disobedience, and disruptiveness. They break rules and are easily angered. Children with OCD sometimes seem defiant, but that's usually because parents, siblings, and teachers fail to understand their unusual behaviors and beliefs. For example, children can become very angry and stubborn when their parents push them to do homework, get ready for school or bedtime, and interrupt their compulsive routines.

>> **Depression:** Kids with OCD may withdraw from others because they are embarrassed by their symptoms and that withdrawal may be mistaken as depression. On the other hand, kids with OCD may become clinically depressed as a result of or in addition to their OCD. Typical signs of depression include sadness, loss of interest, withdrawal, low energy, appetite changes, and problems with sleep.

>> **Learning disabilities:** Kids with OCD can look like they have problems learning because they're not completing schoolwork or paying attention. Therefore, they may have poor grades. Learning disabilities are neurologically based problems and are diagnosed by a school or clinical psychologist.

>> **Autism Spectrum Disorder:** This set of problems involves severe impairment of social interactions and restricted interests. Thus, children with one of these problems may show unusual, keen interest in specific topics, such as airplanes or dinosaurs. Kids with these pervasive developmental disorders also often have trouble with changes and transitions in routines and activities. The rigid interests and routines can sometimes look like obsessions and compulsions.

>> **Tic disorders (including Tourette's syndrome):** Tics are sudden, recurrent motor movements or vocalizations (such as grunts, groans, snorts, words, barks, obscenities) that occur spontaneously and involuntarily. They can be suppressed for a little while but are largely out of the person's control. OCD very often accompanies tics and Tourette's, but most of those with OCD do not have tics or Tourette's. Sometimes compulsive routines in OCD that involve tapping, making certain noises, or saying phrases can seem like tics.

>> **Other disorders:** OCD symptoms can mimic or be confused with other childhood disorders.

- OCD can disrupt eating. Children with OCD may not eat particular foods fearing contamination or even believing that the foods are somehow unlucky or that eating those foods could cause someone else harm. They may also need to line up their foods in strange patterns or orders. These problems with eating need to be carefully differentiated from eating disorders such as bulimia and anorexia. Bulimia and anorexia are serious and require professional treatment.

- Children with OCD can have problems with elimination, including a fear of using public toilets often because of contamination concerns. This issue can result in toileting accidents and be confused with encopresis or enuresis (failure to control bowel movements and urine).

- Selective mutism is a disorder of childhood in which the child does not speak, except to close family members. Though unusual, children with OCD may behave in similar ways because of an obsessional fear of talking to strangers.

- Some children who have been separated from their parents, abused, or neglected develop attachment disorders in which they have trouble becoming securely attached to their caregivers. Kids with OCD may look like they have these problems because they're afraid that showing affection may cause harm or contaminate them or their parents in some way.

WARNING

You can see that the diagnoses of childhood disorders can be quite complicated. If you're concerned about your child, make sure you choose a mental health professional who has experience in child assessment and diagnosis.

TIP

Some professionals are experts in assessment and diagnosis of emotional, neurological, learning, and behavior disorders. These professionals clarify the diagnosis, make specific recommendations, and then refer their clients to others for treatment.

Observing the Effects of OCD

The way OCD plays out in different contexts, settings, and relationships can vary, adding more difficulty to a diagnosis. As a parent, being aware of what's going on with your child in settings both in and out of your home is important. The next three sections show you how OCD affects home life, school performance, and relationships with peers. At least half of all kids with OCD find that one or more of these areas become highly impaired.

Having problems at home

OCD disturbs not only the kids who have it, but all of their family members as well. Morning routines can evolve into disasters. OCD makes kids take too long to wash, dress, eat, or gather materials for the day. When parents start to push or nag, children with OCD get extremely angry and sometimes throw tantrums. Bedtime can also be horrible, with rigid routines and rituals stealing time from homework. These delays also cause children to lose sleep and then feel tired the next morning. Tension, worry, and stress cause many kids with OCD to feel sick to their stomachs and have headaches or muscle aches.

OCD sucks in family members like an industrial strength vacuum cleaner. Parents and/or siblings may become involved in supporting OCD rituals. For example, kids may ask their parents to wash ostensibly contaminated clothes repeatedly. They may demand that meals be served in odd orders or containers. Brothers or sisters may be recruited to check doors and windows. And all family members may be required to provide frequent reassurance. Information about how you can handle all these demands is found in Chapter 21.

On occasion, teachers report that they see none of the problems at school that the parents of OCD kids report seeing at home. When parents hear that their kids are doing just fine at school, they mistakenly assume that their kids are just being defiant. This assumption makes the parents irritated, which only worsens the situation. It's important to realize that OCD can show up only at home and still be OCD.

Experiencing problems at school

Although less common, OCD can appear at school and be minimally obvious at home. When OCD overtakes the mind, school can become a nightmare.

Children with OCD are usually bright and try to be well-behaved. Yet they may get into trouble for not paying attention, not completing work, and being off task. Teachers may not understand what is going on and believe that the OCD child is being disrespectful, uncooperative, and oppositional.

Children with OCD have recurring, distressing thoughts that keep them from paying attention to class work. These kids frequently have fears of making mistakes and are extreme perfectionists. They are tortured by the possibility of errors and, therefore, erase and redo the same problem over and over. This over concern often keeps them from completing assignments.

Those children with fears about contamination may worry obsessively about getting sick from touching objects or other children. They may demand frequent bathroom breaks to wash. They may also refuse to participate in required classroom activities (such as cleaning up or collecting papers) due to fear of contact with dirt or germs.

Furthermore, children with OCD often have additional disorders, such as depression, attention deficit disorder, or tic disorders, which also interfere with learning.

Having difficulties with friends

Children with OCD are often isolated from others. They may have unusual rituals or behaviors, causing other children to tease or ridicule them. Full of fear, they are often victims of bullying.

Obsessions and compulsions take considerable time. Children with OCD don't always have time to make and keep friends. Repetitive thoughts and rituals keep OCD children prisoners of their minds and outcasts among peers.

Finding the Right Help for Your Child

If you have a child who may have OCD or another disorder that is causing problems at home or at school, you must become informed and educated about the services in your area. Chapter 7 describes the various types of professionals that may help diagnose and treat children with OCD.

TIP

Check out the International OCD Foundation on the internet for lists of therapists trained in OCD treatment for kids near you.

The good news is that research indicates that the first line of treatment for childhood OCD is CBT. Medications can be considered when risks and benefits are carefully weighed and follow-through is sufficient. Chapter 21 illustrates how these treatments can be applied to children.

The bad news is that some mental-health professionals lack training and experience in the delivery of these research-backed, effective treatments. Finding a good therapist for your child depends on you doing some work. Talk to others, get referrals from your health-care provider, and then call providers and ask questions. If a provider does not answer phone calls, that's not a great sign. Here are some questions you may want to ask:

>> Are you willing to cooperate with my child's physician, teacher, or school counselor?

>> Are you willing to provide extra sessions, longer sessions, or sessions out of the office?

>> Do you offer exposure and response prevention (ERP) with children?

>> Do you have training and experience in CBT for OCD?

>> Do you work with children or adolescents?

>> Will you develop work to complete outside of the therapy?

If you are satisfied with the answers to the preceding questions, then make arrangements to meet with the mental-health professional. Make sure that you feel comfortable and respected.

TIP

Your child may resist going to therapy at first and may even throw a tantrum. After all, confronting fears and worries can be pretty scary. You have to balance your need to protect your child with what is best for your child. If your child needed a shot of antibiotics to treat a bad infection, you wouldn't hesitate to go to a doctor for the shot, even if it meant dragging your kicking, screaming child all the way to the doctor's office. OCD is a treatable disorder. Without treatment, it's likely to get worse and make your family's life more miserable. Be firm and get your child help.

Chapter **21**

Helping Your Child Conquer OCD

Maybe you've thought that your child has OCD, and a professional diagnosis has confirmed your fears. If so, you're probably worried about your child. After all, obsessive-compulsive disorder sounds ominous, if not overwhelming. But take heart, all is not lost. Lots of people have struggled with this problem yet lived fulfilling lives.

TIP

If your child has been diagnosed with OCD, search the internet together for a list of famous people with OCD as a way for both of you to understand that OCD is common and doesn't need to stand in the way of a successful life.

This chapter first explains how important it is to separate the way you view your child from the way you view your child's disorder. Then I give you information about how to negotiate your relationship with your child and your possible role in therapy. I also offer important tips on the delicate dance between providing needed help versus attempting to rescue a child with OCD, however well-intended those attempts may be.

Separating Your Child from OCD

In order to prepare you for the hard work ahead to help your child emerge from OCD, it's important first to understand the difference between OCD and your child; they are not one and the same.

If your child has the measles, you can see the outbreak on their body. Any irritability and bad behavior are easily understood to be a reaction to how uncomfortable they feel. You can get specific medical help and medicines to treat the measles and ease your child's discomfort. When the disease is gone, so is the outbreak, and your child's behavior returns to normal. Through the entire ordeal, you are able to clearly distinguish between what the disease is doing to your child and who your child is as a person.

OCD is expressed not only through the behavior of your child, which you can see, but also through their thoughts, which you can't. Unlike a disease such as the measles or the mumps, OCD is more personal and intimate, meaning that it impacts and is expressed through the personality of the child. Yet, OCD should not *define* the personality of your child.

Take the measles example again. In some ways, OCD is like the measles. Although OCD is not usually caused directly by a virus, a mixture of biological factors does contribute to its development (see Chapter 4). Just as with the measles, *your child clearly did not ask for or desire to have OCD.*

Yet, when OCD afflicts your child, it can seem as though your child is choosing to intentionally act in childish, oppositional, and defiant ways such as:

>> Displaying new, hard-to-explain fears

>> Refusing to get out of the shower

>> Exhibiting an increase in tantrums when thwarted

>> Having difficulty getting ready on time

>> Taking forever to do homework

>> Insisting on elaborate mealtime rituals

On the surface, these behaviors seem easy enough to change, and for many kids without OCD, they are. If your child has OCD, however, demanding immediate cessation of these symptoms is like insisting your child cure themself of the measles — *now!* Change is possible, but much more challenging. The good news is that a child with OCD who works hard has a good chance of substantial, if not virtually complete, recovery.

Think of it this way: Say your child was in an accident that broke their legs. You were told that recovery was possible, but that they might not be able to walk or do much of anything for weeks. Surgery was required to reset the bones and treat other injuries. Then they needed months of physical therapy to fully regain the use of their legs. They worked hard with the physical therapist and today finally walks with only a barely discernible limp. You certainly wouldn't blame them for the accident or for their residual limp. And you'd be darn proud of them for how brave they were during the long, sometimes painful recovery process.

Your child's OCD is no more under their control than being injured in an accident would be. The expressions of OCD that you see are not who your child truly is, just as injuries are not. With time and treatment, your child can emerge from the OCD, like the proverbial butterfly from the cocoon, to be the healthy person they really are deep down inside. That's the child you need to keep your eye on as you both work through their treatment.

REMEMBER

If your child receives a diagnosis of OCD from a mental-health professional, it's important to understand that the OCD is not easily controlled by your child. It's not your fault or your child's fault. Blame and anger only make things worse.

Helping Your Child and Working with the Therapist

If you read this book carefully, you will have a good understanding of OCD and the treatment options that are available for it. You may think you have everything you need to treat your child on your own, but I don't recommend this. Certainly, you play an important role in your child's recovery, but I suggest you enlist the help of an experienced, professional therapist as well. Together, you and your child's therapist can be more effective than either of you working alone.

Throughout my career as both a school and clinical psychologist, I've always loved working with kids who have OCD. Three reasons stand out. First, almost every time, the parents of these kids are kind, loving people who were totally on board with getting help for their kids. Second, the kids are mostly nice, anxious, and smart. After they understand the process, they're willing to go along with exposure and response prevention. Finally, the best part of working with kids who have OCD, is that with persistence, they almost always make tremendous gains. It is incredibly satisfying work.

This section explains the advantages of enlisting a therapist's help and discusses your role in the recovery process. I illuminate the pitfalls to avoid when helping your child, falling into them is easy if you don't know what to look out for. Then I give you some ways to boost your child's chances of a very successful outcome.

Note: My advice assumes that your child is receiving cognitive behavioral therapy (CBT) that probably includes exposure and response prevention (ERP). Refer to Chapters 8 and 10 for more information on these forms of therapy.

Parenting differently and not being the therapist

WARNING

Parents can be loving and supportive to their children with OCD. However, just like doctors cannot be objective enough to care for close family members, parents should not attempt to become their child's therapist. Simply put, parents love their children far too much to be able to have the necessary objectivity for planning and delivering treatment.

As a parent or caregiver of a child with OCD, you know your child more deeply, and under all sorts of circumstances, far better than a therapist who may only see your child a few dozen times. You want help, and when it comes to your child, you ultimately know what's best. *But you may not know how to get there.*

That's because you probably aren't an expert in treating OCD. Furthermore, the treatment of OCD does not always seem to make sense to a layperson. So, it's no wonder many parents feel uncomfortable when a therapist guides their child through exercises like sifting through garbage, walking on cracks, changing up bedtime routines, or wearing different colored socks. Sometimes, children find these tasks frightening and turn to their parents to help. How can anyone expect a parent to turn away from a child who is crying and in obvious distress?

TIP

A good therapist will never make your child do anything that is highly distressing, however, some discomfort will almost always be part of the process. Especially when OCD has become firmly rooted in a child's habitual behavior, therapy may include some tears and occasional tantrums.

Thus, you very well may feel tempted to argue with your child's therapist by suggesting that your child isn't ready or "just can't take it." Or you may undermine the therapist by comforting and reassuring your child every step of the way. These are natural parental instincts at work. And you must work hard to avoid these pitfalls. A few guidelines follow:

>> **Avoid overprotection.** You have to keep your protective instincts in check. After thoroughly checking out your therapist (see Chapter 7 for how to do this), trust that the therapist knows how to treat OCD and trust that your child

will be strong enough to gradually stand up and talk back to OCD. As your child progresses, the fear and anxiety will decrease.

>> **Avoid impatience.** Positive results from treating OCD do not occur instantaneously. With children, the therapist may need a little more time to build up trust. And a few sessions of supportive therapy may be required to establish rapport before the real work begins.

>> **Avoid rescue.** Parents feel sorry for their children with OCD; that's perfectly understandable. And, in fact, kids with OCD may need a little more help and structure at home and at school. However, it is not a good idea to rescue your child from activities such as cleaning up messy art projects, completing assignments on time, or doing chores around the house. Work with a therapist to develop reasonable expectations and then stick with them. Mastering the art of "not rescuing" is likely to take considerable practice.

TIP

Do your homework, make sure you pick a good therapist who is experienced in CBT and the treatment of OCD, and then let the therapist take charge.

WARNING

If, even after checking your child's therapist out carefully, you develop alarming concerns about the therapy, get a second professional opinion before interfering with the therapy. If you feel it's necessary, you can put the therapy on temporary hold while getting that additional opinion.

Managing your emotions

Parenting any child is a difficult job. Parenting a child with OCD can be extremely hard. You don't always know what your child is thinking, and OCD behaviors can be frustrating, irritating, and annoying. At times you no doubt feel sorry for your child and cave in to demands — unfortunately, that only makes OCD worse.

Managing your own emotions will certainly help your child battle OCD. Take some deep breaths and calm down when you get upset. Here are a couple of the common feelings that parents of children with OCD experience and some ideas about what to do with them:

>> **Anger:** Parents can get frustrated or angry because a child with OCD interferes with family life. There may be battles about getting ready to go somewhere, eating, or sleeping. Kids with OCD may demand certain foods, ask their parents to engage in rituals or special cleaning tasks, and have meltdowns for no reason.

It is easy to see how even the most patient parent can get irritable. Another source of frustration for parents comes when their kids seem able to control aspects of their OCD for a while and then suddenly can't. Anger makes the whole situation worse. Try to understand and get help from your child's therapist on how to handle these times. Reminding yourself that the OCD, rather than your child, is at work here may help.

» **Embarrassment:** Kids with OCD can look strange to other people. Imagine a child who starts to scream because a stranger accidentally bumps into them. Or a case in which an unexpected sneeze triggers a frantic rush to a public restroom and elaborate cleansing rituals to decontaminate. Kids with OCD may have peculiar, inexplicable rituals that must be performed in order to go through doorways.

Some children with OCD refuse to sit in car seats, can't climb certain stairs, refuse to dress for gym class, or spend hours mumbling to themselves. The public acting out of obsessions or compulsions can be quite difficult for a parent to handle or understand. Acceptance comes with education about the disorder. Again, it can help to remind yourself that these behaviors are about OCD and are not a reflection on you as a parent.

Working with the therapist

How a therapist structures therapy with your child depends on many factors, such as your child's age, maturity, conversational skills, shyness, and independence. Some therapists have both parents and child together in the office throughout each session. Other therapists break the session up, having the child come in first and following with a summary for the parents. Teenagers are usually seen alone, with parents attending sessions only occasionally.

The bottom line is that therapy is built on a *collaborative, confidential* relationship between the client (child) and the therapist. The child must be comfortable confiding anything to the therapist. In general, parents need to know what is going on and what progress is being made, but it's counterproductive in most cases for them to be privy to all the details. Don't worry that your child may be talking about family embarrassments (such as the last fight you had with your spouse). Good therapists are not judgmental and keep information confidential. Furthermore, most therapists don't believe everything they hear.

TIP

When your child leaves the therapist's office, ask an open-ended question like, "How are you feeling about today's session?" rather than "What did you talk about?" Don't press your child for details about the therapy.

Collaborating on goals

Parents need to collaborate with their child and their child's therapist in setting appropriate goals. OCD is a formidable foe and is best tackled in small, sequential steps. Everyone needs to know what those steps will be and when they are going to occur. In most cases, some kind of exposure trigger list (see Chapter 10) will be developed and times set aside for managing triggers while delaying or preventing compulsions.

Parents can help the therapist by recording their kid's progress. They should also make note of any setbacks and/or distressing, unanticipated resistance shown by their child during this work. Furthermore, parents can usually be good historians and inform therapists about their child's early symptoms and how those have waxed and waned over the years.

Providing appropriate incentives

Everyone, including adults, feel more motivated to keep working on tasks when they can perceive some sort of payoff or incentive for all their hard work. For adults and even some mature teenagers, that payoff may be something intangible, such as taking pride in a job well done. Younger children often need more concrete, clearer rewards, such as special outings, a later bedtime, praise, money, stickers, or other treats. Most therapists who work with children have an array of interesting ideas for incentives that may work with your child.

TIP

Much as rewards may be useful in keeping your child on track, watch out for these pitfalls when designing your child's incentive plan:

>> Don't overemphasize rewards and become excessively enthusiastic about each and every small gain. Kids sometimes learn to resist the pressure they feel when parents get too excited or push too hard — even with incentives.

>> Rewards must not be the centerpiece of your child's OCD treatment plan. They are only a way to nudge along and encourage good, solid effort.

>> Part of your reward plan needs to include ignoring lack of progress, off-task behavior, and even OCD backslides. Let the therapist deal with these issues. You will become too emotionally entangled if you get involved with telling your child to stop OCD behaviors.

>> The younger your child, the more quickly you need to provide small rewards for specific efforts. Older children can be expected to work longer to obtain larger, less frequent rewards. Again, your child's therapist can provide a lot of guidance here.

REMEMBER

Properly-designed reward plans are not bribes. Bribery is involved when parents dangle rewards and incentives in front of their kids with constant reminders and cajoling to obtain them. You don't want to remind your child about the reward plan very often at all.

Giving appropriate reassurance

A common practice among children and adults with OCD is asking other people for reassurance. These questions are often repeated dozens of times every day. Examples of the type of questions asked include:

>> Are the doors locked?

>> Are you and Daddy mad?

>> Are you and Mom going to get divorced?

>> Are you okay?

>> Are we always going to be safe?

>> Do I look sick?

>> Do you still love me?

>> I've had bad thoughts; will I go to hell?

>> Do you think a storm is coming?

>> Do you think I hurt somebody?

>> Is that dish really clean?

I recommend that you collaborate with your child's therapist in developing an automatic response to each of these questions. Also, tell your child ahead of time what the answer will be. Possible examples of such responses that avoid the reassurance trap include:

>> I understand that you're worried, but I can't answer that.

>> That's your OCD talking, what can you say back to it?

>> You have to find the answer for that yourself.

>> There is no answer to that question.

>> You know I can't answer that.

>> Life is full of uncertainties.

>> You know the answer to that.

Perhaps these answers sound like they lack empathy and compassion. However, providing reassurance to an OCD child who asks for it only fuels OCD. Letting your child know that you understand their feelings is fine, but giving reassurance only ends up reinforcing your child's OCD.

REMEMBER

Telling your child in advance what your responses will be helps reduce frustration on everyone's part and allows you as a parent to feel less guilt about not providing the reassurance that's been requested. Remind yourself of the old adage that sometimes you have to be just a little "cruel to be kind."

TIP

Learning to stop giving children reassurance is hard work, but one of the most important parts of helping kids with OCD.

Acting as a coach and a cheerleader

I discourage parents from trying to be therapists to their children with OCD. But, in reality, parents are obviously involved and must take on some role. After all, parents spend many hours a day with their children. Parents should ideally act as coaches. Not as mean coaches who scream, discourage, and push, nor as coaches who overly praise and cajole. Rather, parents should be fair and kind coaches who motivate through noticing progress and keeping a positive focus, while setting reasonable limits on OCD. Table 21-1 provides some ideas on what coaches should and shouldn't say.

TABLE 21-1 **Bad Coach/Good Coach**

Child's Behavior	Bad Coaching Response	Good Coaching Response
Cuts showers down to three per day from six.	Fine, but when are you going to shower like everybody else in the world — once a day!?	Nice work, I see you've cut your showers down. What's your plan now?
Refuses to engage in an ERP exercise one day.	You'll never get better that way. Have you forgotten about the movie you can earn?	Maybe tomorrow will go better.
Says, "I'm not going to therapy anymore. I hate therapy."	If you go, I'll take you out for ice cream. And besides, I've already paid for it. You have to do this!	I know it's hard, but it's just what we all decided to do. There isn't really a choice here.
Child with contamination fears is able to clean up dog poop in the backyard and not wash for an hour.	Wow! That's so great! I can't believe you managed to do that! You are terrific. It looks like you've just about licked your OCD! Let's go and buy you that new video game you've wanted for so long. I'm so proud of you!	Wow, that looked hard. You must feel proud of yourself. I think you'll be ready for the next step soon. Would you like to pick out your reward from the list?
Child yells at parent for interrupting a bedtime ritual.	Who will ever marry you if you do these weird things all the time? Be normal! I can't stand it when you act crazy like this. Stop it!	I know you're frustrated, but we can't give in to your OCD mind. I want you to try and be more respectful.

As you can see in Table 21-1, bad coaches and good coaches behave differently. Bad coaches criticize, whereas good coaches refrain from criticism. Bad coaches go over the top with praise, cajoling, and reminders about incentives. Other times, they let their anger go out of control.

Good coaches praise with restraint and don't focus too much on rewards. Good coaches are leaders and role models for emotional control. They also set reasonable limits on their kids and their kids' OCD. Finally, they express positive expectations, but without undue pressure. Your child's therapist can help you figure out how to do all of that because it isn't always easy!

TIP

Parenting is a tough job. Parenting a child with OCD can be even more challenging. You are human and may become frustrated. You might even lose your temper from time to time. Forgive yourself, apologize to your child, and use the opportunity to figure out under what circumstances you get the most frustrated. Take another deep breath and try to hold it together next time.

Explaining OCD to Family, Friends, and Schoolmates

Children with OCD work desperately hard to keep people from knowing about their problem. Only rarely do they fully succeed. And when others do see their OCD behaviors, they often fail to understand what's going on. All too often the net result is that the child with OCD experiences a lack of understanding, teasing, and social rejection. Feeling ostracized can lead to depression, anxiety, and failures in school.

So, the questions become whom to tell, what to tell, and how to tell others about OCD. Unfortunately, there are no hard and fast rules. However, consider the following points:

>> **Brothers and sisters:** There's no way that brothers and sisters living in the same household won't at some time and in some way know that their sibling has OCD, or at least some pretty odd behaviors. Sometimes brothers and sisters feel angry because they fear what others will think of them for having a sibling with OCD. They may also feel angry or jealous about the attention paid to the OCD or the fact that their sibling seems to get away with behaviors that they can't. And other times, they worry about catching the OCD.

Acknowledging all of these feelings is important, yet limits must be set on how anger and jealousy get expressed.

Explaining what OCD is all about is equally important. First, tell siblings of the child with OCD that OCD is no one's fault. Explain that the brain of the child with OCD misfires for various reasons. Further note that OCD is treatable, nothing to feel ashamed about, and that you can't "catch" OCD from someone else. Finally, try to spend a little special time with the siblings who don't suffer from OCD.

>> **Relatives and close family friends:** Many people do not understand OCD very well. If your friends and family really want to be helpful, suggest that they educate themselves about OCD; reading this book is one way they could do that. However, if they don't want to spend that much time, you can at least explain a few things.

Tell them the same things that siblings need to know: OCD involves a misfiring of the brain; it's usually very treatable; and it's not contagious. If relatives or close friends are directly involved with childcare, you probably want to explain how treatment works in more detail so they don't inadvertently get in the way of what you're trying to do. If they show interest in helping, you may suggest that they read Chapter 22.

>> **Schoolmates:** First, check with your child, your child's teacher, and the school counselor to see whether schoolmates are causing any problems, such as teasing or bullying due to your child's OCD. Some children have OCD and don't show much of it overtly at school. In that case, leave it alone. However, if problems do crop up, they can be handled a couple of ways:

- The school counselor may either give a talk about OCD to your child's class or recruit an expert to do so.

- If an individual child is causing problems with bullying and teasing, the counselor can probably deal with that.

Your child's therapist can collaborate with the counselor as well. What's important is to protect your child from becoming victimized.

TIP

OCD can easily affect your child's relationship with siblings, friends, and relatives. Help your child realize that any teasing or rejection is really about a misunderstanding of OCD, not about your child. Work with your child to fight back against the OCD.

Getting More Help at School

In a few cases, OCD interferes significantly with learning and achievement in school. Here are a few examples of problems that could crop up:

>> A child with contamination fears may struggle to touch classroom supplies, be in close contact with peers, or have a need to wash regularly. This may be disruptive to the classroom and the child's ability to concentrate.

>> A child may have rituals that they believe must be performed in the morning before school, which causes them to be frequently tardy or absent.

>> A child with perfectionism may not be able to finish assignments on time because of a need to recopy or reread material.

>> Any child with OCD may be consumed by obsessions and be unable to pay attention. When they are not able to complete compulsions, their frustration can be disturbing to the classroom.

Usually, accommodations can be made for a while in the regular classroom. These accommodations may include providing a little extra time to complete tests or written work, seating the child near the front of the class to help with focus, and allowing extra breaks to check in with the counselor. A child's therapist will no doubt want to be consulted on all of these accommodations and will help the school team provide needed help without inadvertently reinforcing the OCD. For instance, it would not be appropriate to allow a child with contamination fears large blocks of time to spend washing or cleaning. That would take away from learning time and let OCD take charge.

If accommodations are not sufficient and a child lags behind, a multidisciplinary evaluation can be requested. The purpose of the evaluation is to gather information about the best ways to help the child function academically, socially, and emotionally. This evaluation may include gathering information from caregivers and teachers. In addition, psychological and educational assessment may be completed, usually by a school psychologist.

TECHNICAL STUFF

Children with OCD who require more help may get services through what is called a 504 plan or through an Individualized Education Plan (IEP). Those with 504 plans will stay in the regular classroom and get accommodations that fit their needs. Children who have IEPs may also stay in the regular classroom for all or part of the day, but usually get more services.

Chapter 22

Helping Family and Friends Cope with OCD

Tackling OCD takes a team, and every team needs a coach, sometimes more than one. If you're interested in helping a friend or family member overcome OCD, understand that it is not an opponent for the faint of heart or a single individual, no matter how brave. That's why I don't advocate a pure self-help approach in this book.

It's not that people can't help themselves, but maintaining the focus, drive, and objectivity required to tackle OCD is easier and more effectively done with the help of others. For most OCD sufferers, which help includes one or more mental-health professionals as well as possibly friends or family. For a few, that help may come only from friends or family members who serve as "coaches."

This chapter tells you what you need to know if you're interested in helping a friend, loved one, child, or relative who suffers from OCD. It explains the task that lies ahead, including figuring out whether you're the right person to do the job and knowing what to look out for. This chapter gives you tools to help assess your coaching capabilities as well as techniques for effective coaching.

Discerning What It Takes to Be Supportive

One of the trendier terms in mental health, business, personal development, and physical fitness circles nowadays is "coach." When you think of the word "coach," you think of someone who listens, watches, provides feedback, models behavior, and instructs. That's a good analogy for the role that a friend or family member may play in helping someone with OCD. But there are two important points I want to clarify before I get into the nitty-gritty of coaching:

>> **You don't have to be a professional to be a coach.** You don't need any sort of professional degree or license. Family and friends who agree to serve as coaches may be of great value in helping someone implement a game plan for fighting OCD.

>> **Your role is to help implement, not develop, a treatment plan.** Unless those acting as coaches are trained and licensed mental-health professionals, they should not be responsible for *developing* an actual treatment plan for OCD. What I'm discussing in this chapter is helping your friend or family member carry out a treatment plan that has been developed in cooperation with a therapist.

To be an effective coach, you need to understand the game that's being played. In this case, which means you need to become educated about OCD. Of course, I recommend reading this book; it really does provide a whole lot of information about OCD. It's also a good idea to find out about the specific type of OCD the person you're helping has. (See Chapter 2 as well as relevant chapters on specific types of OCD.)

Whatever type of OCD the person you care about has, your coaching will likely focus on helping that person to implement exposure and response prevention (ERP). ERP is explained fully in Chapter 10, and that chapter should be read carefully. There, you not only see what ERP is, but also can see lots of examples, as well as advice on troubleshooting.

In brief, ERP involves guiding someone through a series of steps that involve encountering triggers for the OCD. The exposures usually start out fairly easy and become sequentially more difficult. However, they don't always go in any particular order; it depends on what the therapist and person decide to tackle. Although to a layperson some of the triggers may look silly or easy, for a person with OCD they may feel like trying to reach the peak of Mt. Everest.

People with OCD must go through each exposure, one at a time. It's most helpful if they stay with that trigger until their distress levels (what I'm calling Ugh

Factor Ratings) come down a little. For example, imagine you're helping your friend Pete with contamination OCD. Pete fears shaking hands and feels compelled to wash his hands for an hour if he happens to be forced into a hand-shaking encounter.

The first exposure may involve Pete agreeing to briefly shake hands with someone who has just washed up. Pete's next exposure may call for him to not wash his hands for one full hour. Your role as coach is to assist in that process. Read on to discover how to do that right.

Understanding how OCD challenges you

Good coaches know which side they're on. If you're coaching a friend or relative with OCD, you take the side of that person and you work against the OCD. Sounds pretty obvious, doesn't it?

But sometimes OCD makes people act in ways that hook you into working against them. That happens when OCD hijacks someone's mind so much that the person fears and resists treatment of the OCD (see Chapter 6 for examples of such resistance).

Naturally, as a coach and helper, you want to see the person fight OCD with unbridled zeal and enthusiasm. Your intense desire to help may cause you to push, pressure, and prod your friend to increase effort and fight harder. If you see signs of hesitation or reluctance, you may want to confront, cajole, and conquer your friend's reluctance. That's a good idea, right?

Actually, it isn't. Psychologists now know that confronting and pressuring people to change typically causes them to dig in their heels and resist changing all the more. They may run from such "help" and avoid treatment entirely. Thus, if you push too hard, you actually end up serving your friend's OCD mind, not your friend.

Coaches don't coach people who don't want to be coached. They wait for people to seek their services. If resistance pops up, it's important to accept that position. Tell your friend or relative that you're ready to help when they want it — not one minute before that.

TIP

The more you can accept people for who and where they are now, the more likely they are to accept the idea of making changes.

Assessing whether you're the right person to coach

Not everyone is born to coach. You may care a great deal about your friend or relative; yet you may not be the right person to help implement OCD treatment. So how do you know if you'd be a good coach? Here are a few considerations:

>> **Compassion:** You have to realize that OCD is a disorder that's not caused by weakness of character or malicious intentions. The person with OCD truly suffers and needs your empathic support (but not so much that you assuage and reassure).

>> **Humor:** It really helps if you can laugh with the person you're coaching. Obviously, you don't want to laugh *at* the person you're coaching but rather at some of the humorous moments that pop up. Some exposure tasks can get a little silly, and it's okay to laugh so long as you're laughing together.

>> **Temperament:** ERP requires great patience. Those with OCD can also test your mettle. If you're easily frustrated or have a short fuse, you probably ought to cheer from the sidelines rather than coach on the playing field.

>> **Time:** Coaching takes time. Depending on the case, ERP may consume a few hours each week for quite a few weeks or as much as a full day or two each week over a shorter time period. Sometimes ERP is scheduled to occur on a daily basis. Be clear about how much time is being asked of you and be certain you can commit without feeling resentful.

TIP

Think about how you and your life fit into the role of a coach. Don't volunteer if you aren't pretty sure you can follow through. It's okay just to be a supportive bystander.

Knowing your limits

Decades ago, OCD was thought to be a largely untreatable condition. Even today, sometimes OCD comes in a highly treatment-resistant mode. Although the odds are good that treatment will help, it can be difficult and require a lot of time and energy.

Don't take responsibility for the success or failure of the treatment plan. If you feel too personally involved, you may need to back off. You are facilitating, not taking over.

Know your own limits. If your frustration runs too high, it's time to back off. You can still care and even cheerlead a little from the sidelines.

Applying Appropriate Coaching Techniques

If you choose to be a coach, you may become part of a team that includes your friend or relative, probably a mental-health professional, and perhaps other coaches. All of you will likely meet together and collaborate on the game plan. Feel free to toss out a few of your own ideas but realize that responsibility for designing the game plan lies with the professional and the one who has OCD.

If you feel uncomfortable with any aspect of the ERP plan, express that discomfort. You don't want to agree to something that doesn't resonate with you. You may discover that the therapist uses some professional jargon that you don't follow. If that happens, don't hesitate to ask questions, it doesn't mean you're stupid. Sometimes professionals lapse into using shorthand that others shouldn't be expected to know.

Recognizing OCD's dirty tricks

As a coach (or supportive family member or friend), keep your eye on the ball. In this case, the opponent (OCD) is always trying to steal the ball. One way OCD tries to overtake the coach is by enticing the coach or other people to help perform checking or rituals or to provide reassurance. For example:

>> A father repeatedly reassures and reasons with his daughter who has superstitious OCD (see Chapter 17). He patiently explains that numbers have no power over events and that certain symbols and words cannot cause harm. He feels gratified when she feels temporarily relieved, not realizing how much fuel he has provided for her superstitions.

>> A mother agrees to rewash the dishes and rerun the laundry for her son who has contamination OCD (see Chapter 13). The mom goes along because her son becomes distraught if she doesn't.

>> A teenager has their parents chanting certain prayers with him before bed. If they don't do them "just so," they demand that they repeat the prayers. The parents comply so that the teen goes to bed without screaming at them. Again, a simple act of kindness does nothing but make OCD stronger.

>> A woman worries about her appearance. She repeatedly asks her husband whether she looks okay, whether her wrinkles are deeper, and whether he still finds her attractive. He wants her to feel better and consistently reassures her that he thinks she's beautiful. He doesn't realize that he's simply feeding his wife's OCD.

>> Another person may have obsessions about closing up the house after leaving for work. That person calls a spouse or even a neighbor to check again. A half-hour later, the brief relief from the reassurance fades, then the obsessions return, and the person needs to find someone else to check the house.

>> Someone who repeatedly checks to see that appliances are off before going to bed may ask a concerned family member to check one more time. Rather than get into a squabble, that family member gives in. Unfortunately, giving in does not help the person with OCD. Rather, it empowers OCD. Although the person with the OCD feels temporarily assuaged and reassured, OCD doubts quickly return and grow stronger than ever.

REMEMBER

Providing reassurance to a person with OCD fuels OCD. That's because getting reassurance feels good temporarily, thus it reinforces the obsessions that started the cycle.

Furthermore, coaches must refrain from helping the person actually carry out checking or rituals. They also need to avoid reasoning with the person, no matter how rational doing so seems. OCD doesn't go away with reasoning; rather, it deepens. With permission from the person with OCD, coaches can also inform therapists about other friends or family members who are unwittingly feeding the OCD. The therapist can help design strategies to help everyone stop this vicious cycle.

Coaching with kindness

You've seen sports movies that portray really mean, arrogant coaches; sometimes they succeed and pull off miracles. But OCD coaching doesn't work with anything other than a kind, supportive approach. The next sections discuss how to coach with kindness.

Refraining from criticizing

ERP involves hard work. Some of the steps provoke a lot of distress and anxiety. The last thing people with OCD need to hear is that they aren't doing things right.

I'm not saying that you can't provide a little corrective feedback, but any such messages must be worded carefully and gently. For example, instead of saying, "You didn't wait the full 30 minutes before washing," you could say, "You made it 20 minutes; that's good. The step calls for 30 minutes, and I'll bet you can get there next time."

Most people with OCD are quite intelligent, and they didn't ask to have OCD. The person you're coaching is probably working hard to get to a better place. Criticism undermines confidence.

Providing encouragement

It's not only okay, but also useful to express belief in your friend's or relative's ability to tackle OCD. A small dose of persuasion can do wonders too, but only if it is used judiciously. You want to encourage and help the person to maintain a focus on each goal. But if you let your encouragement turn into pressure, it can be like trying to take a mountainous hairpin curve at high speed, you can easily fly off the edge of the road.

Leaving decision-making alone

People with OCD frequently ask for advice on what to do, when to do it, and how to do it; it's actually part of their OCD. If you're the coach, don't fall for this one. You want to keep firmly in your mind that part of good OCD treatment is to keep decision-making in the hands of the person with OCD.

For example, a woman with shaming OCD may worry that she'll shout obscenities in public, or even worse, at church. Her exposure task is to go to a movie while actively focusing on and thinking about obscenities. She may ask you whether she should leave the movie if her anxiety becomes too great. Don't make that decision for her. It's okay to tell her that the general principle is to stay with an exposure until distress comes down some, but how long she actually does so is always completely her decision to make.

Eliminating surprises by asking for permission

As a coach, keep in mind that treatment should be predictable and under the control of the person with OCD. Thus, if an exposure calls for your friend to smear motor oil on their arm, you don't want to surprise them by unexpectedly sullying their arm with oil. Rather, you should discuss the step and ideally allow them to do the dirty work. If they just can't bring themself to do it and *asks* you to, then you can. Their next step can then involve doing it herself.

Furthermore, you want to be sure you're both on the same page. Perhaps you're working with someone who has just so (symmetry) OCD. Don't feel like you can go into their home and mess up their alphabetized cans or make a mess of the carpet fringes without first getting permission. When granted, go for it, have a blast.

Those who have OCD don't give up their fundamental rights when they undergo treatment. Coaches can be effective only when they allow the people that they are helping to control the steps being taken.

Avoiding arguing at all costs

Coaching is tricky business. Sometimes the person you're coaching will suddenly balk and declare themself unable to complete the next exposure. Perhaps you've actually seen them successfully do exposures that appear quite similar to the one they're resisting. Under such circumstances, you may be tempted to argue and convincingly demonstrate that their perspective is flawed. But whether they're right or wrong doesn't really matter.

A good coach doesn't take the bait. A good coach simply says, "You're ready when you're ready. You tell me when that is." Accept the position of the person you're helping and even express a little empathy.

You could easily think I'm saying that you should never disagree with the person you're helping, but that's not quite true. I'm saying that you should avoid *arguing* at almost any cost. You can express disagreement if you do so ever so gently — whether directly or with a question. Following are a few ways to express disagreement if you think doing so may be useful:

>> "I hear you saying that you feel you're at an impasse. And clearly, you're only ready when you're ready. However, I wonder whether that's your OCD mind talking. What do you think?"

>> "I know you feel rather hopeless right now. I'd feel frustrated, too, if I were in your shoes. Have you felt hopeless at other times and felt more hopeful later?"

>> "You're right; the OCD does seem to be in charge right now. However, I do believe in you, and I suspect you're going to find a way to get where you want to be."

Sometimes you word your disagreement beautifully, and your friend or relative still manages to argue back. When that happens, it's best to let go of the issue and allow the therapist to deal with it.

Coaches are not therapists. It is not up to you as a coach to force the person you're coaching to stick with the treatment plan. You can express encouragement and belief in the person but arguing is always counterproductive.

Sidestepping the word "should"

Dr. Albert Ellis was a psychologist who virtually made a career out of railing against the word "should." He aptly noted that there are few behaviors that people absolutely "should" or "should not" do. Obviously, most of us would argue that murder, stealing, and abuse belong on the "should not" do list. However, people have a strong proclivity to use the word "should" in an array of situations that really don't call for the harsh, judgmental tone the word conveys.

Most of the time, other words or phrases do the job of "should" without sounding so evaluative. If you plan to coach someone with OCD, start monitoring your use of the word "should." Try substituting other phrases, such as, "It would be better if . . .," "I suspect you'd want to . . .," or "It would be nice if . . . ." The bottom line is that you don't want to tell those with OCD how they "should" feel, what they "should" be ready for, or what they "should" do. Check out the following list of some "should" statements, along with some improved ways of stating things:

> **"Should" statement:** You should stay with this step for at least 30 minutes.
>
> **Improved statement:** It has been 23 minutes. Just seven more to go. See if you can hang in there.
>
> **"Should" statement:** You shouldn't feel that way.
>
> **Improved statement:** I can tell you're feeling upset.
>
> **"Should" statement:** You shouldn't wash your hands so much. They're starting to bleed!
>
> **Improved statement:** I know it's hard, but it would help if you could stick with the plan of reducing that handwashing.
>
> **"Should" statement:** You shouldn't worry about numbers all the time; that's really silly.
>
> **Improved statement:** I suspect you don't enjoy getting hooked by those number superstitions. It would be nice if you could work a little longer on this number repetition exercise.

TIP

Don't beat yourself up for occasionally lapsing into using the word "should." I'm sure you can find instances where I use it; it's ingrained in the human psyche. But you "should" try to lessen your usage and, in general, avoid being judgmental.

Keeping difficult emotions in check

Watching someone you care about struggle with OCD can be frustrating. OCD is neither logical nor rational. When you see people being irrational, you may want to shake some sense into them. You may feel angry, upset, or distressed.

Try to appreciate the fact that the person you're coaching is likely to be consumed with fighting OCD and doesn't understand your turmoil. Furthermore, if you express your distress, things will only get worse. Read the earlier section in this chapter, "Knowing your limits," if you find yourself overwhelmed with negative emotions.

Developing alternatives to reassurance

In the section "Recognizing OCD's dirty tricks," I note that reassurance, assuaging, and giving into OCD demands only gives the OCD part of someone's mind more fuel. But how do you *not* reassure someone you care about who is in distress and begging for reassurance?

In fact, you'll probably find yourself unable to stop giving reassurance at first. Most kind people are programmed to provide reassurance to those who are in distress and ask for it. That's probably not a big problem for the average person. But OCD changes the game.

Work with the person you're coaching and the therapist on this issue. Everyone needs to know that you plan to respond differently from here on out. I recommend designing a list of automatic responses — ones that you can memorize and use reflexively. Table 22-1 provides a few examples of reassurance requests that may be asked of you and some reassurance-busting responses.

TABLE 22-1   **Reassurance Requests and Reassurance Busters**

OCD Type	Reassurance Request	Reassurance Buster
Contamination	Do you think this table was wiped clean enough?	There's always a chance that germs remain anywhere, including on this table.
Checking and doubting	Do you think that bump we hit was a person?	Remember that your therapist said to say that it's always possible you did hit someone. Beyond that, I don't know.
Shaming	Will I go to hell?	I don't know. Maybe.
Checking and doubting	Are you still attracted to me?	You know I can't answer that for you.
Shaming	Do you think I'm a pedophile?	I can't answer that.
Superstitious	Do you think that hearse will bring us bad luck?	Who knows?

TIP

Your list of reassurance busters needs to be planned in advance and agreed upon by the therapist and the person you're coaching. These are not pulled out as a surprise. And they're not intended to be sarcastic. Feel free to use judicious humor, but not disrespect.

6
The Part of Tens

Manage OCD symptoms quickly.

Check out ways to calm down.

Set up steps for post OCD.

Discover more than you ever wanted to know about dirt.

Chapter **23**

Ten Quick OCD Tricks

A variety of chapters in this book give you detailed, comprehensive plans for dealing with your OCD. But sometimes you just want to make it through a minute, an hour, or a day. This chapter gives you some quick tips for dealing with your OCD. Use these tips to ease your journey.

Breathing Better

Breathing strategies can help you manage difficult feelings. Whether your feelings involve fear, anxiety, sadness, or urges, concentrating on your breath can decrease the intensity of your distress. Focusing on breathing allows you to settle down anywhere, anytime.

First, take a deep breath through your nose. Notice the air going into your nostrils and flowing into your lungs. Fill the lower part of your lungs first by expanding your abdomen and your diaphragm. Hold that breath for a slow count of five. Then slowly release the air to a slow count of eight.

Many people find that making a slight hissing noise through their lips helps them slow down the exhalation. Continue breathing this way for five or six breaths. Notice how the breathing affects your feelings. Deep, slow breathing is a great alternative to other ways of trying to avoid feelings through compulsions.

Considering a Delay

Especially if you're early in the process of working on your OCD, stopping your compulsions may seem to border on the absurd or the impossible. That's okay, you can build up slowly. For now, just delay.

In other words, put off your compulsive behavior (such as handwashing, chanting, arranging things, or cleaning) for two or three minutes. Next, try to make it a bit longer, 10 or 15 minutes. Later, try delaying for half an hour, then an hour. Give yourself credit for each and every delay. Soon you'll find yourself ready for full-blown exposure and response prevention.

Distracting Yourself

Although not an ideal strategy in the long run, distracting yourself during early ERP can help you get through the first steps. Try focusing on another competing activity, such as

>> Eating

>> Going for a walk

>> Knitting

>> Scrolling through social media

>> Reading

>> Playing a game on your phone

After a while, I recommend that you drop your distraction strategies. But distraction can help get you started.

Accepting Discomfort

The OCD mind attempts to avoid discomfort of almost any kind all the time. The mind also labels discomfort as *terrible* and *unacceptable*. However, these attempts to avoid discomfort at all costs inevitably create even more discomfort in the long run.

Instead, open up a little room for discomfort in your life. When you feel distress, notice it and merely study it for a while, as though you were going to write a report about emotional upset. Remind yourself that some discomfort is inevitable in life. As you embrace negative feelings, you'll find that they paradoxically lessen their hold on you and your life.

Doing Jumping Jacks and More

Research has consistently shown that exercise helps just about everything health related. Stop what you're doing. Right now. If you are able, get up and do 25 jumping jacks, 10 push-ups, and/or 25 sit-ups. Do you feel anxious while you are exercising? Or out of breath?

Exercise is not compatible with negative thinking in most cases. Any kind of exercise that requires concentration takes the focus off of you and your problems. That includes obsessions and compulsions. Make exercise a go-to strategy for coping.

WARNING

Don't rely on exercise too much to deal with your OCD. Exercise is important but can also become a compulsion if used exclusively to combat obsessive urges. Furthermore, some people who have obsessive concerns about health may become anxious when exercising. If that is the case for you, exercise can become an exposure.

Realizing It's Not You, It's Your OCD

OCD is not the same thing as who you are. OCD takes control of your brain and compels you to do things you don't like or want to do. OCD makes you feel that these actions are necessary, but you wouldn't choose to do them on your own. So, it's important to remind yourself that you are not full of doubt, uncertainty, and avoidance of all risks — that's your OCD mind talking. As you step back and realize that it's just your OCD mind, you'll gain strength, confidence, and resolve.

Making Flashcards

When you're mired in the throes of an episode of OCD urges, thinking rationally and remembering what you're supposed to do is pretty hard. Therefore, I suggest that you write out a few ideas on some flashcards. Consider the following possibilities:

>> Bad feelings eventually pass; just give them some time.

>> Having bad thoughts doesn't make me a bad person.

>> I've experienced this before and lived through it.

>> The longer I delay a compulsion, the better off I'm going to be.

>> Thoughts are just thoughts; just because I think something doesn't make it true.

Getting Support

As you're working on your OCD, you'll experience your share of both successes and difficult times. When you feel discouraged, alone, or down, seeking some support is never a bad idea. One great place you can go almost anytime is online. I don't have any particular online support group to recommend to you; you need to explore and find one that feels like a good fit.

Various online networks offer encouragement, education, and advice. Of course, they're not a substitute for professional help, but they can support your efforts. Always take great care in terms of revealing personal information and data online that can reveal your identity.

WARNING

The internet and social media can be a great source of information and misinformation. Beware. Sources such as NAMI (National Alliance on Mental Illness) and the International OCD Foundation are reliable.

Minding Meditation

Having a meditation practice can enhance your life in addition to helping manage your OCD. Learning meditation takes regular practice and time. In meditation, you allow thoughts and feelings simply to occur. You are aware without judgement. You spend time noting what goes through your mind and how your body feels.

If you meditate when experiencing obsessions, you may find it easier to put just a bit of distance between you and your thoughts and feelings. Your level of distress will likely go down. So, it's perfectly fine to use meditation as a way of handling OCD.

WARNING

Like other temporary distractions, meditation should not become a compulsive reaction to your obsessive urges. It can bring you temporary peace but does not replace the active work of dealing directly with trigger situations.

Strolling through Nature

Having a bad day? Get outside. Better yet, find a park. Walk around, smell the smells, look up through the trees, and let nature help you heal.

Walking in nature won't cure you of OCD, but it can make you feel better and more up to doing the work you need to do. Take a few deep breaths and relax.

Chapter **24**

Ten Steps for After You Get Better

Obsessive-compulsive disorder (OCD) seriously damages the quality of the lives of those who suffer from it. Many people with OCD report that much of their day focuses on their obsessions and compulsions that involve cleaning, fears of contamination, checking on safety, and various superstitious worries and behaviors. Their OCD slams the door on more positive pursuits such as hobbies, recreation, charitable work, and social connections, most of what makes a life feel full and worthwhile.

However, the odds are high that you'll be able to substantially reduce the hold that OCD has over your life. Assuming you do, you'll have time and resources that you haven't had available to you in many years. You may find this new freedom confusing and not know what to do with it. This chapter gives you ten ideas for filling up the void.

Forgive Yourself

Most people with OCD tend to berate themselves for having the disorder in the first place. Making matters worse, they beat themselves up after they've improved from the OCD, often believing they have wasted years mired in their OCD and should be punished for doing so.

Being angry with yourself only keeps you from finding peace. Finding a way to forgive yourself is important. First, remember that you did not ask for your OCD. OCD is a complicated problem with many causes (see Chapters 4 and 5 for more information about the causes of OCD). For many decades, no effective treatments even existed for OCD — proving just how formidable a foe OCD can really be.

You had to work hard to battle your OCD. If you have experienced significant success, you deserve praise, not punishment. Therefore, when you notice self-punishing thoughts going through your head, try answering back with one of these self-forgiving phrases:

>> I am not the same as my OCD.

>> I didn't ask for my OCD, but I did battle it well.

>> I've made great progress; beating myself up will only make me backslide.

>> If a friend of mine worked hard on their OCD, I'd praise them, not pummel them.

>> It's time to focus on future successes, not past struggles.

Search for Meaning

Many sufferers from OCD report that they feel as though their lives have no meaning outside of dealing with their OCD. But again, if you experience even partial success in battling your OCD, the possibility for discovering new meanings begins to emerge.

Think about what you want to be remembered for; it probably goes beyond your OCD. Do you want to be remembered for your clean house or your kind heart? You may find sources of meaning and ways you'd like to be remembered by considering the following possibilities:

>> Advancing knowledge

>> Being generous

>> Being grateful

>> Helping others who are less fortunate

>> Improving the environment

>> Taking care of rescue animals

>> Teaching others

In addition, honor your personal faith. Believe in something larger than yourself or your OCD.

Strengthen Family Ties

OCD has a way of creating rifts in families. Friends and relatives of those with OCD often become frustrated and upset because they don't understand the disorder. And those who have OCD feel unfairly maligned and misunderstood.

If you've managed to overcome much of your OCD, it's time to mend those fences. Try having a monthly potluck with all family members invited. If you live some distance away, arrange family reunions every couple of years. If your family is willing to listen, you may want to explain OCD to them or suggest that they read this book. If your family is reasonably close, they may consider the value of family therapy; it can help. If you don't have a family, or your family is uninterested in reengaging, read the following section on finding friends.

Find Friends

Your OCD may have dominated so much of your time and attention that you weren't able to develop good friendships. And finding friends, especially as an adult, can be difficult. People are busy with their jobs and immediate families.

Yet, the value of having a circle of friends is considerable. People with the support of friends tend to be much healthier, happier, and fulfilled. Friends give you a source of advice, enjoyable times, and encouragement.

Though the task may sound challenging, you can find friends if you work at it. Consider joining a neighborhood association and actively participating. Search for continuing education classes (see the section "Learning New Skills") and talk with your fellow classmates during breaks or after class. You can find social support groups at churches, synagogues, and mosques. Participate in politics. Be creative; you can do this.

Reach Out to Others with OCD

If you've gone through exposure and response prevention therapy (ERP, see Chapter 10), you could make a great coach for someone else. Look for OCD support groups in your area. You can find them in your local newspaper or on the internet (be sure to check out the International OCD Foundation).

Go to one of these support groups and tell them about your successes. You can also offer to coach. If someone takes you up on the offer, be sure to first read Chapters 10 and 22.

WARNING

Don't try to serve as a therapist for someone; that's the job of a mental-health professional.

Help Others

You can help people who don't suffer from OCD, too! The benefit of helping someone else is reciprocal — you feel good and so does the person you're helping. The possibilities are endless, depending on what skills and interests you have, where you live, and what needs stand out in your community. Some suggestions for ways to help others include:

>> Working with the American Cancer Society

>> Joining Big Brothers or Big Sisters and mentoring a child

>> Helping kids with their homework through Boys and Girls Clubs

>> Judging a school science fair

>> Serving as a docent at a local museum

>> Teaching English as a second language

>> Teaching someone to read (whether a child or an adult) at your local community college

>> Working with the local food bank

You can also go to www.volunteermatch.org. You enter where you live and your interests, and they match you up with available opportunities.

Engage in Exercise as a Lifestyle

OCD takes up so much time that the thought of making time for exercise feels as likely as a cow jumping over the moon. But if you have reduced your OCD, you now have available time that you haven't had in years. Now is the time to take advantage of it and fill what used to be consumed by obsessions and compulsions with something much more positive — exercise!

The benefits of exercise abound. They include improved health, better sleep, increased energy, enhanced moods, and feeling more in control of your life.

WARNING

If you haven't exercised regularly in quite some time, be sure to check with your doctor before you start an exercise regimen. Don't keep checking over and over but do get your doctor's clearance.

Your options for exercise are numerous, but I suggest that you seek a mix of aerobic exercise (exercise that increases your heart rate) and anaerobic exercise (exercise focused on strength training). Many health clubs offer personal trainers who can design an individualized exercise plan. You can either carry out the plan on your own or, if you're lucky enough to be able to afford it, have your personal trainer work with you on a regular basis.

Learn New Skills

Another great way to put new, hard-won time to use is to learn a new skill. New skills keep your brain sharp and enhance your sense of mastery. You may even find that they help you in the workplace. Either way, learning is fun.

Consider taking classes online or at your local community college or university department of adult continuing education. The costs are usually reasonable. The choices are amazing — you can find classes on photography, writing, travel, dance, assertiveness, meditation, history, art, poetry, or birdwatching.

Pursue Hobbies

What's a hobby? Hobbies are activities that you enjoy and that typically are not all that serious. A hobby can involve almost anything at all. You can look into arts and crafts, scrapbooking, painting, pottery, games (such as bridge, scrabble, or chess), gardening, aquariums, model railroads or airplanes, music, or genealogy.

Collections can also be hobbies but be careful if you tend to collect too much; you don't want to develop a related hoarding disorder.

The point of pursuing hobbies is that they can provide you with considerable enjoyment that you haven't experienced in quite a while. You may need to try a variety of hobbies in order to find one that fits you. Many hobbies are hard to appreciate until you take them out for a test ride.

Find Healthy Pleasures

Pursuing pleasures is not only enjoyable, but good for you, too. Numerous studies have shown that including a healthy dose of pleasures in your life decreases chronic pain, improves overall health, decreases risk of heart attacks, combats stress, and increases life expectancy. What pleases you is a rather idiosyncratic enterprise. Of course, hobbies (see the preceding section) may please you, but other pleasurable activities may include eating a great meal; going to movies; reading great books; reading less-than-great, trashy books; taking long walks; and playing with your dogs.

WARNING

Ben Franklin advised about the need for moderation in all things. So, if you love ice cream, great, just don't make it your main pleasurable pursuit. However, most people's scales tilt toward too little pleasure, especially people with OCD.

Chapter **25**

Ten Dirty Little Secrets about Dirt

D irt has a bad name. Those with OCD (especially the contamination type) often view dirt as their arch enemy. They view each speck of dust with disdain and fear. But as the saying goes, you should "know thy enemy." Read on to find out more about dirt.

Defining Dirt

The word "dirt" (or "dirty") generally has negative connotations. Dirt is filthy, squalid, obscene, corrupt, or malicious. Sometimes the term "dirt" refers to unseemly information about someone. Other times it is used to describe excrement, unsanitary conditions, dust, and general uncleanness. Soil is also a form of dirt, but obviously has more positive meanings. Soil allows us to grow crops. Soil consists of humus and disintegrated bits of rock. So, dirt isn't always a bad thing.

Living Dirt

Soil isn't simple, bland, or inert. Soil contains an entire ecosystem in a constant state of change. A square yard of soil can contain several hundred worms. Furthermore, bacteria, actinomycetes (disease-producing bacteria), fungi, micro-algae, nematodes (roundworms, protozoa, and other organisms live, grow, and die in soil.

Digging Dirt

Preschoolers can spend hours digging in the dirt, and parents spend hours cleaning it up. At least a little dirt may actually help build up immune systems in children and protect them from getting allergies, asthma, and autoimmune diseases. Kids who have pets, a big family, or attend daycare in the first year of life are at lower risk of having allergies and asthma than kids brought up in pristine environments. Bet you didn't know that.

Dirt Just Isn't What It Used to Be

Don't take dirt for granted. Although scientists have developed super seeds that can increase food production across the world, people continue to starve. The main reason? Poor dirt. Over the years, nutrients have been taken from the soil and not put back. Without good soil, improvements in agriculture do little to increase the food supply to poor countries.

Chimps Who Eat Dirt

Although babies and toddlers often eat dirt, parents usually try to discourage the practice. However, in nature, chimpanzees have been observed eating dirt before and after eating certain plants. Researchers have found that the mixture of dirt and leaves boosts the chimps' immunity to malaria. Neither the dirt nor the leaves by themselves confer any anti-malaria properties.

Speaking of Washing Off Dirt

Frequent handwashing was a recommendation during the COVID pandemic. A survey was conducted prior to the pandemic regarding handwashing habits. Participants were asked in 2019 (pre-COVID) whether or not they remembered to wash before eating, after using the bathroom, or after coughing, sneezing, or blowing their noses. The same survey was completed in June 2020 during the COVID pandemic. Rates of reported handwashing, as expected, were higher in the 2020 sample. However, only 75 percent of participants reported handwashing routinely in these situations.

The American Society for Microbiology studied the hand-washing habits of 7,836 bathroom-goers in New York, Chicago, Atlanta, New Orleans, and San Francisco. Apparently, handwashing is down since the previous study done in 1996. Less than half the men and slightly more than half the women observed washed their hands after using the public bathrooms. Overall, only 49 percent washed their hands compared to 60 percent in 1996. The researchers also asked people on the phone whether they washed their hands after using the bathroom. Of those who answered, 95 percent reported that indeed they do wash every time — an obvious exaggeration of the truth. Although this research was conducted prior to COVID, the results are still interesting and likely predict what will happen when people return to their previous habits.

Building with Dirt

People have used dirt as a building material for thousands of years. Clay, sand, and straw are mixed to form adobe bricks. Sometimes dung is even used instead of straw — apparently using dung repels insects. An adobe wall can make a surprisingly durable structure, which is fireproof and insulated. Adobe structures have survived earthquakes and hundreds of years of exposure to the elements.

People Who Eat Dirt

Everyone consumes a little dirt — probably quite a few pounds of it over a lifetime. No matter how thoroughly you wash your veggies, a little dirt remains. However, some people actually eat dirt intentionally because, well, umm, they say they like it!

Apparently, pregnant women are especially prone to this practice, which goes by the name of *geophagy*. Typically, they are most drawn to consuming clay. Why they crave clay is an open question. However, speculations include that dirt, and especially clay, contains various critical minerals such as iron, magnesium, and calcium; all of which may be needed in greater abundance during pregnancy. Furthermore, some clays contain kaolin, which used to be a major ingredient in some medications for upset stomachs. Apparently, many white clays are, thus, especially good at calming episodes of morning sickness.

So, am I recommending that you start chowing down on dirt or clay? Well, not really. See the next sections for some of the potential downsides to geophagy.

Kids Who Eat Dirt

Mud pie. Really. Most kids eat dirt from time to time. In fact, it's considered quite normal for a toddler to ingest about 500 mg of dirt in one sitting. In case you haven't been around a toddler, they pretty much stuff everything they find into their mouths such as dirt, paper, dog food, or dust. For the most part, this practice is harmless. But there are some exceptions. If you live on top of a landfill where nuclear waste, products with lead, gasoline, pesticides, old batteries, spent bullets, or other toxic waste products have been discarded, it's best not to let your young child eat dirt. Furthermore, if you have animals that use your garden or lawn for elimination, the dirt may contain some contaminates that could hurt your child. For the most part, letting little ones explore in a safe place, like clean sand, is a better idea.

Pica

A compulsion exists that causes kids to eat dirt that's *not* okay, as opposed to "normal" dirt eating (see the preceding section). This compulsion is called pica. *Pica* is the persistent eating of things that are *not* food. The word pica comes from the Latin word for magpie, a bird that picks up and eats anything.

In order to be diagnosed with pica, a child must eat non-food items for longer than a month and in a greater-than-normal quantity. In fact, the child's eating habits must be really out of the ordinary. Many young children eat stuff that they pick up from the floor in the normal course of learning and crawling. To be diagnosed with dirt pica (also known as geophagy — see the section "People Who Eat Dirt"), a child must eat about 1 gram or more of dirt a day. Other substances that are ingested during bouts of pica include leaves, stones, paint, plaster, string, hair, insects, cigarette butts, animal droppings, or cloth. Yum.

Index

A

accidents
  bodily function, 238, 244, 302
  childhood development of OCD, 74
  doubting and checking OCD, 226, 228–229
  hit-and-run OCD, 222–223
acral canine lick, 50
ADDs (attention deficit disorders), 56, 303
ADHD (attention deficit hyperactivity disorder), 300
adult development of OCD, 70, 76
affective balance, 149
aggressive obsessions and compulsions, 32–33, 237
  childhood OCD, 75
  cognitive behavioral therapy, 123
  common obsessions and compulsions, 33
  example of, 135–137
  fear of hurting someone, 33, 35–36, 75, 91–92, 113–114, 135–137, 166
  fear of losing control, 237–239
  first therapy session, 113–114
  imaginal exposure, 166
  neurotransmitters, 67
  parenting OCD, 35–36
Alzheimer's disease, 67
American Journal of Psychiatry, 191
American Psychologist, 149
American Society for Microbiology, 345
Amitriptyline, 188
amygdala, 61–64
Anafranil (Clomipramine), 16, 188
anorexia, 301
antipsychotic drugs, 293
anxiety and anxiety disorders
  in childhood, 300
  common disorders, 44
  discontinuation syndrome, 188
  exercise, 333

hoarding disorder, 281–282
honesty with doctor, 183
medication, 189
meditation, 158
negative reinforcement process, 78–79
neurotransmitters, 67
OCD vs., 24
shaming OCD, 241
suspending judgment about emotions, 153–154
symptoms of, 44
trigger list for ERP, 169
Anxiety For Dummies, 24, 44
arranging expression of "just so" OCD, 11, 23, 250–252
  books, 252
  carpet fibers and fringe, 252
  clothes, 253
  example of, 80
  exposure and response prevention, 258–259
  food, 27, 252
  money, 252
  ordinary arranging vs., 70
  perfectionism, 82
attachment disorders, 302
attention deficit disorders (ADDs), 56, 303
attention deficit hyperactivity disorder (ADHD), 300
attentional balance, 149
atypical antipsychotics, 293
autism spectrum disorder, 53, 301
avoidance, 212–213
  contamination OCD, 30
  doubting and checking OCD, 227
  negative reinforcement, 78
  perfectionism, 82, 132
  subtle forms of, 179
axons, 65–66
Azrin, Nathan, 284

B

BDD. *See* body dysmorphic disorder

Beck, Aaron, 14

bestiality, 238

bipolar disorder, 45, 184

Bipolar Disorder For Dummies, 45

bladder control, fear of loss of control over, 238, 244

bodily functions
  fear of loss of control over, 237–239, 244–246
  problems with elimination in childhood, 302

body dysmorphic disorder (BDD), 46–47
  common compulsions, 46–47
  common obsessions, 46

bowel control, fear of loss of control over, 238, 244

brain, 59–67
  communication, 65–67
    axons, 65–66
    dendrites, 65–66
    glia, 65
    neurons, 65–66
    neurotransmitters, 66–67, 187
    synaptic clefts, 66
  genetics, 60
  research into, 60–61
  structures and function, 61–65
    amygdala, 61–64
    cortex, 61–64
    hippocampus, 62–64
    response to danger, 62–65
    taking in information, 62
    thalamus, 61–64

brain surgery, 65

breathing
  breathing meditation, 156–159
  obsession with, 36
  relaxation strategy, 177, 331

Buddhism, 149

bulimia, 301

buying
  compulsive, 57
  superstition, 282

C

Canadian Journal of Psychiatry, 187

CBT. *See* cognitive behavioral therapy; exposure and response prevention

Celexa (citalopram), 188

childhood OCD, 297–305, 307–318
  bad experiences, 73–75
    accidents, 74
    illness, 73–74
    stress, 74–75
    trauma, 75
  childhood rituals, 70–71
  development of, 69–76
  effects of, 302–304
    problems at home, 302–303
    problems at school, 303
    problems with friends, 304
  explaining, 316–317
    to family, 317
    to friends, 317
    to schoolmates, 317
    to siblings, 316–317
  getting help at school, 318
  imitating parents with OCD, 75–76
  misguided parenting, 71–73
    inappropriate media, 72
    modeling misguided thinking, 72–73
    overprotecting, 73
    seeking perfection, 73
    too much information, 71–72
  other childhood disorders vs., 300–302
    anxiety and anxiety disorders, 300
    attachment disorders, 302
    attention deficit hyperactivity disorder, 300
    autism spectrum disorder, 301
    bodily function problems, 302
    conduct disorders, 301
    depression, 301
    eating disorders, 301
    learning disabilities, 301
    oppositional defiant disorder, 301
    selective mutism, 302

impulse control disorders *(continued)*
    motor tics, 53–54
    neurotransmitters, 67
    suggested competing response, 289
    touching vs., 276
    vocal tics, 54
  Tourette's syndrome, 53–55, 60, 283–293
    changing thinking, 290–293
    in childhood, 301
    Habit Reversal Training, 284–289
    medication, 293
    neurotransmitters, 67
  trichotillomania, 28, 49–50, 283–294
    changing thinking, 290–293
    defined, 283
    Habit Reversal Training, 284–289
    medication, 294
    suggested competing response, 289
inadequacy, 96, 103
inconsistency, wariness of, 90
Individualized Education Plans (IEPs), 316
insurance, 111–112, 184, 191, 232
International OCD Foundation, 41–42, 107, 110, 304, 334

J

Jacobsen, Edmund, 285
Journal of Biological Psychiatry, 187
"just so" ("just right") OCD (symmetry), 18, 249–259
  arranging expression of, 11, 23, 250–252, 258–259
    books, 252
    carpet fibers and fringe, 252
    clothes, 253
    example of, 80
    exposure and response prevention, 258–259
    food, 27, 252
    money, 252
    ordinary arranging vs., 70
    perfectionism, 82
  in childhood, 250
  co-existing with other forms of OCD, 250
  common obsessions and compulsions, 34
  compulsions, 23

delusional thinking, 26
ego-dystonic and ego-syntonic, 251
examples of, 35, 74, 255–257
hoarding, 282
impulses, 27
irrational nature of obsessions or compulsions, 26
perfectionism, 82
repeating expression of, 252–253, 258–259
shifting attention (set shifting), 251
symmetry, 34–35, 167–168, 249–252, 258–259
treatments and help for, 254–258
  exposure and response prevention, 258–259
  rethinking emotional responses, 256–258
  rethinking self-image, 255–256

K

kleptomania, 57

L

lapses, compared to relapses, 196–197
learning disabilities, 301
Lexapro (escitalopram), 188
litigation, 115
Luvox (fluvoxamine), 188

M

mania, 44
mantras, 156
MAO inhibitors, 188
medication, 181–189. *See also names of specific medications*
  childhood OCD, 304
  discontinuing, 17, 183, 194–195
  example of, 185
  exposure and response prevention and, 195, 214
  honesty with doctor, 182–183
  Imipramine, 188
  impulsive problems, 293–294
  PANDAS, 300
  physical exam, 182
  prolonging treatment, 199
  reasons for using, 183–185

S

V

victimhood, 97
videos, in imaginal exposure, 165–166
virtual reality (VR), in imaginal exposure, 165–166
VolunteerMatch, 340
vomiting, 238–239, 245–246

W

walking meditation, 158–159
Wallace, B. Alan, 149
Washington Post, 265
wood knocking, 27
worries and fears, 8–10, 88–92
   of being unable to stand the treatment, 92
   of doing something against your will, 92
   doubt, 10
   of getting sick or dying, 90–91
   of going crazy, 88–89
   of hurting someone, 33, 35–36, 75, 91–92, 113–114, 135–137, 166
   of inconsistency, 90
   of losing control, 237–239
   of loss of control over bodily functions, 237–239, 244–246
   of missing OCD, 90
   of risk and uncertainty, 9–10, 89–90
   shame, 9
   that therapy doesn't work, 92

Y

Yale-Brown Obsessive Compulsive Scale (Y-BOCS), 115

Z

Zoloft (sertraline), 188

About the Author

Laura L. Smith, PhD is a clinical psychologist. She is a past president of the New Mexico Psychological Association. She has considerable experience in school and clinical settings dealing with children and adults who have obsessive compulsive disorder, anxiey, depression, anger, and personality disorders. She completed specialized training and was certified by the Behavior Therapy Training Institute of the International OCD Foundation. She has presented workshops on cognitive therapy and mental health issues to national and international audiences. She recently completed *Anxiety and Depression For Dummies Workbook*, 2nd Edition and *Anger Management For Dummies*, 3rd Edition.

Dr. Smith has worked on numerous publications together with her husband Charles Elliott, PhD, who is now retired. They are coauthors of *Anxiety for Dummies*, 3rd Edition; *Depression For Dummies*, 2nd Edition; *Quitting Smoking & Vaping For Dummies*; *Borderline Personality Disorder For Dummies*, 2nd Edition; *Child Psychology & Development For Dummies*; and *Seasonal Affective Disorder For Dummies* (all published by Wiley).

Dedication

I dedicate this book to my family and friends, who too many times get neglected during these writing projects. To my husband, who is still my favorite editor, and my dog, Oliver, who keeps me company in my office while I write. In addition, to the heroic readers with OCD, I want you to know that help is available. I hope this book gets you started on the journey to feeling better and overcoming OCD.

Author's Acknowledgments

In my 20 years writing for Wiley, I am continuously impressed by the support and guidance of their talented crew. Thank you to Kelsey Baird, acquisitions editor, for her advice and encouragement during the initial planning for the book. Development editor Tim Gallan is always available to respond to my repeated queries and keeps me from wandering astray. Joseph Bush is a superb and detail-oriented technical editor (who is almost always right). Kristie Pyles, senior managing editor, stays in the background keeping everyone on task. Finally, thank you to the careful editing of copy editor Kelly Henthorne.

A loving acknowledgment to Charles Elliott, coauthor of the first edition of *OCD For Dummies*. Throughout his unintended retirement, he has remained helpful, optimistic, and always available for encouragement, handholding, and editing.

Publisher's Acknowledgments

Acquisitions Editor: Tracy Boggier

Editorial Project Manager:
Carmen Krikorian, Michelle Hacker

Development Editor: Jennette ElNaggar

Copy Editor: Kelly Dobbs Henthorne

Technical Editor: Becky Stidham, LCSW

Art Coordinator: Alicia B. South

Production Editor: Tamilmani Varadharaj

Cover Image: © Melinda Podor/Getty Images